ADVANCES IN
HUMAN GENETICS 14

CONTRIBUTORS TO THIS VOLUME

G. Battistuzzi

Department of Haematology
Royal Postgraduate Medical School
University of London
London, England

**Andre Boué and
Joëlle Boué**

Unité de Recherches de Biologie Prénatale
INSERM U.73
Paris, France

Jan L. Breslow

Children's Hospital Corporation and
Harvard Medical School
Boston, Massachusetts

James F. Crow

Laboratory of Genetics
University of Wisconsin
Madison, Wisconsin

Carter Denniston

Laboratory of Genetics
University of Wisconsin
Madison, Wisconsin

Alfred Gropp †

Institut für Pathologie
Medizinische Hochschule
Lübeck, West Germany

L. Luzzatto

Department of Haematology
Royal Postgraduate Medical School
University of London
London, England

Larry J. Shapiro

Department of Pediatrics and
  Biological Chemistry
School of Medicine
University of California at Los Angeles
Los Angeles, California

Vassilis I. Zannis

Children's Hospital Corporation and
Harvard Medical School
Boston, Massachusetts

A Continuation Order Plan is available for this series. A continuation order will bring delivery of
each new volume immediately upon publication. Volumes are billed only upon actual shipment.
For further information please contact the publisher.

ADVANCES IN HUMAN GENETICS 14

Edited by

Harry Harris

Harnwell Professor of Human Genetics
University of Pennsylvania, Philadelphia

and

Kurt Hirschhorn

Herbert H. Lehman Professor and Chairman of Pediatrics
Mount Sinai School of Medicine of The City University of New York

PLENUM PRESS • NEW YORK AND LONDON

The Library of Congress cataloged the first volume of this title as follows:

Advances in human genetics. 1—
  New York, Plenum Press, 1970—
    (1) v. illus. 24-cm.
    Editors: V. 1—   H. Harris and K. Hirschhorn.
  1. Human genetics—Collected works.I. Harris, Harry, ed. II.Hirschhorn, Kurt, 1926—
    joint ed.
QH431.A1A32   573.2'1   77-84583

ISBN-13: 978-1-4615-9402-4   e-ISBN-13: 978-1-4615-9400-0
DOI: 10.1007/978-1-4615-9400-0
©1985 Plenum Press, New York
Softcover reprint of the hardcover 1st edition 1985
A Division of Plenum Publishing Corporation
233 Spring Street, New York, N.Y. 10013

ARTICLES PLANNED FOR FUTURE VOLUMES

Biochemical Defects in Immunodeficiency • *Rochelle Hirschhorn*
Neonatal Lethal Chondrodystrophies • *Jurgen Spranger and P. Maroteaux*
Advances in Prenatal Genetic Diagnosis • *John C. Hobbins and Maurice J. Mahoney*
Malformation Syndromes Caused by Single Gene Defects • *Judith G. Hall*
DNA Polymorphisms in Man • *Ray White*
The Genetics of Alcohol and Aldehyde Dehydrogenases • *Moyra Smith*
The Human Argininosuccinate Synthetase Locus and Citrullinemia • *Arthur L. Beaudet and William E. O'Brien*
Chromosomes and Neoplasia • *Janet Rowley*
Mutations in Man • *James N. Neel and Michael Skolnick*
The Molecular Genetics of the Major Histocompatibility Locus • *Jack L. Strominger*
Genetic and Physiological Aspects of Granulocyte Dysfunction • *Bernard M. Babior*
The Genetic and Biochemical Aspects of Primary and Late Onset Lactase Deficiency • *Gebhard Flatz*
The Processing of Lysosomal Enzymes and Its Genetic Implications • *William S. Sly*

CONTENTS OF EARLIER VOLUMES

Contents

Chapter 2

Mutation in Human Populations

James F. Crow and Carter Denniston

Chapter 3

Genetic Mutations Affecting Human Lipoprotein Metabolism

Vassilis I. Zannis and Jan L. Breslow

Chapter 4

Glucose-6-Phosphate Dehydrogenase

L. Luzzatto and G. Battistuzzi

Chapter 5

Steroid Sulfatase Deficiency and the Genetics of the Short Arm of the Human X Chromosome

Larry J. Shapiro

Chapter 1

Cytogenetics of Pregnancy Wastage

André Boué and Joëlle Boué

Unité de Recherches de Biologie Prenatale
INSERM U.73
Paris, France

Alfred Gropp*

Institut für Pathologie
Medizinische Hochschule
Lübeck, West Germany

---

*Alfred Gropp died October 22nd, 1983. This chapter is dedicated to his memory (A. B. and J. B.)

INTRODUCTION

During the last two decades, the important progress that has been made in the control of human reproduction, in medical care during pregnancy and the neonatal period, and more recently in *in vitro* fertilization (Schlesselman, 1979; Biggers, 1981) has focused interest on the understanding of the causes of the high mortality rate among human conceptuses before, during, and shortly after birth. It has been recognized that chromosomal abnormalities are among the most important causes of this high mortality rate, and thus couples with a history of pregnancy wastage are now frequently referred to a geneticist for counseling.

ESTIMATION OF PREGNANCY WASTAGE

For a given couple, it is difficult to estimate the probability of conception of a living newborn. Thus, demographers have defined "fecund-

1

ability" as the probability of producing a full-term infant per menstrual cycle during which intercourse occurred. Different demographic studies collected by Short (1979) show that at the age of 20–30 years, fecundability ranges from 21 to 28%. Thus, human fecundability is very low when compared to the fertility of domestic mammals.

From the results of studies using different methodological approaches it has been shown that this low fecundability can be explained by a high rate of intrauterine mortality occurring in the period from fertilization until delivery.

Using a statistical model, Roberts and Lowe (1975) postulated a 78% loss of all human conceptions, most of them occurring before the first missed period.

A 4-year followup study of 3084 pregnancies in the Hawaiian island of Kauai from the first missed menstrual period showed that 23.7% of these presumed conceptions failed to result in a live birth and that the mortality was largely concentrated in the early months of pregnancy (French and Bierman, 1962).

The detection of elevated human chorionic gonadotropin (hCG) by RIA for the β subunit of hCG allows the diagnosis of early pregnancy after implantation 8–9 days after fertilization. In a prospective study of normal women (Edmonds et al., 1982) 118 pregnancies were diagnosed on biochemical criteria, 67 of which had increased hCG levels but no clinical pregnancy; of the remaining 51 pregnant women, six had clinical abortions. Thus the postimplantation pregnancy loss rate was 62%.

Prior to these studies, the work of Hertig had shown not only the high rate of early embryonic mortality, but also that a high percentage of these embryos were abnormal. Thus the causes of early embryonic wastage were mainly linked to zygotic defects and not to maternal factors. In

Table I. Simple Morphological Results of an Analysis of 1000 Consecutive Spontaneous Abortions[a]

Pathological ova with absent or defective embryos	489
Embryos with localized anomalies	32
Placental abnormalities	96
Anatomically normal ova with macerated embryos	146
Total	763
Anatomically normal ova with nonmacerated embryos	74
Uterine abnormalities	64
Others	99
Total	237

[a] From Hertig and Sheldon (1943).

Table II. Incidence of Morphological Abnormalities in Relation to the Developmental Age of the Abortus

Study		Incidence of abnormalities at given developmental age		
		≤4 weeks	5–8 weeks	9–12 weeks
Mikamo (1970)	Number of abortuses	48	61	81
	Number of abnormal abortuses	48	40	10
	Percent abnormal abortuses	100	65.6	12.3
Miller and Poland (1970)	Number of abortuses	83	122	177
	Number of abnormal abortuses	73	71	56
	Percent abnormal abortuses	88	58	32

a study of 34 early fertilized ova from 1 to 17 days, 13 showed some degree of abnormality (Hertig and Rock, 1949). In a morphological study of 1000 spontaneous abortions about three-fourths showed abnormalities (Hertig and Sheldon, 1943) (Table I).

Other pathological studies on abortuses (Mikamo, 1970; Miller and Poland, 1970) confirmed the findings of Hertig and showed that the frequency of abnormality was related to the developmental age, approaching 90–100% in early specimens arrested during the first month after fertilization (Table II) and decreasing when developmental arrest occurred later.

These studies showed that intrinsic zygotic defects are the main causes of early embryonic losses and spontaneous abortions. The discoveries that congenital malformation syndromes may result from chromosome anomalies led to cytogenetic studies seeking the etiology of fetal wastage.

EVALUATION OF THE INCIDENCE OF CHROMOSOME ABNORMALITIES

The main problem has been the collection of specimens allowing cytogenetic surveys at different stages of development. Investigation of human abortions (spontaneous or induced) have provided the largest amount of data, followed by surveys of perinatal deaths and more recently by the analysis of some data of prenatal diagnosis. Unfortunately, the collection of embryonic losses of the first 2 weeks of development is nearly impossible.

Spontaneous Abortions

Most spontaneous abortions (about 90%) occur during the first trimester of pregnancy. In these abortions the developmental age of the embryo is generally less than 8 weeks, and a prolonged *in utero* retention follows embryonic death.

A large number of publications have reported chromosome abnormalities in spontaneous abortions. Most of the studies published in the 1960s were analyzed by Carr (1971b) in his article in the second volume of this series. Since then, surveys based on the cytogenetic analysis of hundreds of specimens have been published, and these furnish the basis of this chapter (J. Boué and Boué, 1973a; Carr and Gedeon, 1978; Creasy et al., 1976; Hassold et al., 1980a; Kajii et al., 1980; Lauritsen, 1976; Warburton et al., 1980a; Meulenbroek and Geraedts, 1982).

The manner in which specimens are collected is an important factor that is sometimes difficult to clarify. It can be estimated that the number of induced abortions included in the large surveys is low, which is not the case in some of the earlier studies.

Many spontaneous abortions (especially the earlier ones) occur at home and do not necessitate hospitalization (Stevenson et al., 1959). Specimens collected either at home by the patient or in the hospital reflect different ways of sampling.

There are also differences in the distribution of gestational ages at abortion and especially in the percentage of older fetuses in some studies. From the followup studies after amniocentesis for prenatal diagnosis, which are usually performed at the beginning of the second trimester pregnancy (16–17 weeks gestational age), the incidence of late spontaneous abortions is low, 1.5–2% of the pregnancies in progress at the time of amniocentesis. In some abortion surveys, the number of abortuses with a gestational age of 18 weeks and more exceed 20% of the specimens collected, which is far more than expected from clinical studies.

This may explain the differences in the total frequencies of chromosome abnormalities among the studies. In order to minimize the bias in selection, different criteria were used to calculate the incidence of chromosome abnormalities.

Abortions During the First Trimester

In some surveys in which pathological examination of abortuses was performed, the incidence of chromosome abnormalities was evaluated according to the developmental age (Mikamo, 1970; J. Boué and Boué, 1973a). Anatomical studies have demonstrated that the duration of development is a reliable criterion for the classification of specimens. An estimation of the stage of development attained by the specimen is based on pathological examination, which comprises a detailed macroscopic description of the abortus and a microscopic study of the placenta (Philippe, 1974).

When embryonic formation exists, the age of the embryo is estimated by the stage of embryogenesis it has attained, rather than by its size, which is usually modified by maceration.

Detailed histologic examination of the placenta, including an appreciation of the degree of maturity of the villi and their blood vessels, permits the determination of the stage of development (Philippe and Boué, 1969).

Table III shows that the incidence of chromosome abnormalities is greater than 60% in abortuses of a developmental age less than 7 weeks and then decreases.

In other studies the incidence of chromosome abnormalities was evaluated in relation to the gestational age of the abortus calculated as the time from the first day of the last menstrual period to the day of abortion. This age is usually easy to determine but is highly dependent on the long and variable time of *in utero* retention, which in many cases is longer (mean time 6–7 weeks) than the developmental age of the embryo (mean age 4–5 weeks).

Table IV gives the results of four surveys (Creasy *et al.*, 1976; Kajii *et al.*, 1980; Hassold *et al.*, 1980a; Warburton *et al.*, 1980a) that showed that in abortuses of 8–16 weeks gestational age the incidence of chromosome abnormalities was about 50% and then decreased.

The rate of abnormalities in the earliest abortions (less than 8 weeks) is surprisingly low. These results are in contradiction with the increased incidence observed in studies based on developmental age either in spon-

Table III. Incidence of Chromosome Abnormalities in Spontaneous
Abortuses in Relation to Developmental Age[a]

Developmental age, weeks	Number of abortuses analyzed	Chromosome abnormalities	
		Number	Percent
2	23	18	78
3	374	258	69
4	203	125	61.6
5	139	85	62.2
6	302	211	69.9
7	56	27	48.2
Total, weeks 2–7	1097	724	66
8	36	8	
9	42	6	
10	14	7	
11	8	1	
12	8	3	
Total, weeks 8–12	108	25	23

[a] From J. Boué and Boué (1973a).

taneous abortions or in induced abortions, which showed that the highest frequencies are observed in embryos less than 8 weeks of development, and also in contradiction with the studies on morphological abnormalities in abortuses (Table II). Among the different ideas put forth to explain these discrepancies is the suggestion by Warburton *et al.* (1980a) that the low rate was the result of a trend to retain specimens with abnormal chromosomes *in utero* for several weeks after implantations. It is also possible

Table IV. Frequency of Chromosome Anomalies by Gestational Age in Four Series of
Spontaneous Abortions

Week of gestation	Percent chromosomally abnormal[a]			
	Geneva (Kajii et al., 1980; $N = 395$)	Honolulu (Hassold et al., 1980a; $N = 997$)	London (Creasy et al., 1976; $N = 893$)	New York (Warburton et al., 1980a; $N = 876$)
0–7	36.1	30.8	—	14.0
8–11	57.1	43.0	50.4	49.2
12–15	46.0	51.6	44.1	39.1
16–19	27.7	39.7	21.4	18.5

[a] N, Total number of karyotyped abortuses.

that abortions occurring in early pregnancy are more frequently linked to maternal factors, especially of hormonal origin.

Late Abortions

In two surveys a large number of late abortions were collected. The rates of chromosome abnormalities at gestational ages over 20 weeks were 11.7% (Creasy *et al.*, 1976) and 6.6% (Warburton *et al.*, 1980a).

Induced Abortions

Apparently, systematic cytogenetic analysis of induced abortuses may represent a better approach to evaluating the true incidence of chromosome abnormalities at a given developmental age, which in this case corresponds to the gestational age (minus 14 days).

There were, however, also methodological problems in the identification of recovered tissues. When efforts were made to identify fragments from the embryo itself, specimens with normal karyotype were selected (Kajii *et al.*, 1978).

In two important surveys cytogenetic examinations were made in both the embryo itself and its chorionic villi, but in most cases only tissues of the chorionic villi were analyzed. Kajii *et al.* (1978) found a chromosome abnormality in 4.5% of 469 successfully analyzed abortuses of 4–9 weeks of developmental age. Yamamoto and Watanabe (1979), using a direct chromosome technique, successfully analyzed 1250 abortuses of 3–10 weeks of developmental age and found an incidence of 6.4% of abortuses with abnormal chromosomes. The percentages are higher in the earlier abortuses (Table V).

Table V. Incidence of Chromosome Abnormalities in Induced Abortuses in Relation to Developmental Age[a]

Developmental age, weeks	Number of abortuses analyzed	Chromosome abnormalities	
		Number	Percent
3–4	108	10	9.3
5–6	570	37	6.5
7–8	389	25	6.4
9–10	130	7	5.4

[a] From Yamamoto and Watanabe (1979).

Table VI. Chromosome Studies in Infants Dying during the Perinatal Period[a]

Status	Number studied	Abnormal karyotype	
		Number	Percent
Macerated stillbirth	112	13	11.6
Nonmacerated stillbirth	340	13	3.8
Early neonatal death	824	41	5.0
Total	1176	67	5.7
Cases with severe congenital malformations[b]	143	41	28.6

[a] Data from Machin and Crolla (1974), Kuleshov (1976), Sutherland et al. (1978).
[b] Data from Machin and Crolla (1974), Sutherland et al. (1978).

Perinatal Deaths

Some cytogenetic surveys were performed on infants who died during the perinatal period, stillbirths, or early neonatal deaths (Machin and Crolla, 1974; Kuleshov, 1976; Sutherland et al., 1978). Chromosome abnormalities were found in about 6% of the cases. The incidence is higher in macerated stillbirths (11.6%) and when cases with severe malformations are selected (28.6%) (Table VI).

Given the difficulties inherent in these types of studies (collection of specimens, tissue culture, etc.), it is remarkable that most of them are in agreement and emphasize the importance of chromosome abnormalities in pregnancy wastage. Figure 1 combines the results of the evaluation of intrauterine mortality and of the cytogenetic surveys. Even though data on the first 2 weeks of zygotic development are scarce, it is clear that the incidence of intrauterine mortality decreases from the first weeks of development until term and that the incidence of chromosome anomalies decreases in the same way.

TYPES OF CHROMOSOME ABNORMALITIES

Analysis of cytogenetic surveys done on early spontaneous abortions, late spontaneous abortions, and perinatal deaths shows that in each type of pregnancy wastage the relative frequency of the different types of chromosome abnormalities reported in the different studies is similar. These results reflect a phenomenon characteristic of the human species, with the same frequency in different parts of the world. Table VII sum-

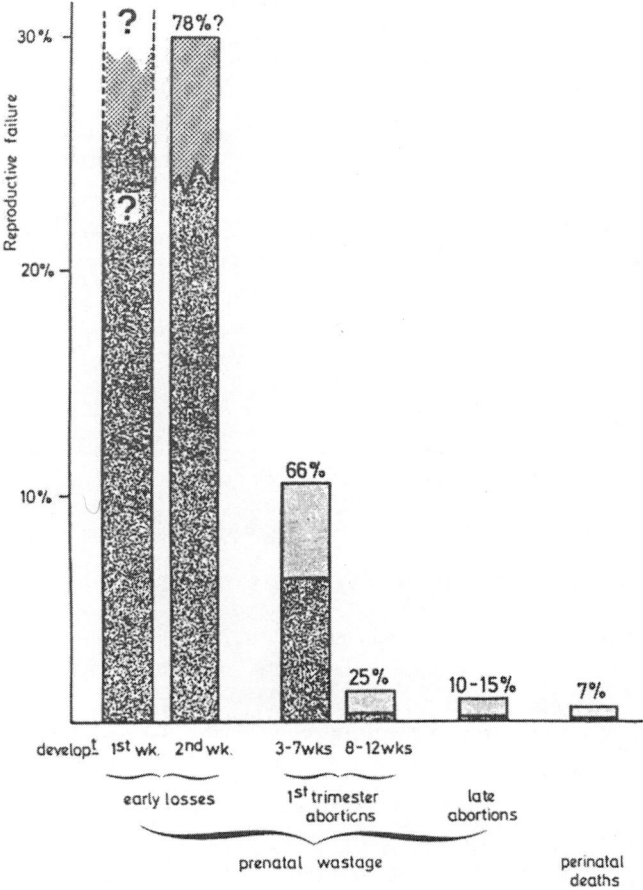

Fig. 1. Evaluation of mortality at different stages of development of conceptuses, and percentages of chromosome anomalies.

marizes the results of some important surveys. Autosomal trisomies are by far the most frequent and represent more than 50% of the observed abnormalities.

Autosomal Trisomies and Monosomies

In abortion surveys more than 1000 autosomal trisomies have been identified by banding techniques (Table VIII). With the exception of chromosome 1, trisomies involving all of the autosomes have been

Table VII. Frequency of the Different Types of Chromosome Anomalies in Abortuses and
Perinatal Deaths

	Percent of all anomalies		
	Spontaneous abortions[a]	Induced abortions[b]	Perinatal deaths[c]
Numerical anomalies			
Monosomy X	20	11	18[d]
Autosomal monosomies	Extremely rare	—	—
Autosomal trisomies	52	53	50
Triploidies	16	11	5
Tetraploidies	6	6	—
Structural anomalies	4	3	16
Percent of chromosome anomalies among entire material	50–60	6.5	5.5

[a] Total of 2085 karyotyped abortuses. J. Boué et al. (1975), Carr (1977), Creasy et al. (1976), Hassold et al. (1980a), Kajii et al. (1980), Warburton et al. (1980a).
[b] Five to ten weeks gestational age; 1250 karyotyped abortuses. Yamamoto and Watanabe (1979).
[c] Total of 1176 observations. Machin and Crolla (1974), Kuleshov (1976), Sutherland et al. (1978).
[d] Including other sex chromosome anomalies.

observed, but their relative frequencies differ widely: some have been rarely observed (trisomies 3, 5, 6, 11, 12, 17, and 19); in all surveys trisomy 16 represents about one-third of all the autosomal trisomies, followed by trisomies of the acrocentric chromosomes (385/1036 autosomal trisomies, 37.2%). Thus, a high percentage of trisomies is found in chromosomes with heterochromatic polymorphic centromeric regions and there may exist a causal relationship between the presence of these heterochromatic polymorphisms and the occurrence of nondisjunction (Meulenbroek and Geraedts, 1982).

The difference in the frequencies of various autosomal trisomies may reflect (1) differences in the rates of nondisjunction for each chromosome pair, (2) differences in the rate of loss of conceptuses before the pregnancy is recognized by the mother, or (c) an association of both causes.

Double autosomal trisomies also occur in abortuses. Table IX shows that the observed distribution of the two extra autosomes is not different from that expected on the basis of the frequencies observed in single autosomal trisomies. Thus, it appears that the two events leading to double autosomal trisomies are independent, but it is unknown whether the two

Table VIII. Autosomal Trisomies in Abortuses[a]

Trisomy	Number	Percent	Trisomy	Number	Percent
1	—	—	13	63	6.1
2	53	5.1	14	51	5.0
3	8	1	15	75	7.2
4	26	2.5	16	326	31.4
5	1	1	17	7	1
6	3	1	18	51	4.9
7	46	4.4	19	1	1
8	37	3.6	20	28	2.7
9	33	3.2	21	89	8.6
10	22	2.1	22	107	10.3
11	2	1			
12	9	1	Total	1064	

[a] Compiled from surveys of J. Boué et al. (1976a), Carr and Gedeon (1978), Creasy et al. (1976), Hassold et al. (1980a), Kajii et al. (1980), Therkelsen et al., (1973), Warburton et al., (1980a), Meulenbroek and Geraedts (1982).

aberrations result from different nondisjunctions in the same gamete or from a nondisjunction in each of the gametes that participated in the formation of the zygote.

In late abortions or in surveys of perinatal death the autosomal trisomies observed are mainly 13, 18, and 21, with trisomy 18 being the most frequent.

Table IX. Distribution of the Extra Chromosomes in Trisomies and Double Trisomies[a]

Chromosome group	Trisomies		Double trisomies	
	Number	Percent	Number observed	Number expected
A (1–3)	23	2.8	3	1.8
B (4–5)	18	2.2	1	1
C (6–12)	142	17.2	17	10.9
D (13–15)	170	20.6	8	13.2
E (16–18)	277	33.6	14	21.5
F (19–20)	15	1.8	0	1.1
G (21–22)	178	21.6	21	13.8
Total	823	—	32[b]	—

[a] Compiled from J. Boué and Boué (1973a), Hassold et al. (1980a), and Kajii et al. (1980).
[b] Thirty-two observations of double trisomies make 64 extra chromosomes.

In contrast to the high frequency of autosomal trisomies, especially in abortion surveys, autosomal monosomies have been rarely reported. There have been a few observations of monosomy 21. Since the mechanisms of nondisjunction may lead either to a gamete with an extra chromosome or to one lacking a chromosome, it can be expected that the same number of fertilizations have occurred leading either to autosomal trisomies or to autosomal monosomies. The very early loss of conceptuses with autosomal monosomies seems to be the most likely explanation of the observed differences in abortion surveys and is supported by the experimental data on mice (see below, Table XXVII and Fig. 4).

The sex ratio among trisomic abortions as a whole in five cytogenetic studies of spontaneous abortions (Hassold *et al.,* 1983) was significantly greater than 1.0, but not as high as the estimates of sex ratio for chromosomally normal abortions (approximately 1.30). However, large differences in sex ratio were observed among individual trisomies. In trisomy 16, the sex ratio was 1.01. In trisomy 9, the excess of female specimens (sex ratio 0.29) seems to be the result of a very early selection against male trisomy 9 conceptuses. In trisomy 21, the increased sex ratio among liveborns (1.28) is also observed in abortuses with trisomy 21 (1.67). There is no evidence of a differential selection based on sex in trisomy 21.

Mechanisms of Nondisjunction and Epidemiologic Studies

Using fluorescent markers of chromosome polymorphism, it has been possible to trace the exact mechanism of trisomic conceptuses in (1) liveborn subjects with trisomy 21 (Mikkelsen, 1982) and (2) trisomic spontaneous abortions (Lauritsen, 1976; Niikawa *et al.,* 1977; Hassold *et al.,* 1980a; Meulenbroek and Geraedts, 1982). Table X shows the data from these studies. In spontaneous abortion material, the observations were pooled for trisomy 16 and for acrocentric chromosomes (Jacobs, 1981b). All four possible meiotic errors (paternal and maternal, meiosis I and II) have been observed, but in the great majority of cases the error occurred at the first maternal meiotic division. If the incidence of the different types of errors is the same for all autosomal trisomies, and of course for the autosomal monosomies that are their counterpart, about two-thirds of the most frequent anomalies in humans are the result of an

Table X. Origin of the Extra Chromosome in Autosomal Trisomies

	Maternal		Paternal	
	First meiosis	Second meiosis	First meiosis	Second meiosis
Trisomy 21[a]	66.2%	12.7%	14.0%	7.0%
Trisomy 16[b]	73.3%	6.6%	13.3%	6.6%
Trisomies of acrocentric chromosomes[c]	63.4%	4.9%	7.3%	2.4%
	19.5%[d]		2.4%[d]	

[a] Liveborn infants, 228 observations (Mikkelsen, 1982).
[b] Spontaneous abortions, 30 observations (Lauritsen, 1976; Meulenbroek and Geraedts, 1982).
[c] Spontaneous abortions, 41 observations (Niikawa et al., 1977; Hassold et al., 1980a; Meulenbroek and Geraedts, 1982).
[d] First or second meiosis.

error in the first meiotic divison of the oocyte. The data came from very small series and a greater number of observations is needed to determine if such differences exist for all the autosomal trisomies in both liveborn and aborted trisomies and particularly those involving autosomes without polymorphisms.

As pointed out by Chandley (1981), man appears unique among all investigated mammalian species in showing such high levels of chromosomal aneuploidy among its early zygotes.

Recently, Mirre et al. (1980), studying prophase I of meiosis in oocytes from 16- to 25-week-old fetuses, showed that there are basic differences between human and mouse oocytes during meiotic prophase. In the mouse oocyte, each of the two nucleoli has a fibrillar center containing the ribosomal genes originating from one of the paired chromosomes. In the human oocyte, a given fibrillar center may contain not only the ribosomal genes from two paired nucleolar chromosomes, but also those from two or even three bivalents. This situation could favor the occurrence of chromosomal nondisjunction.

Delays in fertilization have been suspected as being involved in the origin of trisomic conceptuses, but the fact that errors are frequently encountered in the first meiotic division of the oocyte is not in favor of this hypothesis (Chandley, 1981).

The existence of spermatozoa with abnormal chromosome constitution was demonstrated initially by chromosome fluorescent markers

(Pearson *et al.*, 1973) and more recently by direct chromosomal analysis of human spermatozoa after *in vitro* fertilization of zona-free hamster eggs (Martin *et al.*, 1982).

In the chromosomal analysis of 1000 spermatozoa from 33 normal men (Martin *et al.*, 1983), an aneuploidy was observed in 5.2%. The frequencies of hyperhaploid and hypohaploid sperm complement were not significantly different and all chromosome pairs were involved.

The maternal age effect associated with nondisjunction in man was first demonstrated for Down syndrome by Penrose (1933). This has been largely confirmed since the onset of cytogenetic studies and extended to the two other autosomal trisomies (13 and 18) observed in livebirths.

Cytogenetic surveys of spontaneous abortions have also shown the influence of maternal age on the incidence of autosomal trisomies (Table XI). However, in abortuses, although the mean maternal age is increased for the trisomies as a whole, there are variations with respect to individual chromosomes (J. Boué *et al.*, 1975; Hassold *et al.*, 1980*b*; Kajii *et al.*, 1980). There is a striking maternal age effect associated with trisomies involving an acrocentric chromosome and with double trisomies; the same effect is also observed in some of the small nonacrocentric chromosomes (18 and 20).

There is a limited number of observations for trisomies 17 and 19. For trisomy 16 the mean maternal age is only moderately elevated. For trisomies of the A, B, and C groups of chromosomes, the mean maternal

Table XI. Maternal Age in Relation to the Different Types of Chromosome Anomalies in Abortion Surveys[a]

Karyotype	Kajii *et al.* (1980) (N = 614)	Hassold *et al.* (1980*a*) (N = 999)	J. Boué *et al.* (1975) (N = 1337)	Lauritsen (1976) (N = 255)
Normal	28.9	27.0 (32.0)[b]	27.5 (30.6)[b]	27.1 (28.2)[b]
45,X	25.8	26.9	27.5	26.6
Trisomy	31.9	29.8	31.2	28.7
Double trisomy	37.9	35.4	35	—
Triploidy	28.6	26.5 (29.9)[b]	27.4 (30.4)[b]	25.7 (27.6)[b]
Tetraploidy	27.5	28.4	26.8	26.7
Structural anomalies	26.7	25.9	27.0	—

[a] *N*, Number of observations.
[b] Paternal age.

Table XII. Mothers with Two Abortions Karyotyped. Combined Results[a]

First abortion	Number of women	Second abortion			
		Normal	Trisomy	Other abnormal	Translocation
Normal	115	95	9	11	0
Monosomy	18	8	6	4	0
Trisomy	51	16	30	5	0
Polyploidy	16	7	7	2	0
Translocation	7	0	0	1	6

[a] From Warburton et al. (1982).

age is generally increased, but the effect is less pronounced than for trisomies of the acrocentric chromosomes.

It has been postulated that decreasing maternal selection against affected conceptuses with advancing maternal age may explain the increased maternal age in trisomies of the acrocentric chromosomes, mainly in trisomies 21 (Aymé and Lippman-Hand, 1982). This hypothesis is not supported by the previous epidemiologic studies on abortion (J. Boué et al., 1975) and the recent prospective studies of Hook (1983), which showed that whether a conceptus with trisomy 21 is spontaneously aborted or is delivered at term does not depend on the age of the mother.

In all studies, no paternal age effect has been demonstrated for any of the chromosome abnormalities. These results are in agreement with the recently published studies of paternal age in prenatally diagnosed trisomies (Hook and Cross, 1982; Roth et al., 1983), which did not confirm the findings of Stene et al. (1981).

Among other possible factors studied for a possible effect on the rate of nondisjunction during gametogenesis, x-ray irradiation has been suspected. The evidence that maternal radiation exposure is associated with an increase of Down syndrome (Alberman et al., 1972a) has been extended to chromosomally abnormal abortions (Alberman et al., 1972b) and a correlation has been observed between paternal occupational radiation exposure and chromosomally abnormal abortions (J. Boué et al., 1975).

In some surveys, two consecutive abortions from the same woman have been karyotyped (J. Boué and Boué, 1973b; Hassold, 1980; Warburton et al., 1982; D. Warburton, personal communication). The combined results are shown in Table XII. There is a significant concordance between the chromosome status of the first and that of the second abortions studied. When the first abortus has a trisomic karyotype, the subsequent abortus also frequently has a trisomic karyotype. The extra chromosomes involved in these two trisomies are different in most cases.

These data seem to indicate that certain couples have a higher risk of producing trisomic conceptions and thus of nondisjunction occurring during gametogenesis.

Epidemiologic studies on these couples have been unable to confirm the existence of a gene that results in meiotic nondisjunction (Alfi *et al.*, 1980). Environmental factors that may act on early reproductive loss make such studies very difficult.

Phenotypic Expressions of Autosomal Trisomies

Due to the existence of several types of autosomal trisomies, it has been difficult to collect enough material to describe the phenotypic characteristics of each trisomy in early abortions.

A common feature is the hypoplasia of the trisomic placentas showing an underdeveloped trophoblast, with lack of villous structural uniformity and severe vascular hypoplasia. In about 50% of the cases, large isolated intravillous cytotrophoblastic cells were observed and in some cases it was possible to trace their migration from the epithelium into the stroma (Philippe and Boué, 1969; Honoré *et al.*, 1976).

There are variations in embryonic development:

1. In most of the rarely observed autosomal trisomies (mainly trisomies 2, 6, 11, 19, and 20) no embryonic formation was detected. The conceptuses were blighted ova, which reflected a developmental arrest at 3 weeks.
2. Trisomies 16 looked like blighted ova and were characterized by a chorionic vesicle of 2–3 cm, a small amnion of 5 mm, and a tiny embryonic formation of less than 1 mm arrested at the embryonic disc stage.
3. In trisomies 4, 5, 7–10, and 22, disorganized embryos of a developmental age of 25–35 days were generally observed. At microscopic examination, it could be seen that some embryonic cell

types of the embryo underwent early necrosis, whereas others, such as conjunctival cells, were more resistant; these survived and grew into an undifferentiated mass, which caused a secondary disorganization of the embryo (J. Boué et al., 1976b). Similar aspects were also observed in some trisomies 21.

4. In trisomies 13–15 the embryonic development reached 40–45 days. In both trisomies 13 and 14, underdeveloped nasal processes and cyclocephalia were observed, which resembled the features of Patau syndrome.

5. Trisomies 21 aborted during the first trimester had a developmental age of 6–7 weeks. Gross abnormalities were rarely observed.

In trisomies that lead to late abortions and perinatal deaths, trisomies 13, 18, and 21, the phenotypic characteristics had the main features of the same trisomies found in living subjects (Stephens and Shepard, 1980). For instance, the typical finger deformity of the Edwards syndrome is constant in all fetuses with trisomy 18 and eventually allows a diagnosis at ultrasound examination (J. Boué et al., 1982).

Hook (1983) studied the rate of spontaneous fetal deaths in trisomies 13, 18, and 21 that were diagnosed prenatally and whose mothers had declined selective abortion (Table XIII); a significant proportion of these trisomies led to intrauterine mortality. This may explain the discrepancy between the incidence of these trisomies at the time of amniocentesis and the incidence in liveborn infants.

Table XIII. Proportions of Spontaneous Fetal Deaths Following the Prenatal Diagnosis of a Chromosome Abnormality[a]

Abnormality detected	Number of diagnoses	Proportion of fetal deaths, %
47, +21	73	30.1
47, +18	25	68.0
47, +13	7	43.
47, XXX	39	0
47, XXY	37	8.1
47, XYY	33	3.
45, X	12	72.
Balanced structural anomaly	71	2.8

[a] From Hook (1983).

Sex Chromosome Aneuploidies

Monosomy X

In all the cytogenetic surveys of spontaneous abortions, monosomy X represents 15–25% of the chromosome abnormalities. The majority have a pure 45,X karyotype, in opposition to the observations of living patients with Turner syndrome, in whom mosaicism is frequently detected.

The mechanisms leading to the 45,X karyotype remain unknown. In aborted material, it has not been possible to demonstrate which sex chromosome is lacking and to confirm if, as in living subjects with monosomy X, the sex chromosome lacking is of paternal origin in 75% of the observations.

One interesting finding has been the association of monosomy X abortuses with a young maternal age: in all the published surveys the mean maternal age is (1) either identical to the maternal age of the control group with abortuses having normal karyotype (Table XI) or (2) as in the New York survey (Warburton *et al.,* 1980*b*), lower for mothers of monosomy X abortions (normal karyotype, 26.8 ± 6.6 years; monosomy X, 23.8 ± 5.0 years).

Phenotypic Expression

The phenotype of monosomy X abortuses allows one to suspect the diagnosis in many cases by a macroscopic examination alone.

In early abortions, in two-thirds of the collected cases the specimen consists of an intact, closed amniotic sac 50–80 mm in length (6 weeks of development) with a well-defined umbilical cord ending in a small mass with the remnants of macerated embryonic cells. The placenta is usually invaded by large subchorial thromboses. In other cases, the appearance of the placenta is the same but a macerated embryo of a developmental age of 6 weeks exists; histological examination frequently reveals a horseshoe kidney.

In late abortions, the phenotype is characterized by generalized edema, hygroma on each side of the neck, and horseshoe kidneys (Singh and Carr, 1966, 1967) similar to the findings in the Bonnevie–Ullrich syndrome.

Other Sex Chromosome Aneuploidies

In abortion surveys, no 47,XYY karyotype has been reported and 47,XXX and 47,XXY karyotypes have been rarely observed. From these few observations, it is difficult to estimate the prenatal loss of conceptuses with these karyotypes.

The data collected by Hook (1983) confirmed the low incidence of late fetal deaths due to 47,XXX, 47,XXY, and 47,XYY conceptuses and the frequency of late fetal deaths in the 45,X conceptuses (Table XIII).

Errors of Chromosome Haploid Sets

The first descriptions of an abnormal karyotype in spontaneously aborted embryos were triploidies (Penrose and Delhanty, 1961; Delhanty et al., 1961). Later, the association of a triploid karyotype with partial hydatidiform mole was recognized (Atkin and Klinger, 1962; Makino et al., 1964). The correlation of cytogenetic and morphological studies distinguishes two distinct syndromes: (1) triploid partial moles and (2) diploid complete moles (Philippe and Boué, 1969; Carr, 1969; Vassilakos et al., 1977; Szulman and Surti, 1978). More recently, cytogenetic studies have shown that the complete mole has a paternally derived genome with no maternal chromosome contribution (Kajii and Ohama, 1977; Jacobs et al., 1978b). Another error involving a chromosome haploid set described in humans is represented by benign ovarian teratomas, which contain two identical haploid complements derived from the host (Linder et al., 1975).

Triploidy

Triploidy is a common numerical anomaly occurring in 15–20% of spontaneous abortions with abnormal karyotype (Carr, 1971a; J. Boué et al., 1975; Creasy et al., 1976; Hassold et al., 1980a; Kajii et al., 1980; Meulenbroek and Geraedts, 1982).

Triploid conceptuses were also observed (1) in cytogenetic studies of induced abortions: in the 1250 karyotyped abortuses of the Yamamoto and Watanabe series (1979) the incidence of triploid specimens was 0.7%;

Table XIV. Karyotypes of Triploid Abortuses

Study	69,XXX	69,XXY	69,XYY	68,XX	68,XXY −22	≥70
J. Boué et al. (1975)	57	92	7	2	—	4
Carr (1971a)	13	9	—	—	—	3
Creasy et al. (1976)	18	18	1	—	—	2
Jacobs et al. (1982)	31	64	1	2	1	5
Kajii et al. (1980)	11	16	—	—	—	2
Lauritsen (1976)	9	5	—	—	—	—
Warburton et al. (1980a)	23	25	1	1	—	1
Total	162	229	10	5	1	17

(2) in prenatal diagnosis performed at 16–18 weeks of gestation; and (3) even after *in vitro* fertilization (Lopata, 1980; Steptoe *et al.*, 1980).

Only a few triploid conceptuses have survived until term as stillborn infants or as infants who died in the immediate postnatal period (Wertelecki *et al.*, 1976; Gosden *et al.*, 1976; Fryns *et al.*, 1977).

From these data it has been estimated that triploidy occurs in about 1% of recognized human conceptions, but is observed in only one of 10,000 livebirths.

Cytogenetic Studies.   According to the constitution of the gonosomes, three types of triploidies are distinguished (Table XIV): 69,XXY, the most frequent; 69,XXX; and 69,XYY, which has been rarely observed. The small number of abortuses with 69,XYY constitution may be explained by the fact that this karyotype leads to very early developmental arrest and that such cells do not grow well in tissue culture (A. Boué, personal observations).

Observations of nearly triploid karyotypes have been reported (Table XIV). The occurrence of two different chromosomal errors leading to a double anomaly explains these karyotypes: (1) 68,XX, associated with the error leading to a monosomy X; (2) 68,XXY minus an autosome and, (3) 70,XXX or 70,XXY plus an extra autosome, associations with the errors giving autosomal monosomy or trisomy. These observations, which are not so rare (5.5% of the triploidies were associated with another chromosome error), confirm the high frequency of chromosome errors in human zygotes.

The origin of the supernumerary set of chromosomes results from different mechanisms: chromosome nonreductions either in the first or in the second maternal meiotic division (digyny), or in the first or in the second paternal meiotic division (diandry), or dispermy. It has been possible to document these mechanisms using different approaches: (1) XYY sex chromosome complement indicates an extra set of paternal origin, the possible mechanisms being either diandry (meiosis II) or dispermy; (2) heteromorphic fluorescent regions in some chromosomes have been used as markers, first by Uchida and Lin (1972) and Jonasson *et al.* (1972) and then in other series of studies (Kajii and Niikawa, 1977; Lauritsen *et al.*, 1979; Jacobs *et al.*, 1982; Meulenbroek and Geraedts, 1982). (3) HLA typing of cells of triploid abortuses (Couillin *et al.*, 1978) allows the identification of the extra set of chromosomes.

Table XV shows the results of five series of studies. About three-fourths of triploid abortuses have two paternal haploid sets. In some cases, it was possible to demonstrate clearly that dispermy was the mechanism, but in other cases it was not possible to distinguish diandry from dispermy. A diploid sperm resulting from failure of the second meiotic division seems a rare event and it can be estimated (Jacobs *et al.*, 1978a) that two-thirds of triploidies result from dispermy.

The results of sex chromatin analysis show that X-inactivation in triploid cases is variable. In abortuses, two-thirds of the triploid speci-

Table XV. Mechanisms of Triploidy

	Lauritsen *et al.* (1979)	Kajii and Niikawa (1977)	Couillin *et al.* (1978)	Jacobs *et al.* (1982)	Meulenbroek and Geraedts (1982)	Total	
Dispermy	6	5	2	41	4	58	
Dispermy or diandry MI	1	2	9	16	—	28	90
Dispermy or diandry MII	0	2	2	—	—	4	(72.6%)
Digyny MI	5	1	—	8	2	16	
Digyny MII	0	—	—	13	—	13	34
Digyny MI or MII	—	—	5	—	—	5	(37.4%)
Total	12	10	18	78	6	124	

Table XVI. Sex Chromatin Findings in Cells of Triploid Specimens

Specimens	Karyotypes	Sex chromatin		
		Negative	Single positive	Double positive
Abortions[a]	69,XXX	—	38	16
	69,XXY	48	27	—

[a] From Fryns et al. (1977).

mens with XXY or XXX complement have two active X chromosomes, and in the remaining one-third only one X is active (Table XVI). These results were obtained in primary cultures from embryonic or chorioamniotic tissues, but in all fibroblast cell lines initiated from triploid embryos (XXY or XXX) the two X chromosomes were active irrespective of the situation in primary cultures (J. Boué, unpublished work).

The evidence for two active X chromosomes was confirmed by the determination of isozymes of glucose-6-phosphate dehydrogenase (Weaver et al., 1975) and by a gene dosage effect (Junien et al., 1976).

Androgenesis

The first cytogenetic surveys on spontaneous abortions showed that the "classic" hydatidiform complete moles without amniotic sac and embryonic formation have a diploid and, in 90% of the cases, an apparently female karyotype (Carr, 1969; J. Boué and Boué, 1973a).

Using fluorescent markers, Kajii and Ohama (1977) found that the chromosome complement, though apparently normal female 46,XX, consisted of two sets of paternally derived chromosomes without any maternal chromosome contribution. These first observations were confirmed by Jacobs et al. (1978b) with fluorescent markers and by Yamashita et al. (1979) with HLA markers. The paternal origin of the two sets of chromosomes was extended to the less frequent diploid moles with 46,XY complement (Surti et al., 1979).

In the case of 46,XX moles, Kajii and Ohama (1977) suggested two possible mechanisms for such androgenesis: fertilization of an "empty egg" by (1) a diploid spermatozoon resulting from failure of meiosis II, or by (2) a haploid spermatozoon that duplicates in the ovum to restore the diploid number. The fact that moles with 46,YY karyotype have not been found may be due to nonviability of moles with this karyotype. The results of Jacobs *et al.* (1980) using chromosomes and enzymatic markers (PMG 1) suggest that a haploid spermatozoon duplicating in the ovum is the more likely possibility. In studies of 46,XY moles (Ohama *et al.,* 1981) only paternal markers were detected, but with both homozygous and heterozygous chromosomal polymorphisms, indicating the entry of two spermatozoa (an X and a Y).

One issue remains open: the loss of the maternal haploid set. It may be lost before or at the time of penetration of the spermatozoon or at the time of the first mitotic division.

Since studies on the mechanisms of triploidy have shown the existence of maternal nonreduction at the first or second meiotic division producing a diploid oocyte, the counterpart may exist giving a diploid polar body and an anucleate oocyte.

The recent study of Wallace *et al.* (1982) shows that complete moles contain exclusively maternal mitochondrial DNA, suggesting the fertilization of a mature anucleate ovum.

Although androgenesis seems to be the most frequent event leading to hydatidiform mole, there have also been two observations of 46,XX moles in which both a paternal and a maternal genome were detected (Jacobs and Hassold, 1980; P. Couillin and J. Boué, unpublished observation).

The results of sex chromatin analysis show that in 46,XX moles X-chromosome inactivation is present. This situation can be compared to the parthenogenetic ovarian teratoma, in which a late-replicating X has been demonstrated (McCaw and Latt, 1977). In these two types of chromosome abnormalities with an apparently normal 46,XX karyotype the two X chromosomes are identical, and yet, according to the Lyon hypothesis, X-inactivation occurs.

Tetraploidy

Observed in about 5% of the chromosome abnormalities found in abortuses, tetraploidy has been occasionally reported in a liveborn infant (Golbus *et al.,* 1976; Pitt *et al.,* 1981).

The sex chromosome complements of all reported human tetraploidies have been either XXXX or XXYY. Tetraploidy is a postconceptional event resulting from a failure of cell cleavage at the first mitotic division, the 46 chromosomes dividing to create 92 chromosomes in the same undivided cell. The observations of abortuses with 94 chromosomes in which the extra chromosome was duplicated [i.e., 94,XXXX, 16+, 16+ (J. Boué and Boué, 1973a; Kajii et al., 1980)] are explained by the same event occurring in a trisomic zygote, and thus confirm the mechanism.

The results of sex chromatin analysis show that 92,XXYY tetraploidies are chromatin negative and that 92,XXXX tetraploidies have two Barr bodies.

Recently Sheppard et al. (1982) reported an aborted tetraploid conceptus in which one maternal and three paternal chromosome contributions were demonstrated, in favor of a trispermic origin. This specimen was macroscopically a complete mole.

Phenotypic Expression

During the last decade cytogenetic studies associated with pathological analysis have allowed the distinction of different syndromes among the molar pregnancies and their possible malignant sequelae. Thus, comparison with previous descriptions must be made with caution, as they include mixed populations incorporating different molar syndromes.

Complete Hydatidiform Moles.   The complete trophoblastic hyperplasia or complete hydatidiform mole is characterized by rapidly progressing, generalized vesicular change of all the placental villi and widespread gross trophoblastic hyperplasia of both layers, cyto- and syncytiotrophoblast. There is no amniotic sac with membranes, no embryonic formation, and no cord or evidence of fetal placental circulation.

These moles are associated with a diploid karyotype, mainly 46,XX, the chromosomes being paternally derived.

There have been previous observations of hydatidiform moles with a coexistent fetus, but in a recent observation (Fisher et al., 1982) it has been shown that it was a twin pregnancy with an androgenetic complete mole and a fetus with a diploid karyotype derived from both parents.

Human Triploidy: Partial Moles with Embryonic Formation.   This morphological entity is observed in the majority (86%) of triploid abortuses (Philippe et al., 1980; Szulman et al., 1981) and is characterized by a specimen with a large amniotic sac with membranes, a cord, and an embryonic formation. The placenta shows partial and focal trophoblastic hyperplasia and hydatidiform changes.

Scalloping of the villi is a highly characteristic feature of triploid moles and so is the formation of trophoblastic inclusions or microcysts.

Irrespective of the gestational age at abortion, the developmental arrest of the embryos occurs at 4–6 weeks in most cases, but there are wide variations, from early arrests at 3 weeks to stillborn infants at term.

In abortuses, the malformations seen in the embryos were mainly those of the central nervous system: cyclocephaly, absence or anomaly of the hypophysis, failure of closure of the neural groove, and craniorachischisis or spina bifida (Giroud et al., 1973; J. Boué et al., 1976b). Specimens aborted during the second trimester usually had minor malformations.

At term, the clinical syndrome of triploidy is also associated with placental lesions, partial hydatidiform changes, and different types of malformations. Among these the most frequent are low birthweight, cranial bone abnormalities associated with central nervous system abnormalities, and genital anomalies. A nearly constant malformation is syndactyly (Wertelecki et al., 1976; Gosden et al., 1976; J. Boué, personal observations; Blackburn et al., 1982).

In about 15% of triploid conceptuses, the same phenotypic expressions of the embryos were found, but the pathological examination of the placentas showed a normal or hypoplastic trophoblast without macroscopic villous enlargment (Szulman et al., 1981).

Recently, the histopathologic examination of triploid abortuses was investigated in correlation with the parental origin of the additional haploid complement (Jacobs et al., 1982). It was shown that the development of partial hydatidiform mole is highly correlated with the mechanism of origin of the triploidy. Most partial moles are paternally derived triploids, and maternally derived triploids corresponding to digyny II are nonmolar.

In correlation with these findings, the mean gestational age of triploid abortuses with two paternal sets of chromosomes is generally longer (122 ± 34 days) than in triploid abortuses with two maternal sets (74 ± 25 days).

The placental pathological findings observed in both complete and partial moles correlate highly with the.presence of two paternal haploid sets, but in the case of a partial mole, the effect may be diluted by the presence of a maternal haploid complement (Surti et al., 1979). It is interesting to note that when explants of hydatidiform moles or of triploid chorionic tissues are grown in tissue culture it is possible to observe *in vitro* circlelike proliferation of cells starting from explants, reproducing, in a two-dimensional plane, the aspects of swelling villi (A. Boué *et al.,* 1980).

The partial mole syndrome with a long *in utero* retention time is associated with high hCG levels and sometimes preeclampsia.

The most important point pertains to malignant or residual trophoblastic disease. Patients with spontaneous abortions of partial triploid moles had a rapid return to normal of hCG titers, and from different followup studies (Philippe *et al.,* 1980; Szulman and Surti, 1982; Lawler *et al.,* 1982*a*) there has been no case of metastatic disease following a partial mole pregnancy. Thus, malignant sequelae seem to arise only from complete hydatidiform moles.

Tetraploidy. The abortus consisted of a small chorionic vesicle often without amniotic membranes with a developmental age of 2–3 weeks. Embryonic formations were never observed.

Epidemiology

Triploidy and Tetraploidy. From the results of abortion surveys done in different parts of the world, no secular, seasonal, geographic, or racial variations have been observed in the incidence of triploidies and tetraploidies. No maternal or paternal age effects have been detected (Table XI).

It seems that delays in fertilization may have some influence on the occurrence of polyploidies. Different types of delays may be observed: aging of spermatozoa in the female genital tract, delay in release of mature oocytes (intrafollicular overripeness or preovulatory aging), and aging of ova released normally but fertilized late (intratubal overripeness or postovulatory aging). All three mechanisms are possible in human beings; the first and third are related to sexual activity and the second to anomalies in ovulation.

Even though it is extremely difficult to establish that a delay in fertilization occurs involving aging of gametes, analysis of the questionnaires filled out by parents at the time of an abortion has offered some material for speculation.

A significant increase in the frequency of polyploidy was observed when ovulation occurred after the 14th day. The average interval found in the first part of the cycle was 14.95 days for normal karyotypes and 15.0 days for trisomies. For polyploidies, the interval is markedly longer: 17.06 days. This delay may reflect an anomaly of ovulation leading to intrafollicular overripeness.

It is difficult to demonstrate delay between ovulation and fertilization. Only those cases in which a temperature curve was available and in which the dates of intercourse seemed sufficiently reliable were selected for analysis. In 24 observations, there were intervals of 2 days or more before and after the probable date of ovulation and the possible day of fertilization (J. Boué et al., 1975).

It has been suggested that some drugs might produce conditions favoring the occurrence of accidents leading to triploidies. An increased frequency of polyploidy was noted by Carr (1970) after steroid contraceptive treatment. Subsequent studies (J. Boué et al., 1975; Alberman et al., 1980) did not confirm these findings.

An increase in the frequency of polyploidy in abortuses was observed in pregnancies after ovulation-inducing therapy and especially after hCG (Table XVII) (J. Boué et al., 1975). These findings can be compared to the experimental studies of Takagi and Sasaki (1976) in mice (Table XVII), in which the incidence of digynic triploidies was significantly increased after superovulation with hCG treatment.

More recently, in a cytogenetic epidemiologic study of induced abortions (Yamamoto et al., 1982), it was shown that triploid formation was

Table XVII. Frequency of Abortuses with Polyploidy

From pregnancies after ovulation stimulation (hCG)[a]	Control	After stimulation
Number of abortuses karyotyped	1374	61
Polyploidy ($3n$ and $4n$)	216 (15.7%)	17 (27.9%)
Digynic triploidy after superovulation (hCG) in mice[b]	Control	Superovulated
Number of embryos karyotyped	1406	421
Polyploidy ($3n$ and $4n$)	67 (4.7%)	86 (20.4%)

[a] J. Boué and Boué (1975).
[b] Takagi and Sasaki (1976).

related to drug consumption. In the group of women receiving analgesics or antipyretics before the time of fertilization the frequency of triploid abortuses was 3/58 (5.2%) compared to 6/1136 (0.5%) in the untreated group.

The mechanisms leading to triploidy seem more sensitive to environmental factors that may act on the maturation of the oocytes.

Hydatidiform Moles. Some etiologic factors have been associated with hydatidiform moles that may explain the occurrence of an anucleate ovocyte.

First, this event seems more frequent at extreme reproductive ages, in women under 20 or over 40. Then, in small series of studies containing a total of 112 mothers in whom chromosome polymorphisms were studied, four women with a balanced structural rearrangement were detected. (Kajii and Ohama, 1977; Lawler et al., 1982b). Such a rearrangement may interfere with the segregation of chromosomes at meiosis I.

But the most striking etiologic problem is the geographic variation in the incidence of molar pregnancies, in opposition to all the other chromosome abnormalities responsible for pregnancy wastage, which have a similar incidence in all parts of the world.

In developed Western countries, hydatidiform moles are rarely observed (less than one in 2000 pregnancies), and it seems that during recent decades there has been a decrease in this frequency (E. Philippe, personal communication). However, hydatidiform moles occur in one pregnancy out of about 200 in Japan, more so in some Southeast Asian countries (Indonesia, the Philippines), and in one pregnancy out of about 400 in some West African countries (Senegal, Ivory Coast).

These geographic variations suggest environmental factors mostly linked to socioeconomic conditions. P. A. Jacobs (personal communication) also observed that the incidence decreases in women belonging to a high-risk ethnic group but born in a developed country.

To explain these variations, different hypotheses may be posed:

1. Environmental causative factors affect (directly or indirectly) the meiotic process in women and increase the incidence of anucleate oocytes. This is illustrated by the incidence of hydatidiform moles in women with balanced structural chromosome rearrangements.

2. The incidence of androgenesis is the same in all female populations, but the time of elimination of these abnormal eggs is different and influenced by environmental factors. This is supported by the fact that in

induced abortion studies, small eggs with all the characteristics of hydatidiform moles (karyotype and histological) have been collected. In countries where the incidence of hydatidiform moles is high, most of the population is immunocompromised and thus the recognition of a foreign cell is not as efficient as that in a population with high living standards.

3. It is also possible that there is an interaction of these factors.

Mosaicism

Different cytogenetic surveys of spontaneous abortions, induced abortions, and perinatal deaths have reported different incidences of mosaicism. Comparison of these results has also been possible with mosaic trisomies (Hassold 1982). The level of mosaicism varies in different surveys: several studies failed to identify any mosaics among spontaneously aborted trisomic conceptions (Lauritsen, 1976), others reported low levels, 1.6% (J. Boué and Boué, 1973a; Kajii et al., 1980), and some surveys reported levels of 5% or more (Creasy et al., 1976; Warburton et al., 1978; Hassold et al., 1980a). The distribution of the extra chromosomes involved is similar in nonmosaic and mosaic trisomies, trisomy 16 being the most frequent.

The detection of mosaicism depends on methodological factors, some of which are encountered in all cytogenetic analyses, i.e., the number of cells analyzed; others are related to the type of material in spontaneous abortion studies. While maternal cell contamination may be excluded by the high number of male specimens in these mosaics, the origin of the zygotic tissue does not exclude a result from *in vitro* changes in culture of these tissues (Kajii et al., 1980). Almost all the tissue samples from mosaic trisomies have been set up from amnion and chorion and not from the embryo itself, and *in vitro* change cannot be excluded.

Two interesting observations have been made:

1.The data of Hassold (1982) suggested that the extra chromosome in mosaic trisomies has a meiotic origin, the normal line developing after fertilization. In the mosaic trisomy group the mothers have the same mean maternal age as the mothers of the nonmosaic trisomic specimens.

2. The process leading to mosaicism does not occur with the same frequency among the different trisomies (Stene and Warburton, 1981).

The frequency of mosaicism is elevated among nonacrocentric trisomies (37 of 409 trisomic abortuses, 9%), and is very unusual among the acrocentric trisomies (one in 229 trisomic abortuses) (Hassold, 1982).

Structural Anomalies

The frequency of structural chromosome rearrangements involved in pregnancy wastage, the different types of rearrangement that are observed, and the question of their inheritance or *de novo* appearance have been evaluated in different ways.

1. *Cytogenetic studies of pregnancy wastage.* Unbalanced structural rearrangements have been detected in only 3–6% of the chromosomal abnormalities found in abortuses. But the data of seven surveys collected by Jacobs (1981a) show an increase of unbalanced rearrangements in abortuses compared to the incidence in population studies. A similar increase has been observed in perinatal death surveys (Table XVIII). In a series of 37 unbalanced rearrangements observed in abortuses, about one-half were inherited and the other half appeared *de novo* (J. Boué and Boué, 1973a).

2. *Cytogenetic studies of couples with recurrent abortion.* Table XIX shows the results of different European surveys of couples with two or more spontaneous abortions. A balanced structural rearrangement has been found in one member in 7.2% of these couples.

Table XVIII. Incidence of Structural Chromosome Rearrangements

Population studied	Number	Balanced rearrangements		Unbalanced rearrangements	
		Number	Percent	Number	Percent
Newborn (seven surveys[a])	59,452	113	0.19	31	0.05
Abortuses (seven surveys[a])	5,726	16	0.28	88	1.54
Perinatal deaths (three surveys[b])	1,176	5	0.4	6	0.5

[a] From Jacobs (1981a).
[b] Data from Machin and Crolla (1974), Kuleshov (1976), Sutherland *et al.* (1978).

Table XIX. Incidence of Structural Chromosome
Rearrangements in Couples with Recurrent (≥2) Abortions[a]

	Number of couples studied	Couples with balanced structural rearrangements	
		Number	Percent
Barcelona	32	6	17.8
Gent	96	8	8.3
Leiden	67	9	13.4
Padova	145	14	9.6
Paris	315	16	5.1
Prague	115	89	7.8
Rotterdam	148	14	9.6
Strasbourg	217	6	2.8
Zurich	96	7	7.3
Total	1231	89	7.2

[a] European studies. Antich et al. (1980), Matton et al. (1980), Geraedts and Klasen (1980), Bortotto et al. (1980), Turleau et al. (1979), Subrt (1980), Sachs (1980), Stoll et al. (1980), Schmid (1980).

The analysis of the frequency of the different types of structural anomalies in these couples compared to the frequency in newborn surveys shows a 20-fold increase of these anomalies. Different types of rearrangement are involved in this increase (Table XX).

In the recent study of Schwartz and Palmer (1983) structural chro-

Table XX. Frequency of Structural Chromosome Rearrangements

Types of rearrangements	In newborn surveys[a]		In couples with recurrent abortions[b]		Increase
	Number	Percent	Number	Percent	
Robertsonian	52	0.087	20	0.89	×10
Reciprocal	52	0.087	39	1.75	×20
Inversion	9	0.015	13	0.58	×40
Others	—	—	8	—	—
Total	113	0.19	80	3.58	×20

[a] Total of 59,452 individuals.
[b] Total of 2232 individuals.

Table XXI. Ascertainment of Structural Rearrangements in 152 Couples
Referred for Prenatal Diagnosis

Rearrangements	Infant with unbalanced anomaly	Abortions or sterility		Others	Total
		Number	Percent		
DqDq	5	22	71	4	31
DqGq	21	4	14	3	28
Reciprocal	30	31	40	16	77
Inversions	2	14	64	6	22
Total	58	71	45	29	158

mosome rearrangements were found in ten of 137 couples (7.3%) experiencing only first trimester abortions and no chromosome abnormalities were found in the groups with fetal wastage occurring later.

3. *Analysis of the ascertainment of the anomaly in parents* carrying a balanced structural rearrangement who are referred for a prenatal diagnosis. Table XXI shows the ascertainment in 152 couples studied in our laboratory; 45% were ascertained by a history of recurrent abortions.

Some particular aspects of pregnancy wastage can be studied in relation to the types of structural rearrangements.

Robertsonian Translocations.   Studies on the segregation of the rearranged chromosomes in families with Robertsonian translocations (Hamerton, 1970) have shown that the risk of a heterozygous mother having an affected child is greater than that of a heterozygous father. Similar results were observed in data collected from prenatal diagnoses (European Collaborative Study, A. Boué and Gallano, 1984). From the data collected in spontaneous abortion material, it was observed that when the unbalanced Robertsonian translocation was inherited in spontaneously aborted fetuses the carrier was the mother in most of the cases (Table XXII). These observations seem to exclude the hypothesis of frequency differences of early losses of unbalanced fetuses in relation to the sex of the carrier of the balanced translocation.

These finding in humans can be compared with the observation made in the progeny of mice heterozygous for Robertsonian translocation chromosomes (see page 36).

Reciprocal Translocations.   Some aspects of the consequences of reciprocal translocations have been studied in couples referred for pre-

Table XXII. Inherited Unbalanced Robertsonian Translocations

		Parent carrying the balanced translocation	
Survey	Anomaly	Mother	Father
Liveborn progeny	DqDq	1	1
(Hamerton, 1970)	DqGq	16	4
	GqGq	2	—
Prenatal diagnosis	DqGq	25	—
(A. Boué et al., 1983b)	GqGq	3	—
Spontaneous abortions	DqDq	6	1
(Boué and Boué, 1981)	DqGq	5	—
	GqGq	—	—

natal diagnosis (European Collaborative Study, A. Boué and Gallano, 1984).

The frequency of unbalanced fetuses was correlated with the method of ascertainment of the anomaly in the family. Results in Table XXIII clearly show that when the structural anomaly was ascertained through a history of recurrent abortions, the risk of detecting an unbalanced fetus in prenatal diagnosis was low (3.8%) compared with the risk in the group where the anomaly was ascertained through an infant with an unbalanced karyotype (21.6%).

Some characteristics of reciprocal translocations ascertained through a history of recurrent abortions were compared to those ascertained through an unbalanced malformed infant:

The distribution of break points on the chromosomes is not significantly different from the expected random distribution when the trans-

Table XXIII. Risk of an Unbalanced Fetus in Relation to the Ascertainment of the Anomaly in the Family[a]

	Unbalanced infant	Spontaneous abortion	Other anomaly
Reciprocal translocations	50/232	7/184	15/197
	(21.6%)	(3.8%)	(7.6%)
Inversions	6/11	0/21	1/100
	(54%)		(1%)

[a] From A. Boué et al. (1983b).

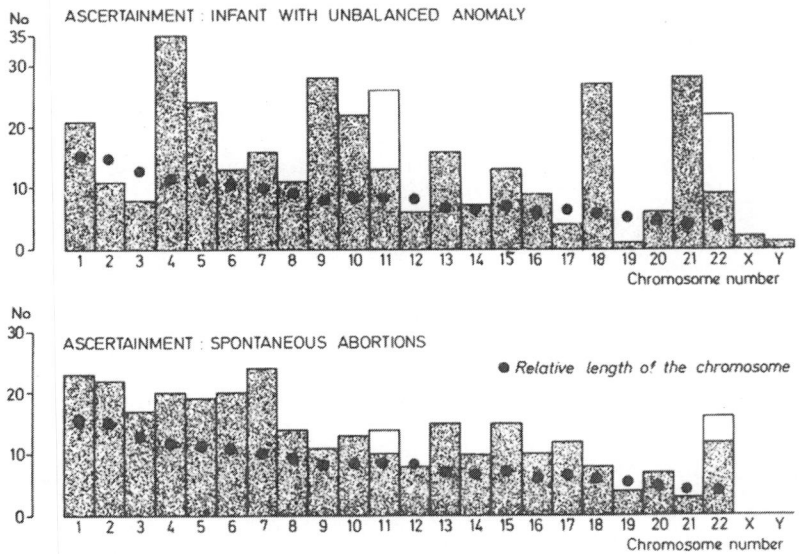

Fig. 2. Distribution of the chromosomes involved in reciprocal translocations in relation to the method of ascertainment of the anomaly in the family. The numbers of observations for each chromosome are compared to the random distribution calculated according to the relative length of the chromosome (black dots). Due to the number of 11;22 translocations the white column represents the total number of observations collected for chromosomes 11 and 22 and the grey column the number of observations if only one 11;22 observation is taken in account.

location has been ascertained through prenatal wastage (European survey) (Fig. 2). These results are in contrast with the nonrandom distribution when the anomaly was ascertained in unbalanced infants. Similar results were observed previously by Aurias *et al.* (1978) and Daniel (1979).

The potential chromosome imbalance in these translocations was measured in units, assuming that the haploid human karyotype consists of 300 bands (Aurias *et al.*, 1978); for example, the short arm of chromosome 6 measures six units.

When the anomaly was ascertained through a history of recurrent abortions, the total length of chromosome segments that can be involved in the imbalance is longer (mean imbalance, 5.95 units) than when the anomaly was ascertained through an unbalanced infant (mean imbalance, 3.56 units) (Fig. 3).

Inversions.   Few data have been collected on chromosome inversions and their consequences on prenatal wastage.

In the collaborative studies on prenatal diagnosis, most of the inversions were ascertained through a history of recurrent abortions and in this group the total potential imbalance is much longer (9.36 units) than in the inversions ascertained through an infant with the unbalanced anomaly (four families only; mean imbalance, 3 units).

The structural anomalies responsible for recurrent abortions generally have a greater possible chromosome imbalance, which leads in most cases to early arrest of development.

Combining different studies, Lippman-Hand and Vekemans (1983) showed that in couples with recurrent abortions, females are more likely than males to be carriers, reflecting the fact that structural rearrangements that are compatible with fertility in the female may be associated with sterility in the male. This seems to be the case in 13q14q Robertsonian translocations.

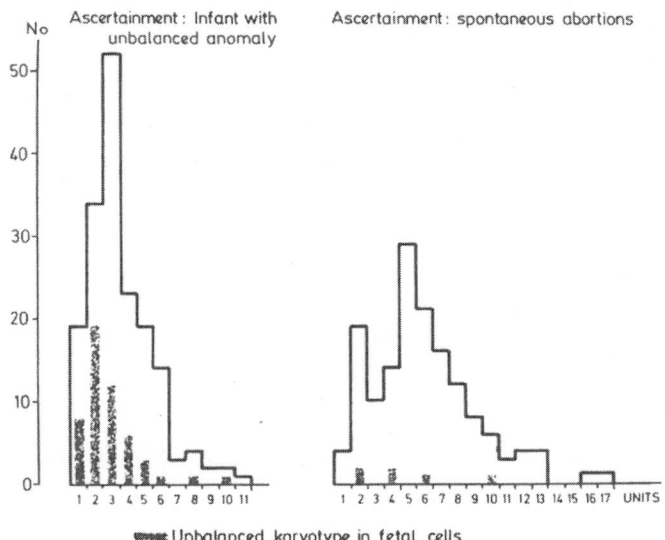

Fig. 3. Distribution of the length of the potential chromosome imbalance in reciprocal translocations in relation to the method of ascertainment of the anomaly in the family. The grey columns represent the number of observations of unbalanced karyotypes in prenatal diagnoses performed in these families (in some families more than one prenatal diagnosis has been performed; see Table XII).

ANIMAL MODEL FOR MEIOTIC NONDISJUNCTION AND EXPERIMENTALLY INDUCED MONOSOMY AND TRISOMY

Many of the problems related to the developmental pathology of zygotic and fetal aneuploidy, as discussed in the previous sections, are amenable to systematic investigation in a mouse model of autosomal monosomy and trisomy (Gropp, 1982). The experimental design is based on the occurrence and controllability of meiotic nondisjunction in a breeding system with Robertsonian (Rb) heterozygosity (Gropp et al., 1975; Gropp and Winking, 1981). It has been established in the mouse by introduction of Rb chromosomes from wild mice into laboratory strains using selective backcross breeding procedures.

In principle, the purpose of an animal model for human disease is to fill gaps of clinical knowledge, to elucidate or to ascertain mechanisms difficult to assess in man, and to improve the understanding of a clinical problem by providing a background of systematic knowledge. Along these lines, it is the aim of this section to supplement the previously discussed clinical issues with observations made in the mouse model on (1) disorders of meiotic segregation in individuals heterozygous for Rb chromosomes, (2) the conditions and the chronological order of prenatal loss and elimination of monosomic and trisomic zygotes, and (3) the developmental profiles of specific trisomies, since trisomy represents the most frequent type of prenatal disorder in man.

Model for the Study of Meiotic Malsegregation and Preferential Segregation of Rb Chromosomes

In the house mouse *(M. m. domesticus),* as in some other mammalian species, Robertsonian (Rb) variation due to centric whole arm translocation is a frequent type of chromosome rearrangement, and is an important mechanism of evolutionary karyotype diversification. A great and almost unlimited reservoir of metacentric Rb chromosomes with different arm compositions exists in regional races of commensal and wild-living populations of the house mouse in Central and Southern Europe (Gropp and Winking, 1981; Gropp et al., 1983) and is available for introduction by backcross breeding into laboratory strains. Genetically, there

XXIV. Rates of Malsegregation (Nondisjunction) of Males Heterozygous for a Single Rb Metacentric (Rb/+) Chromosome

Designation (arm composition)	Chromosome arm counts in male meiotic metaphase II, %					Nondisjunction rates calculated on the basis of percentage of $>20 \times 2^a$	Number of MII cells scored
	<19	19	20	21	>21		
Rb(1.3)1Bnr/+	—	8	85	7		14	400
Rb(4.6)2Bnr/+	—	10	79	11		22	300
Rb(5.15)3Bnr/+	—	13	73	14		28	300
Rb(11.13)4Bnr/+	—	12	74	14		28	400
Rb(8.12)5Bnr/+	2	3	93	2		4	300
Rb(9.14)6Bnr/+	1	5	89	5		10	300
Rb(16.17)7Bnr/+	1	2	95	2		4	300
Rb(10.11)8Bnr/+	—	4	95	1		2	600
Rb(4.12)9Bnr/+	—	5	91	4		8	400
Rb(1.10)10Bnr/+	—	2	96	2		4	400
Rb(3.8)2Rma/+	0.5	9	81.5	9		18	200
Rb(6.13)3Rma/+	—	4.3	92.3	3.3		6.6	300
Rb(4.15)4Rma/+	—	11	78	11		22	300
Rb(10.11)5Rma/+	—	6.6	86.2	7.2		14.4	600
Rb(2.18)6Rma/+	—	7	84.7	8.3		16.3	300
Rb(9.16)9Rma/+	—	11.7	80	8.3		16.6	300

[a] This calculation avoids errors by overrepresentation of hypomodal cells due to artificial chromosome losses (Gropp and Winking, 1981).

is evidence for perfect arm homology between metacentric Rb chromosomes derived from wild mice and the acrocentrics contributed in laboratory-bred hybrids by the laboratory mouse. However, cytological disorders of meiosis, with nondisjunction of the chromosomes involved in the formation of metacentric/acrocentric trivalents, or of multivalents of higher order, are frequent in the gametogenesis of male and female hybrids heterozygous for Rb chromosomes derived from wild mice (Gropp and Winking, 1981). Table XXIV shows that the actual rates of meiosis I nondisjunction, as calculated from chromosome arm counts in meiotic metaphase II plates, are highly variable in heterozygous males with Rb metacentrics of different arm compositions. The variation comprises a range from very low values up to 28% unbalanced products of anaphase I malsegregation. A similarly broad variation of meiotic anaphase I malsegregation is found in oocytes of different Rb heterozygotes, but if the same heterozygous conditions are compared in males and

Table XXV. Comparison of Rates of Meiotic Anaphase I Malsegregation
(MII Evaluation) in Male versus Female Single Rb Metacentric
Heterozygotes

Spermatocytes			Oocytes	
n	Rate of nonmodal MII,[a] %	Rb/+	Rate of nonmodal MII,[a] %	n
400	14	Rb(1.3)1Bnr	58	103
400	28	Rb(11.13)4Bnr	34	77
300	4	Rb(16.17)7Bnr	34	83
300	7	Rb(6.13)3Rma	34	69
300	22	Rb(4.15)4Rma	50	85
300	16	Rb(4.17)13Lub	61	66
300	4	Rb(8.17)1Iem	33	102

[a] Calculated by doubling the hyperhaploid MII counts.

females (Table XXV), most malsegregation rates are found to be 3–4 times higher in females. The rates of meiotic malsegregation presented in Tables XXIV and XXV were confirmed by karyotype evaluations of the postzygotic progeny derived from the unbalanced products of meiotic nondisjunction. The considerable variation of the risk of malsegregation among different heterozygotes might be explained by structural differences that presumably exist in the pericentric regions of Rb metacentrics where a spatial adjustment is necessary in the meiotic prophase (Gropp and Winking, 1981). On the other hand, the reasons for the higher risk of female versus male heterozygotes in producing first meiotic anaphase nondisjunction remain obscure.

A further feature observed in many of the female but not in the male Rb heterozygotes is a distorted transmission of the rearranged Rb chromosome to the balanced products of the meiotic divisions, and thus to the balanced offspring. Table XXVI shows that such distortion leads to a higher representation of segregation products without the Rb chromosome in the balanced progeny, which corresponds to a sort of meiotic drive against the rearranged chromosome. Transmission distortion in some males (see Table XXVI) is an exception due to *t*-mutants on chromosome 17, as in the Rb13Lu8 metacentric. Segregation distortion occurs also in man, as shown by Hamerton (1970) and A. Boué *et al.* (1984). However, in man the drive goes in the opposite direction, i.e., in favor of the rearranged chromosome, and the phenomenon is not unfrequent in the male sex, which poses greater problems of explanation than in the female, where the conditions of an unequal first meiotic division make preferential inclusion or exclusion of a special chromosome in the polar body understandable.

It appears that meiotic malsegregation in the mouse is mostly caused by first meiotic anaphase nondisjunction. Second meiotic anaphase malsegregation has been observed, but its frequency is low, although exact evaluations do not exist.

Thus, the use of the Rb mouse model for meiotic nondisjunction induced by structural heterozygosity shows (1) variability of rates depending on the composition of the rearranged chromosome, (2) considerably higher rates in female versus male heterozygous carriers of the same Rb chromosome, and (3) a phenomenon of meiotic drive, which leads in the mouse, in contrast to man, to a higher representation of the rearranged chromosome in the progeny.

Table XXVI. Transmission of the Rb Metacentric Chromosome in the Balanced Progeny of Single Rb Metacentric Male and Female Heterozygotes[a]

Male				Female		
n	Percent heterozygous	Percent homozygous	Balanced progeny	Percent heterozygous	Percent homozygous	n
271	48	52	Rb(1.3)1Bnr	36	64	261*
154	52	48	Rb(5.15)3Bnr	36	64	83*
132	52	48	Rb(11.13)4Bnr	49	51	108
154	52	48	Rb(8.12)5Bnr	51	49	160
151*	59	41	Rb(16.17)7Bnr	38	62	89*
110	54	46	Rb(10.11)8Bnr	40	60	120*
125	49	51	Rb(4.12)9Bnr	46	54	107
			Rb(1.10)10Bnr	49	51	142
93	44	56	Rb(6.13)3Rma	26	74	62*
124	48	52	Rb(4.15)4Rma	36	64	67*
191	43	53	Rb(10.11)5Rma	33	67	126*
78	42	58	Rb(2.17)11Rma	28	72	99*
214*	88	12	Rb(4.17)13Lub	38	62	181*
96	44	56	Rb(8.17)6Sic	40	60	102*
114	43	57	Rb(8.17)1Iem	47	53	98
103	44	56	Rb(6.15)1Ald	39	61	103*

[a] See Gropp and Winking (1981). Asterisk denotes a significant deviation from 1:1 distribution; in the male deviations as in Rb(4.17)3Lub/+ are attributable to t-mutants.

Model of Multiple Rb Heterozygosity for Production of High Rates of First Meiotic Anaphase Nondisjunction and Evaluation of Prenatal Losses

Errors of meiotic chromosome segregation are responsible for mono-somic and trisomic zygotes. These are subject to selection in the pre- or postimplantation period. The principles of postzygotic selection working against abnormal products of meiotic errors in male and female game-togenesis are summarized in Fig. 4.

Direct evidence for these principles is provided by a design of mas-sive production of aneuploid gametes, both hypohaploid and hyperhap-loid, using backcrosses of mouse hybrids heterozygous for a series of seven independent Rb metacentric chromosomes (Gropp, 1971; Ford, 1972). In this system an almost equal distribution of monosomy and tri-somy is noted among the preimplantation embryos on day 4–4½ (Table XXVII). This is expected since meiotic nondisjunction produces a com-plementary gamete without a special chromosome for every gamete car-rying two copies of it, and prezygotic selection of gametes is most prob-ably negligible. Later in development, at least after day 9, monosomy is no longer found. These results show that the deficiency of monosomic embryos in later gestation is not due to nullisomic gametes being less able to participate in fertilization than euhaploid or disomic gametes. Rather, the deficiency of monosomic embryos is due to impaired viability. It

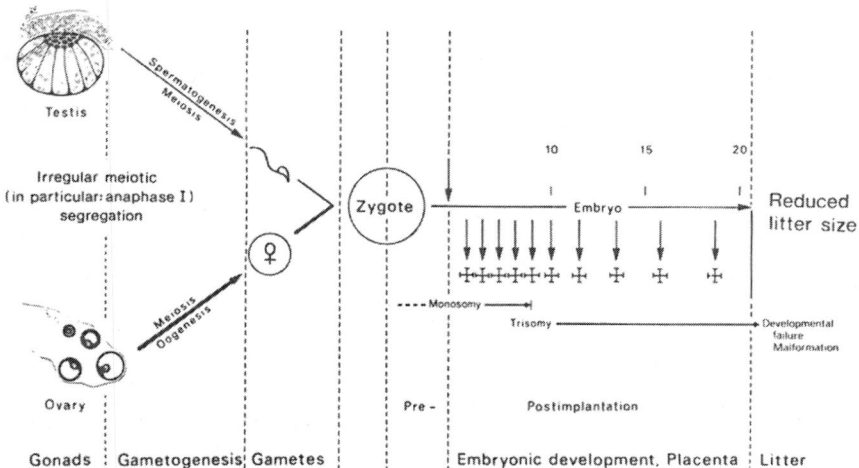

Fig. 4. Principle of the mouse model of segregational meiotic disorders.

Table XXVII. Frequency Distribution of Euploid ($2n = 40$) versus Monosomic/Trisomic ($2n \gtrless 40$) Embryos[a] in the Progeny of Male (Rb1–7Bnr) Heterozygotes[b] × Female NMRI

Stage of development	Day	Number of chromosome arms (hypomodal ← euploid → hypermodal)									Total
		≦36	37	38	39	40	41	42	43	≧44	
Preimplantation embryo	4–4.5	4	2	14	35	74	28	16	1	—	174
Postimplantation embryo	7–8	—	—	—	3	81	30	10	4	—	128
Postimplantation embryo	9–15	—	—	—	3	239	79	14	—	1	336
Postimplantation embryo	19	—	—	—	—	56	2	—	—	—	58
Liveborn young	—	—	—	—	—	58	—	—	—	—	58

[a] Data for male and female F_1 from Gropp (1978) and Ford (1972).
[b] "Poschiavinus" (Tobacco mouse) F_1 with heterozygosity of seven Rb chromosomes, Rb1Bnr/+–Rb7Bnr/+ (Gropp and Winking, 1981).

seems that monosomy 19, i.e., the monosomy of the smallest autosome, is the most rapidly lethal, because it is no longer found by day 4.5 (Magnuson *et al.*, 1982). Other monosomies, such as 5, 12, or 17, survive slightly longer, but it is not yet clear how long they are viable past implantation and before day 7 (see Table XXVII). In contrast, losses of trisomies are barely perceptible before day 10 of fetal development, but they occur more and more frequently after this time.

Developmental Profiles of Monosomy and Trisomy: Principles and Mechanisms of Abnormal Development

General Developmental Aspects of Monosomy and Trisomy

The most suitable experimental strategy for production of specific monosomies and trisomies is based on first meiotic anaphase nondisjunction in a parent doubly heterozygous for two Rb metacentrics with both Rb chromosomes showing partial homology for one of their arms (Fig. 5). Under these circumstances the meiotic quadrivalents in a heterozygous father or mother produce predictable types of unbalanced gametes (Fig. 6). In particular, sufficiently high yields are found of mal-

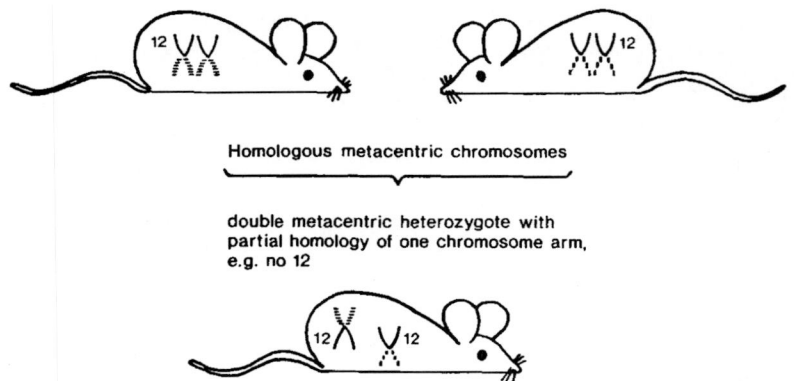

Fig. 5. Design for breeding mice doubly heterozygous for two different Rb chromosomes that share one of their arms (in the present case, chromosome 12).

segregation products with both Rb metacentrics (Fig. 6b) or the complementary condition without such chromosomes (Fig. 6a). They give rise, after fertilization with a chromosomally balanced gamete (Fig. 6c), to the type of monosomy predetermined by the choice of the special double Rb heterozygous combination in one of the parents. This system comprises

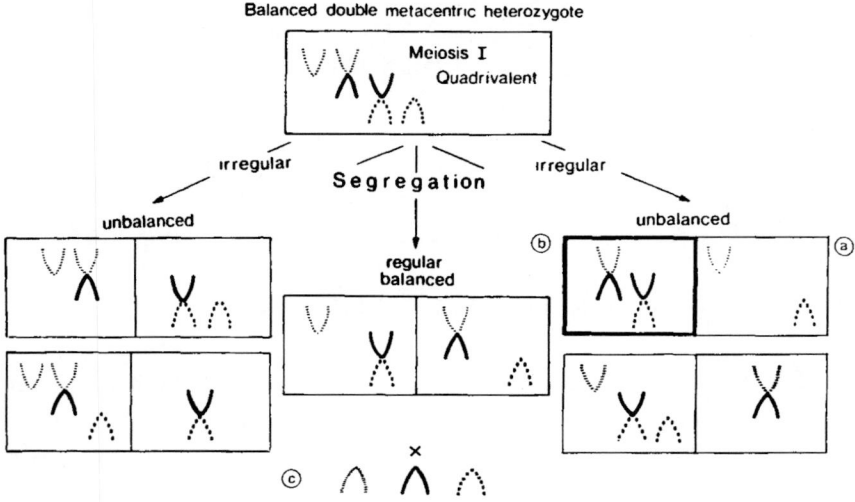

Fig. 6. Breeding design for induction of (a) monosomy and (b) trisomy by nondisjunction of partially homologous Rb metacentric chromosomes. Both (a) and (b) are frequent types of unbalanced segregation products.

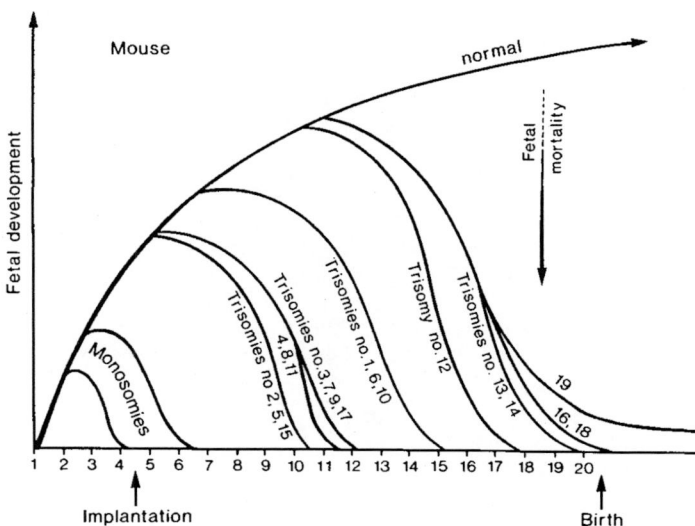

Fig. 7. Developmental profiles of monosomies and trisomies.

all autosomes, but not the sex chromosomes of the mouse. It allows the induction of each one of the 19 autosomal monosomies and trisomies and the establishment of their developmental profiles (Fig. 7).

Lethality of the monosomies is early, as shown in Table XXVII. Studies on specific monosomies have been carried out in the preimplantation period on monosomies 5 and 17 by Dyban and Baranov (1978) and on monosomies 1, 12, 17, and 19 by Epstein and Travis (1979) and Magnuson et al. (1982). It appears that monosomic embryos in the morula and early blastocyst stage have fewer cells than normal or trisomic littermates (Gropp, 1978). Observations on monosomy 19 do not reveal abnormalities on a gross morphological level or in cellular ultrastructure until the time of death (Magnuson et al., 1982). Evidence for dosage effects rather than the haploid expression of lethal genes as cause of early mortality in monosomy is provided by the studies of Magnuson et al. (1982), showing that the loss of monosomy 19, before the late blastocyst stage, occurs at similar rates in inbred and in noninbred strains, and that viable monosomic cells were present in monosomy 19 ↔ diploid chimaeras. Such observations need an explanation like the metabolic complementation of a defect in synthesis.

In contrast, most mouse trisomics (Fig. 7) are viable at least until day 11 or 12, while some others reach the late gestational period. Trisomy

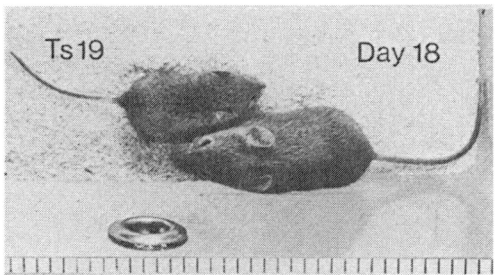

Fig. 8. Trisomy 19 male together with normal littermate on day 18 after birth. Note marked hypoplasia of trisomy 19 individual. The eyelids are open in the trisomy 19 (not seen on the photograph) and in the normal.

19 can survive postnatally (Figs. 7 and 8). The longest documented survival is 27 days after birth. However, the actual developmental profiles of trisomic conditions depend to a large extent on the genomic or strain background. Thus, trisomy 12 shows earlier death (around day 13) on partial BALB/c or C3H background, late death (around days 18–19) on partial C57BL/6J background, and earlier death in pure C57BL/6J genome (unpublished observations).

Gross Phenotype Abnormality

The main abnormalities observed with variable severity in all trisomies are developmental retardation and hypoplasia. Trisomy 19 represents an example of marked hypoplasia with only slight developmental retardation, as shown in Fig. 8 for an individual on day 18 after birth compared with a normal littermate. The individual organs, such as brain, lung, kidneys, and gonads, display similar features of prevalent hypoplasia with slight to moderate retardation. This is shown for the brain in Fig. 9. In contrast, developmental retardation is more marked in some other trisomies, as, e.g., in trisomy 1 (see Fig. 10b), 6, 10, or 12.

Several trisomies with survival until the later fetal stages very often exhibit more or less severe subcutaneous edema and cavital hydrops with first appearance around day 15. Observations from trisomy 19 show that the edematous changes can disappear in the final prenatal period or at least by the neonate stage (Gropp, 1982).

Another major developmental disorder is gross malformation. In the

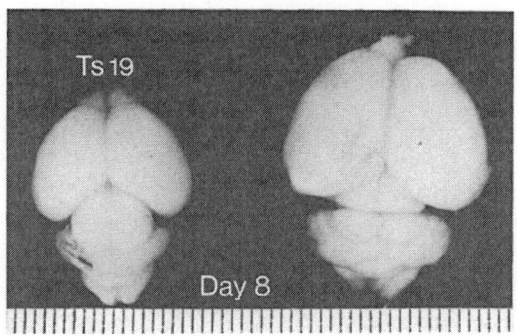

Fig. 9. Brains of (left) trisomy 19 and (right) normal littermate on day 8 after birth. Regular appearance of gross morphology of the brain in trisomy 19, but very marked hypoplasia.

severe form of trisomy 1, holoprosencephaly combined with aprosopia or cyclopia is observed (see Fig. 10c). Exencephaly occurs in several trisomies. It is a constant finding in trisomy 12, less frequent in 14, and rare in 9, 16, and 17. The conclusion from this limited specificity is that the malformation is trisomy-dependent rather than trisomy-specific. A further observation according to which exencephaly invariably includes the rhombencephalic segment of the hindbrain in trisomy 12, while this segment is always closed in trisomy 14, lends support to the assumption that this malformation is caused by temporal disturbances of the morphogenetic processes of organ development (Putz *et al.*, 1980). Apparently, the eventual developmental consequences of chromosome triplication are mediated indirectly by complex disorders of growth and differentiation,

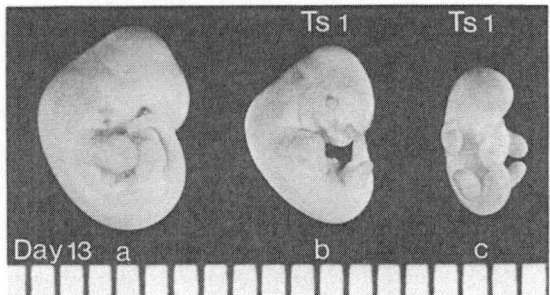

Fig. 10. (a) Normal fetus compared with (b,c) trisomy 1 of the same litter on day 13 of fetal development. (b) Hypoplasia and developmental retardation of trisomy 1 fetus. (c) More severe hypoplasia and developmental retardation together with aprosopia and holoprosencephaly in trisomy 1 fetus.

rather than by direct gene effects. Support for such a concept of incomplete specifity also comes from observations on cleft palate and of cardiovascular malformations. Cleft palate is almost regularly associated with trisomy 13 (Hongell and Gropp, 1982), frequent in trisomy 18, and occasionally found in trisomy 16. It was not observed in our studies in trisomy 19, whereas cleft palate was reported by White *et al.* (1974) in some late trisomy 19 fetuses. Cardiovascular malformations are frequent in several mouse trisomies, such as ventricular septal defect (VSD) in trisomies 10, 12, 14, and 16 at rates above 50%, and "double outlet right ventricle" (DORV) in trisomies 13 and 14 at low rates, but more frequent in trisomy 16. Other cardiovascular malformations are observed in more specific associations, such as pulmonary stenosis (PS) in 86% of trisomy 13, and transposition of the great vessels (TGV) in 13.5% of trisomy 14.

Murine Trisomies As Specific Models for Human Trisomy

Mouse and human trisomy may show, by morphogenetic coincidence, similar developmental disorders. The occurrence of holoprosencephaly and cyclopia with very similar features in the more severe forms of murine trisomy 1 (Fig. 10c) and human trisomy 13 seems to reflect the fact that mammalian embryology follows similar morphogenetic patterns in mouse and man.

A more specific relationship has been claimed to exist between trisomy 16 of the mouse (Fig. 11) and trisomy 21 (Down syndrome) in man

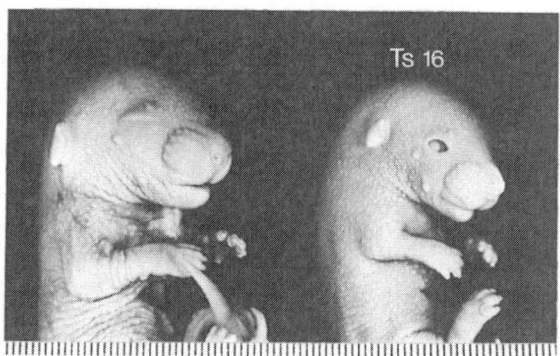

Fig. 11. Trisomy 16 on day 18 of fetal development compared with normal littermate. Note abnormally open eyelid in trisomy 16.

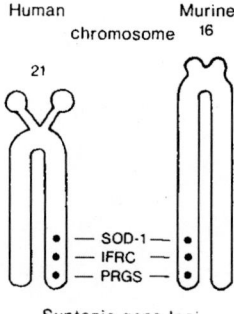

Human   Murine
chromosome   16

21

Fig. 12. Syntenic genes on mouse chromosome 16 and human chromosome 21. SOD-1, Superoxide dismutase; IFRC, interferon receptor protein; PRGS, phosphoribosylglycinamide synthetase.

— SOD-1 —
— IFRC —
— PRGS —

Syntenic gene loci

(Polani and Adinolfi, 1980; Epstein *et al.,* 1981). The narrow but trustworthy basis for such an assumption is the conservation and synteny of at least three gene loci [superoxide dismutase, SOD-1; the interferon receptor protein IFRC; and phosphoribosylglycinamide synthetase, PRGS (Francke and Taggart, 1979; Epstein *et al.,* 1981; C. J. Epstein *et al.,* unpublished work)] on a distal segment of the murine chromosme 16 and the human chromosome 21 (Fig. 12). From the descriptive embryology of murine trisomy 16 (Myabara *et al.,* 1982) it is worthwhile to emphasize the role played by the persistence of a common AV-canal and other cardiovascular disorders (VSD and DORV). Also, the eyelid, which normally closes at day 16–17, is mostly open in trisomy 16 (Fig. 11). In addition, this anomaly is often found associated with degeneration of the ocular lens. On the other hand, persistence of the common AV-canal is a very characteristic finding in Down syndrome, as are lid and lenticular (cataract) anomalies in this syndrome. No genetic homologies can be claimed for these parellelisms, but further studies should broaden the genetic basis of murine trisomy 16 as a natural model for human chromosomal disease, and stimulate embryologic, clinical, and immunologic studies in trisomy 16.

Principles of the Developmental Abnormality Caused by Chromosome Disorders

There are no simple answers to the question of why monosomy and trisomy in the zygote result in abnormal development, and why early or later developmental breakdown is inevitable.

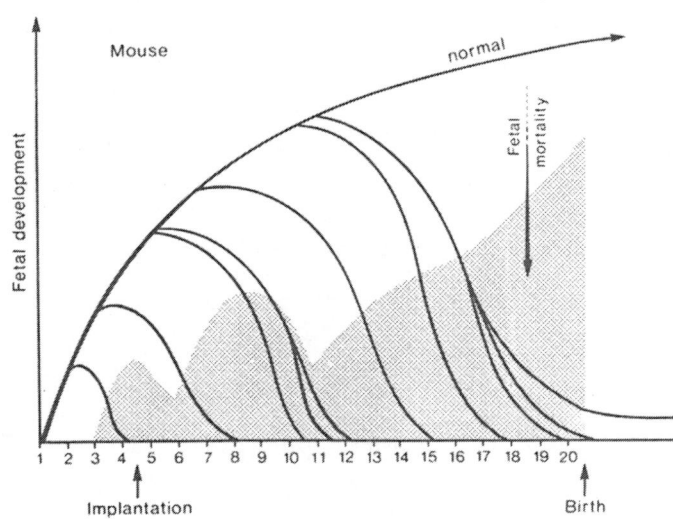

Fig. 13. Critical and vulnerable phases (grey) in relation to developmental profiles of monosomies and trisomies (see Fig. 7).

It may be meaningful to propose three main critical phases that determine the eventual downward course in the development of monosomy and trisomy (Fig. 13). A first and second phase of increased developmental vulnerability coincide roughly with the periods of implantation and organogenesis, respectively, the first of which selecting in particular against monosomies. One has to suppose that death of anlagen in the early developmental phase occurs to a large extent as a consequence of direct as well as indirect gene dosage effects, with metabolic disturbances and impairment of proliferation and differentiation (Epstein *et al.*, 1981; Gropp, 1982).

The origin of gross malformations, such as neural tube defects, craniofacial anomalies, and cardiovascular disorders, falls into the second critical phase (Fig. 13). Stage-, time-, and strain-specific vulnerability of blastemas involved in morphogenesis, on the one hand, and systemic hypoplasia or excessive cell deficiency in specific blastemas, on the other hand, can explain the actual types and the variability of malformations as well as their limited specificity.

Evidence for a third, presumably continuous critical phase (Fig. 13) comes from the observations of late fetal damage associated with severe or at least variably expressed edema in almost all trisomies surviving longer than day 15–16. This probably multifactorial condition is thought to be a consequence of vascular insufficiency in the (trisomic) hypoplastic fetal part of the placenta (Gropp, 1982) as well as of anemia and cardio-vascular anomalies of the fetus as main factors. It is proposed that edema in X0-Turner syndrome as well as in some autosomal errors in man are caused by similar mechanisms. The condition in the mouse might well be considered as an animal model for edema observed in developmental disorders in man.

It appears logical to assume that the different mechanisms of damage to the fetus can overlap each other, and that the superposition of different effects leads to changing patterns in the course of development.

Perspectives for Studies in the Mouse

It is proposed to consider the mouse model of Rb heterozygosity as a useful design for a step-by-step analysis of meiotic errors, zygotic aneu-ploidy, and ensuing developmental disorders (see Fig. 4). The method-ology and the actual accumulation of such knowledge in the animal model will direct new lines of research in man. Clearly, in the field of genetic and, in particular, chromosomal disease, the stimulation pro-vided by the mouse model for human pathology is not merely based on formal analogies. Its impact comes from the similarity of the fundamen-tal mechanisms, and, in at least some instances, from homologies of the genetic material.

CONCLUSION

Cytogenetic studies on spontaneous and induced abortions and on perinatal deaths have demonstrated the great frequency and variety of chromosome abnormalities at conception. These findings were unsus-pected and nearly unbelievable 20 years ago when these studies were started.

Those involved in the cytogenetic studies of pregnancy wastage were the first to be surprised by the variety of the types of chromosome errors observed in human conceptuses. It seems that any theoretically possible error can be observed at conception. Androgenesis was one of these surprises some years ago, and, very recently, another surprise was the observation of two conceptuses with a haploid state among 11 embryos obtained after *in vitro* fertilization (Angel *et al.,* 1983).

Pregnancy wastage represents the main natural means to eliminate the major part (around 99%) of chromosomally abnormal conceptuses, and "the efficiency of the natural process working to reduce the human genetic load can be considered truly remarkable" (Chandley 1981).

Knowledge of this phenomenon is important for the geneticist, the obstetrician, the pediatrician, and all medical practitioners. For example, an increase of the incidence of Down syndrome among younger mothers was recently noticed (Anon, 1983) and some environmental factors were suspected. But, as pointed out by Polani (1983), the effect may be due to an increased rate of survival to term of trisomic fetuses; the incidence of trisomy 21 at conception may be unchanged and the shift could be due to a variety of factors affecting fetal well-being.

The usefulness of an animal model for these studies is clearly demonstrated, and requires a selection of animals with structural rearrangements. In the same species the spontaneous incidence of chromosomal numerical errors should be relatively low. It seems that man in fact appears unique among all investigated mammalian species in showing such a high level of chromosomal abnormality among its early zygotes (Chandley, 1981). The species that have been studied are domestic or laboratory mammals that have been highly selected either by farmers over many centuries or by laboratory workers over decades. What is the situation among wild species and especially among primates?

The high incidence of genomic mutations and of chromosomal mutations (A. Boué *et al.,* 1983*a*) represents the sacrifice that the human species pays for its evolution: "le prix de la vie" (de Grouchy, 1976). Of these innumerable mutations and chromosome anomalies a few have been incorporated into our hereditary pattern and have provided the extensive diversity of the human genome.

REFERENCES

Alberman, E., Polani, P. E., Fraser Roberts, J. A., Spicer, C. C., Eliott, M., and Armonstrong, E., 1972*a*, Parental exposure to X-irradiation and Down's syndrome, *Ann. Hum. Genet.* **32:**195–208.

Alberman, E., Polani, P. E., Fraser Roberts, J. A., Spicer, C. C., Eliott, M., Armstrong, E., and Dhadial, R. K., 1972b, Parental X-irradiation and chromosome constitution in their spontaneously aborted foetuses, *Ann. Hum. Genet. Lond.* **36**:185–194.

Alberman, E., Pharoah, P., Chamberlain, G., Roman, E., and Evans, S., 1980, Outcome of pregnancies following the use of oral contraceptives, *Int. J. Epidemiol.* **9**:207–213.

Alfi, O. S., Chang, R., and Azen, S. P., 1980, Evidence for genetic control of nondisjunction in man, *Am. J. Hum. Genet.* **32**:477–483.

Angel, R. R., Aitken, R. J., Van Look, P. F. A., Lumsden, M. A., and Templeton, A. A., 1983, Chromosome abnormalities in human embryos after *in vitro* fertilization, *Nature* **303**:336–338.

Anon, 1983, The elusive cause of Down's syndrome, *Lancet* **1**:1143–1144.

Antich, J., Clusellas, N., Twose, A., and Codo, R. M., 1980, Chromosomal abnormalities in parents in cases of reproductive failure, *Clin. Genet.* **17**:52.

Atkin, N. B., Klinger, H. P., 1962, The superfemale mole, *Lancet* **II**:727–728.

Aurias, A., Prieur, M., Dutrillaux, B., and Lejeune, J., 1978, Systematic analysis of 95 reciprocal translocations of autosomes, *Hum. Genet.* **45**:259–282.

Aymé, S., and Lippman-Hand, A., 1982, Maternal age effect in aneuploidy: Does altered embryonic selection play a role, *Ann. J. Hum. Genet.* **34**:558–565.

Biggers, J. D., 1981, *In vitro* fertilization and embryo transfer in human beings, *N. Engl. J. Med.* **304**:336–342.

Blackburn, W. R., Miller, W. P., Superneau, D. W., Cooley, N. R., Zellweger, H., and Wertelecki, W., 1982, Comparative studies of infants with mosaic and complete triploidy: An analysis of 55 cases, in: *Dysmorphology, Birth Defects: Original Article Series,* Vol. 18, Part 3B, pp. 251–274.

Bortotto, L., Baccichetti, C., Lenzini, E., Tenconi, R., Delendi, N., and Caufin, D., 1980, Cytogenetic survey of couples with habitual abortion and other reproductive wastage, *Clin. Genet.* **17**:56.

Boué, A., Boué, J., and Couillin, P., 1980, Aspects génétiques des arrêts précoces du développement, *Reprod. Nutr. Dev.* **20**:485–498.

Boué, A. and Boué, J., 1981, Chromosome structural rearrangements and reproductive failure, in: *Chromosome Today,* Vol. 7, (M. D. Bennet, M. Bobrow, and G. M. Hewitt eds.) pp. 281–290, George Allen and Unwin, London.

Boué, A., Gallano, P., Boué, J., Serre, J. L., and Feingold, J., 1983a, Genome and chromosome mutations, balance between appearance and elimination, in: *Issues and Reviews in Teratology* (H. Kalter, ed.), pp. 111–147, Plenum Press, New York.

Boué, A., Gallano, P., *et al.,* 1984, A collaborative study of the segregation of inherited chromosome structural rearrangements in 1356 prenatal diagnosis, *Prenatal Diagnosis* **4**:45–67.

Boué, J., and Boué, A., 1973a, Anomalies chromosomiques dans les avortements spontanés, in: *Chromosomal Errors in Relation to Reproductive Failure* (A. Boué and C. Thibault, eds,), pp. 29–55, INSERM, Paris.

Boué, J., and Boué, A., 1973b, Chromosomal analysis of two consecutive abortuses in each of 43 women, *Humangenetik* **19**:275–280.

Boué, J., Boué, A., and Lazar, P., 1975, Retrospective and prospective epidemiological studies of 1500 karyotyped spontaneous human abortions, *Teratology* **12**:11–26.

Boué, J., Daketse, M. J., Deluchat, C., Ravisé, N., and Boué, A., 1976a, Identification par les bandes Q et G des anomalies chromosomiques dans les avortements spontanés, *Ann. Genet.* **19**:233–239.

Boué, J., Philippe, E., Giroud, A., and Boué, A., 1976b, Phenotypic expression of lethal chromosomal anomalies in human abortuses, *Teratology* **14**:3–20.

Boué, J., Vignal, P., Aubry, M. C., and MacAleese, J., 1982, Ultrasound movement patterns of fetuses with chromosome anomalies, *Prenatal Diagnosis* **2**:61–65.

Carr, D. H., 1969, Cytogenetics and the pathology of hydatidiform degeneration, *Obstet. Gynecol.* **33**:333–342.

Carr, D. H., 1970, Chromosome studies in selected spontaneous abortions. 1: Conception, after oral contraceptives. *Can. Med. Assoc. J.* **103**:343–348.

Carr, D. H., 1971a, Chromosome studies in selected spontaneous abortions: Polyploidy in man, *J. Med. Genet.* **8**:164–174.

Carr, D. H., 1971b, Chromosomes and abortion, in: *Advances in Human Genetics,* Vol. 2. (H. Harris and K. Hirschhorn, eds.), pp. 201–257, Plenum Press, New York.

Carr, D. H., 1977, Population cytogenetics of human abortuses, in: *Population cytogenetics. Studies in humans.* (E. B. Hook and I. H. Porter, eds.), pp. 1–9, Academic Press, New York.

Carr, D. H., and Gedeon, M., 1978, Q-banding of chromosomes in human spontaneous abortions, *Can. J. Genet. Cytol.* **20**:415–425.

Chandley, A. C., 1981, The origin of chromosomal aberations in man and their potential for survival and reproduction in the adult human population, *Ann. Genet.* **24**:5–11.

Couillin, P., Hors, J., Boué, J., and Boué, A., 1978, Identification of the origin of triploidy by HLA markers, *Hum. Genet.* **41**:35–44.

Creasy, M. R., Crolla, J. A., and Alberman, E. D., 1976, A cytogenetic study of human spontaneous abortions using banding techniques, *Hum. Genet.* **31**:177–196.

Daniel, A., 1979, Structural differences in reciprocal translocations, *Hum. Genet.* **51**:171–182.

De Grouchy, J., 1976, Le Prix de la vie, *Arch. Fr. Pediatr.* **33**:841–846.

Delhanty, J. D. A., Ellis, J. R., and Rowley, P. T., 1961, Triploid cells in a human embryo, *Lancet* **1**:1286.

Dyban, A. P., and Baranov, V. S., 1978, Cytogenetics of Mammalian development (in Russian), in: *Problemi Biologii Razvitija,* p. 216, Nauka, Moscow.

Edmonds, D. K., Lindsay, K. S., Miller, J. F., Williamson, E., and Wood, P. J., 1982, Early embryonic mortality in women, *Fertil. Steril.* **38**:447–453.

Epstein, C. J., and Travis, B., 1979, Preimplantation lethality of monosomy for mouse chromosome 19, *Nature* **280**:144–145.

Epstein, C. J., Epstein, L. B., Cox, D., and Weil, J., 1981, Functional implications of gene dosage effects in trisomy 21, in: *Trisomy 21* (G. R. Burgio, M. Fraccaro, L. Tiepolo, and U. Wolf, eds.), p. 155–171, Springer, Berlin.

Fisher, R. A., Sheppard, O. M., and Lawler, S. D., 1982, Twin pregnancy with complete hydatidiform mole (46,XX) and fetus (46,XY): Genetic origin proved by analysis of chromosome polymorphisms, *Brit. Med. J.* **284**:1218–1220.

Ford, C. E., 1972, Gross genome unbalance in mouse spermatozoa: Does it influence the capacity to fertilize?, in: *The Genetics of the Spermatozoon,* (R. A. Beatty and S. Glueck-sohn-Waelsch, eds.), pp. 359–369, University of Edinburgh, Edinburgh.

Francke, U., and Taggart, R. T., 1979, Assignment of the gene for cytoplasmic superoxide dismutase (Sod-1) to a region of chromosome 16 and Hprt to a region of the X chromosome in the mouse, *Proc. Natl. Acad. Sci. USA* **76**:5230–5233.

French, F. E., and Bierman, J. M., 1962, Probabilities of fetal mortality, *Publ. Health Rep.* **77**:835–847.

Fryns, J. P., Van de Kerckhove, A., Godderis, P., and Van den Berghe, H., 1977, Unusually long survival in a case of full triploidy of maternal origin, *Hum. Genet.* **38**:147–155.

Geraedts, J. P. M., and Klasen, E. C., 1980, Chromosomal studies and alpha-antitrypsin phenotypes in recurrent abortions, *Clin. Genet.* **17**:68.

Giroud, A., Deluchat, C., and Boué, J., 1973, Aberrations chromosomiques et malformations embryonnaires dans les avortements précoces, in: *Chromosomal Errors in Relation to Reproductive Failure* (A. Boué and C. Thibault, eds.), pp. 127–142, INSERM, Paris.

Golbus, M. S., Bachrnan, R., Wiltse, S., and Hall, B. D., 1976, Tetraploidy in a liveborn infant. *J. Med. Genet.* **13:**329–332.

Gosden, C. M., Wright, M. O., Paterson, W. C., and Grant, K. A., 1976, Clinical details, cytogenetic studies, and cellular physiology of a 69,XXX fetus, with comments on the biological effect of triploidy in man, *J. Med. Genet.* **13:**371–380.

Gropp, A., 1971, Reproductive failure due to fetal aneuploidy in mice, in: *VII World Congress on Fertility and Sterility,* pp. 326–330, Excerpta Medica, Amsterdam.

Gropp, A., 1978, Relevance of phases of development for expression of abnormality. Perspectives drawn from experimentally induced chromosome aberrations (Life Sciences Report 10), in: *Dahlem Konferenzen,* pp. 85–110, Berlin.

Gropp, A., 1982, Value of an animal model for trisomy, *Virchows Arch. Pathol. Anat.* **395:**117–131.

Gropp, A., and Winking, H., 1981, Robertsonian translocations: Cytology, meiosis, segregation patterns and biological consequences of heterozygosity, *Symp. Zool. Soc. Lond.* **47:**141–181.

Gropp, A., Kolbus, U., and Giers, D., 1975, Systematic approach to the study of trisomy in the mouse. II, *Cytogenet. Cell. Genet.* **14:**42–62.

Gropp, A., Winking, H., Redi, C., Capanna, E., Britton-Davidian, J., and Noack, G., 1983, Robertsonian karyotype variation in wild house mice from Rhaeto-Lombardia, *Cytogenet. Cell. Genet.* **34:**67–77.

Hamerton, J. L., 1970, Robertsonian translocation: Evidence on segregation from family studies, in: *Human Population Cytogenetics* (P. A. Jacobs, W. H. Price, and P. Law, eds.), pp. 64–80, Edinburgh University, Edinburgh.

Hassold, T., 1980, A cytogenetic study of repeated spontaneous abortions, *Am. J. Hum. Genet.* **32:**623–730.

Hassold, T., 1982, Mosaic trisomies in human spontaneous abortions, *Hum. Genet.* **61:**31–35.

Hassold, T., Chen, N., Funkhouser, J., Jooss, T., Manuel, B., Matsuura, J., Matsuyama, A., Wilson, C., Yamane, J. A., and Jacobs, P. A., 1980a, A cytogenetic study of 1000 spontaneous abortions. *Ann. Hum. Genet.* **44:**151–178.

Hassold, T., Jacobs, P., Kline, J., Stein, Z., and Warburton, D., 1980b, Effect of maternal age on autosomal trisomies. *Ann. Hum. Genet. Lond.* **44:**29–36.

Hassold, T., Quillen, S. D., and Yamane, J., 1983, Sex ratio in spontaneous abortions, *Ann. Hum. Genet.* **47:**39–47.

Hertig, A. T., and Rock, J., 1949, A series of potentially abortive ova recovered from fertile women prior to the first missed menstrual period, *Am. J. Obstet. Gynecol.* **58:**968–993.

Hertig, A. T., and Sheldon, W. H., 1943, Minimal criteria required to prove *prima facie* case of traumatic abortion or miscarriage. An analysis of 1000 spontaneous abortions, *Ann. Surg.* **117:**596–606.

Hongell, K., and Gropp, A., 1982, Trisomy 13 in the mouse, *Teratology* **26:**95–104.

Honoré, L. H., Dill, F. J., and Poland, B. J., 1976, Placental morphology in spontaneous human abortuses with normal and abnormal karyotypes, *Teratology* **14:**151–166.

Hook, E. B., 1983, Chromosome abnormalities and spontaneous fetal death following amniocentesis: Further data and associations with maternal age, *Am. J. Hum. Genet.* **35:**110–116.

Hook, E. B., and Cross, P. K., 1982, Paternal age and Down's syndrome genotypes diagnosed prenatally: No association in New York state data, *Hum. Genet.* **62:**167–174.

Jacobs, P. A., 1981a, Mutation rates of structural chromosome rearrangements in man, *Am. J. Hum. Genet.* **33:**44–54.

Jacobs, P. A., 1981b, The origin of chromosome abnormalities in man, in: *Chromosomes Today,* Vol. 7 (M. D. Bennet, M. Bobrow, and G. M. Hewitt, eds.), pp. 271–280, Allen and Unwin, London.

Jacobs, P. A., and Hassold, T. J., 1980, The origin of chromosome abnormalities in spontaneous abortion, in: *Human Embryonic and Fetal Death* (I. H. Porter and E. B. Hook, eds.), pp. 288–298, Academic Press, New York.

Jacobs, P. A., Angell, R. R., Buchman, I. M., Hassold, T. J., Matsuyama, A., and Manuel, B., 1978a, The origin of human triploids, *Ann. Hum. Genet.* **42:**49–57.

Jacobs, P. A., Hassold, T. J., Matsuyama, A. M., and Newlands, I. M., 1978b, Chromosome constitution of gestational trophoblastic disease, *Lancet* **2:**49.

Jacobs, P. A., Wilson, C. M., Sprenkle, J. A., Rosensheim, N. B., and Migeon, B. R., 1980, Mechanism of origin of complete hydatidiform moles, *Nature* **286:**714–716.

Jacobs, P. A., Szulman, A. E., Funkhouser, J., Matsuura, J. S., and Wilson, C. C., 1982, Human triploidy: Relationship between parental origin of the additional haploid complement and development of partial hydatidiform mole, *Ann. Hum. Genet.* **46:**223–231.

Jonasson, J., Therkelsen, A. J., Lauritsen, J. G., and Lindsten, J., 1972, Origin of triploidy in human abortuses, *Hereditas* **71:**168–171.

Junien, C., Rubinson, H., Dreyfus, J. C., Meienhofer, M. C., Ravisé N., Boué, J., and Boué, A., 1976, Gene dosage effect in human triploid fibroblasts, *Hum. Genet.* **33:**61–66.

Kajii, T., and Niikawa, N., 1977, Origin of triploidy and tetraploidy in man: 11 cases with chromosome markers, *Cytogenet. Cell Genet.* **18:**109–125.

Kajii, T., and Ohama, K., 1977, Androgenetic origin of hydatidiform mole, *Nature* **268:**633–634.

Kajii, T., Ohama, K., and Mikamo, K., 1978, Anatomic and cytogenetic studies of 944 induced abortions, *Hum. Genet.* **43:**247–258.

Kajii, T., Ferrier, A., Niikawa, N., Takahara, H., Ohama, K., and Avirachan, S., 1980, Anatomic and chromosomal anomalies in 639 spontaneous abortuses, *Hum. Genet.* **55:**87–98.

Kuleshov, N. P., 1976, Chromosome anomalies of infants dying during the perinatal period and premature newborn, *Humangenetik* **31:**151–160.

Lauritsen, J. G., 1976, Aetiology of spontaneous abortion. A cytogenetic and epidemiological study of 288 abortuses and their parents, *Acta Obstet. Gynecol. Scand. Suppl.* **52:**1–29.

Lauritsen, J. G., Bolund, L., Friedrich, U., and Therkelsen, A. J., 1979, Origin of triploidy in spontaneous abortuses, *Ann. Hum. Genet.* **43:**1–5.

Lawler, S. D., Fisher, R. A., Pickthall, V. J., Povey, S., and Evans, M. W., 1982a, Genetic studies on hydatidiform moles. 1. The origin of partial moles, *Cancer Genet. Cytogenet.* **5:**309–320.

Lawler, S. D., Povey, S., Fisher, R. A., and Pickthall, V. J., 1982b, Genetic studies on hydatidiform moles. II. The origin of complete moles, *Ann. Hum. Genet.* **46:**209–222.

Linder, D., McCaw, B. K., and Hecht, F., 1975, Parthenogenetic origin of benign ovarian teratomas, *N. Engl. J. Med.* **292:**63–66.

Lippman-Hand, A., and Vekemans, M., 1983, Balanced translocations among couples with two or more spontaneous abortions: Are males and females equally likely to be carrier?, *Hum. Genet.* **63:**252–257.

Lopata, A., 1980, Success and failures in human *in vitro* fertilization, *Nature* **288:**642–643.

Machin, G. A., and Crolla, J. A., 1974, Chromosome constitution of 500 infants dying during the perinatal period, *Humangenetik* **23:**183–198.

Magnuson, T., Smith, S. A., and Epstein, C. J., 1982, The development of monosomy 19 mouse embryos, *J. Embryol. Exp. Morphol.* **69**:223–236.

Makino, S., Sasaki, M., and Fukuschima, T., 1964, Triploid chromosome constitution in human chorionic lesions, *Lancet* **2**:1273–1275.

Martin, R. H., Lin, C. C., Balkan, W., and Burns, K., 1982, Direct chromosomal analysis of human spermatozoa: Preliminary results from 15 normal men, *Am. J. Hum. Genet.* **34**:459–468.

Martin, R. H., Balkan, W., Burns, K., Rademaker, A. W., Lin, C. C., and Rudd, N. L., 1983. The chromosome constitution of 1000 human spermatozoa, *Hum. Genet.* **63**:305–309.

Matton, M., Verschraegen-Spae, M. R., De Bie, S., and Van den Wijngaert, T., 1980, Incidence of T. carriers amongst couples with repetitive abortion, after exclusion of any other etiology, *Clin. Genet.* **17**:78.

McCaw, B. K., and Latt, S. A., 1977, X-chromosome replication in parthenogenetic benign ovarian teratomas, *Hum. Genet.* **38**:253–264.

Meulenbroek, G. H., and Geraedts, J. P., 1982, Parental origin of chromosome abnormalities in spontaneous abortions, *Hum. Genet.* **62**:129–133.

Mikamo, K., 1970, Anatomic and chromosomal anomalies in spontaneous abortions, *Am. J. Obstet. Gynecol.* **103**:143–154.

Mikkelsen, M., 1982, Down syndrome: Current stage of cytogenetic epidemiology, in: *Human Genetics,* Part B (B. Bonne-Tamir, ed.), pp. 297–309, Alan R. Liss, New York.

Miller, J. R., and Poland, B. J., 1970, The value of human abortuses in the surveillance of development anomalies, *Can. Med. Assoc. J.* **103**:501–502.

Mirre, C., Hartung, M., and Stahl, A., 1980, Association of ribosomal genes in the fibrillar center of the nucleolus: A factor influencing translocation and nondisjunction in the human meiotic cycle, *Proc. Natl. Acad. Sci. USA* **77**:6017–6020.

Myabara, S. H., Gropp, A., and Winking, H., 1982, Trisomy 16 in the mouse fetus associated with generalized edema, cardio-vascular and urinary tract anomalies, *Teratology* **25**:369–380.

Niikawa, N., Merotto, E., and Kajii, T., 1977, Origin of acrocentric trisomies in spontaneous abortuses, *Hum. Genet.* **40**:73–78.

Ohama, K., Kajii, T., Okamoto, E., Fukuda, Y., Imaizami, K., Tsukahara, M., Kabayashi, K., and Hagiwara, K., 1981, Dispermic origin of XY hydatidiform moles, *Nature* **292**:551–552.

Pearson, P. L., Geraedts, J. P. M., and Pawlowitzki, I. H., 1973, Chromosomal studies on human male gametes, in: *Chromosomal Errors in Relation to Reproductive Failure* (A. Boué and C. Thibault, eds.), pp. 219–229, INSERM, Paris.

Penrose, L. S., 1933, The relative effect of paternal and maternal age in mongolism, *J. Genet.* **27**:219–224.

Penrose, L. S., and Delhanty, J. D. A., 1961, Triploid cell cultures from a macerated foetus, *Lancet* **1**:1261–1262.

Philippe, E., 1974, *Histopathologie Placentaire,* Masson, Paris.

Philippe, E., and Boué, J. G., 1969, Le placenta des aberrations chromosomiques léthales, *Ann. Anat. Pathol.* **14**:249–266.

Philippe, E., Boué, J., and Boué, A., 1980, Les maladies trophoblastiques gestationnelles, *Ann. Anat. Pathol.* **25**:13–38.

Pitt, D., Leversha, M., Sinfield, C., Campbell, P., Anderson, R., Bryan, D., and Rogers, J., 1981, Tetraploidy in a liveborn infant with spina-bifida and other anomalies, *J. Med. Genet.* **1981**:309–311.

Polani, P., 1983, The elusive cause of Down's syndrome, *Lancet* **1**:1340.

Polani, P. E., and Adinolfi, M., 1980, Annotations: Chromosome 21 of man, 22 of the great apes and 16 of the mouse, *Dev. Med. Child Neurol.* **22**:223–225.

Putz, B., Krause, G., Garde, T., and Gropp, A., 1980, A comparison between trisomy 12 and vitamin A induced exencephaly and associated malformations in the mouse embryo, *Virchows Arch. Pathol. Anat.* **368**:65–80.

Roberts, C. J., and Lowe, C. R., 1975, Where have all the conceptions gone?, *Lancet* **1**:498–499.

Roth, M. P., Stoll, C., Taillemite, J. L., Girard, S., and Boué, A., 1983, Paternal age and Down's syndrome diagnosed prenatally: No association in French data, *Prenatal Diagnosis* **3**:327–335.

Sachs, E. S., 1980, Fertility of translocation carriers, *Clin. Genet.* **17**:83.

Schlesselman, J. J., 1979, How does one assess the risk of abnormalities from human *in vitro* fertilization, *Am. J. Obstet. Gynecol.* **135**:135–148.

Schmid, W., 1980, Cytogenetic results in 96 couples with repeated abortions, *Clin. Genet.* **17**:85.

Schwartz, S., and Palmer, C. G., 1983, Chromosomal findings in 164 couples with repeated spontaneous abortions: With special consideration to prior reproductive history, *Hum. Genet.* **63**:28–34.

Sheppard, D. M., Fisher, R. A., Lawler, S. D., and Povey, S., 1982, Tetraploid conceptus with three paternal contributions, *Hum. Genet.* **62**:371–374.

Short, R. V., 1979, When a conception fails to become a pregnancy, in: *Maternal Recognition of Pregnancy,* pp. 377–387, Excerpta Medica, Amsterdam.

Singh, R. P., and Carr, D. H., 1966, The anatomy and histology of XO human embryos and fetuses, *Anat. Rec.* **155**:369–381.

Singh, R. P., and Carr, D. H., 1967, Anatomic findings in human abortions of known chromosomal constitution, *Osbstet. Gynecol.* **29**:806–818.

Stene, J., and Warburton, D., 1981, Evidence for smaller probabilities for trisomic mosaicism for acrocentric than for non acrocentric chromosomes, *Am. J. Hum. Gent.* **33**:484–485.

Stene, J., Stene, E., Stengel-Rukkowski, S., and Murken, J. D., 1981, Paternal age and Down's syndrome: Data from prenatal diagnosis, *Hum. Genet.* **59**:119–124.

Stephens, T. D., and Shepard, T. H., 1980, The Down syndrome in the fetus, *Teratology* **22**:37–41.

Steptoe, P. C., Edwards, R. G., and Purdy, J. M., 1980, Clinical aspects of pregnancies established with cleaving embryos grown *in vitro, Br. J. Obstet. Gynecol.* **87**:757–768.

Stevenson, A. C., Dudgeon, M. Y., and McClure, H. I., 1959, Observations on the results of pregnancies in women resident in Belfast: II. Abortions, hydatidiform moles and ectopic pregnancies, *Ann. Hum. Genet.* **23**:395–411.

Stoll, C., Flori, E., Rumpler, Y., and Warker, S., 1980, Cytogenetic findings in 217 couples with recurrent fetal wastage, *Clin. Genet.* **17**:88.

Subrt, I., 1980, Reciprocal translocation with special reference to reproductive failure, *Hum. Genet.* **55**:303–308.

Surti, U., Szulman, A., and O'Brien, S., 1979, Complete (classic) hydatidiform mole, with 46, XY karyotype of paternal origin, *Hum. Genet.* **51**:153–155.

Sutherland, G. R., Carter, R. F., Baud, R., Smith, I. I., and Bain, A. D., 1978, Chromosome studies at the paediatric necropsy, *Ann. Hum. Genet.* **42**:173–181.

Szulman, A. E., and Surti, U., 1978, The syndromes of hydatidiform mole, *Am. J. Obstet. Gynecol.* **131**:655–671.

Szulman, A. E., and Surti, U., 1982, The clinicopathologic profile of the partial hydatidiform mole, *Obstet. Gynecol.* **59**:597–602.

Szulman, A. E., Philippe, E., Boué, J. G., and Boué, A., 1981, Human triploidy: Association with partial hydatidiform moles and nonmolar conceptuses, *Hum. Pathol.* **12**:1016–1021.

Takagi, N., and Sasaki, M., 1976, Dygynic triploidy after superovulation in mice, *Nature* **264**:278–281.

Therkelsen, A. J., Grunnet, N., Njort, T., Myhre Jensen, O., Jonasson, J., Lauritsen, J. G., Lendsten, J., and Bruun Peterson, G., 1973, Studies on spontaneous abortion, in: *Chromosomal Errors in Relation to Reproductive Failure* (A. Boué and C. Thibault, eds.), pp. 81–93, INSERM, Paris.

Turleau, C., Chavin-Colin, F., and de Grouchy, J., 1979, Cytogenetic investigation in 413 couples with spontaneous abortion, *Eur. J. Obstet. Gynecol.* **9**:65–74.

Uchida, I. A., and Lin, C. C., 1972, Identification of triploid genome by fluorescence microscopy, *Science* **176**:304–305.

Vassilakos, P., Riotton, G., and Kajii, T., 1977, Hydatidiform mole: Two entities, *Am. J. Obstet. Gynecol.* **127**:167–170.

Wallace, D. C., Surti, U., Adams, C. W., and Szulman, A. E., 1982, Complete moles have paternal chromosomes but maternal mitochondrial DNA, *Hum. Genet.* **61**:145–147.

Warburton, D., Yu, C., Kline, J., and Stein, Z., 1978, Mosaic autosomal trisomy in cultures from spontaneous abortions, *Am. J. Hum. Genet.* **30**:609–617.

Warburton, D., Stein, Z., Kline, J., and Susser, M., 1980a, Chromosome abnormalities in spontaneous abortions: Data from the New York City study, in: *Human Embryonic and Fetal Death* (I. H. Porter and E. B. Hook, eds.), pp. 261–287, Academic Press, New York.

Warburton, D., Kline, J., Stein, Z., and Susser, M., 1980b, Monosomy X: A chromosomal anomaly associated with young maternal age, *Lancet* **1**:167–169.

Warburton, D., Hutzler, M., Kline, J., Stein, Z., and Strobins, B., 1982, Recurrence risk for trisomy following trisomic spontaneous abortions; *Am. J. Hum. Genet.* **34**:149A.

Weaver, D. D., Gartler, S. M., Boué, A., and Boué, J., 1975, Evidence for two active X chromosomes in a human XXY triploid, *Humangenetik* **28**:39–42.

Wertelecki, W., Graham, J. M., and Sergovich, F. R., 1976, The clinical syndrome of triploidy, *Obstet. Gynecol.* **47**:69–76.

White, B. J., Tjio, J. H., van de Water, L. C., and Crandall, C., 1974, Trisomy 19 in the laboratory mouse. I. Frequency in different crosses at specific developmental stages and relationship of trisomy to cleft palate, *Cytogenet. Cell Genet.* **13**:217–231; Trisomy 19 in the laboratory mouse. II. Intra-uterine growth and histological studies of trisomics and their normal littermates, *Cytogenet. Cell Genet.* **13**:232–245.

Yamamoto, M., and Watanabe, G., 1979, Epidemiology of gross chromosome anomalies at the early embryonic stage of pregnancy, *Contrib. Epidemiol.* **1**:101–106.

Yamamoto, M., Ito, T., Watanabe, M., and Watanabe, G., 1982, Causes of chromosome anomalies suggested by cytogenetic epidemiology of induced abortions, *Hum. Genet.* **60**:360–364.

Yamashita, K., Wake, N., Araki, T., Ichinof, K., and Makoto, K., 1979, Human lymphocyte antigen expression in hydatidiform mole: Androgenesis following fertilization by a haploid sperm, *Am. J. Obstet. Gynecol.* **135**:597–600.

Chapter 2

Mutation in Human Populations*

James F. Crow and Carter Denniston

Laboratory of Genetics
University of Wisconsin
Madison, Wisconsin 53706

INTRODUCTION

Spontaneous mutation in man was reviewed in this series almost a decade ago (Vogel and Rathenberg, 1975). These authors remarked that mutation rates in general, and human rates in particular, had not been the subject of the extensive, systematic study that might be expected from the importance of the subject. That statement is still true. As mentioned by Vogel and Rathenberg, estimates of human mutation rates depend on large epidemiologic studies of a type that were more popular in the 1940s and 1950s than since. As a result, the values given in still earlier reviews (Penrose, 1961; Crow, 1961) do not differ importantly from those of more recent reviews, including the present one.

Now that mutations can be detected at the necleotide level it will soon be feasible to carry out human mutation studies with a precision comparable to those now routine in experimental organisms. It is already possible to measure mutation rates for small, selected regions of DNA; it should soon be possible to measure the rates for large regions, without the previous limitation to areas in which a mutation has a phenotypic effect. Furthermore, mutation is being used increasingly as a tool for understanding molecular and developmental functions. However, this

* This is paper 2690 from the Laboratory of Genetics, University of Wisconsin, Madison, Wisconsin.

review will not deal with such subjects, nor with environmental mutagens and test systems for detecting them.

We emphasize that there are two quite different problems. One is measuring the amount of change in the DNA from mutation. The second is assessing the impact of mutation on human health and well-being. For the latter, molecular studies of mutation are insufficient and often irrelevant. It is the phenotypic effects of the mutations that matter.

Consequently, we will concentrate on rates of phenotypically detectable mutation, on attempts to assess the impact of mutation on human welfare, and on some evolutionary considerations.

We list here some references to other reviews. The general reviews of human mutation by Vogel and Rathenberg (1975) and Vogel and Motulsky (1979) are detailed and remarkably complete, with extensive bibliographies. For this reason we have omitted many references to earlier work. The United Nations reports (UNSCEAR, 1972, 1977, 1982) contain a wealth of material on spontaneous and radiation-induced mutation, again with extensive bibliographies; see also Vogel (1983). For additional reviews on human effects of radiation and chemical mutagens, see Bora et al. (1982), Denniston (1982), National Academy of Sciences (1972, 1980, 1983), Vogel and Röhrborn (1970), and Hollaender (1971, and succeeding volumes). For population aspects, see Hook and Porter (1981), Morton (1982), and Morton and Chung (1978).

We begin with a general review of human mutation and the estimation of mutation rates.

CLASSES OF MUTATION

Classification by Phenotypic Effect

Mutations can affect any structure or process; hence the range of mutational possibility extends over the entire gamut of morphology, physiology, biochemistry, and behavior. The magnitude or severity of effect ranges from trivial to catastrophic. There are two obvious limitations to the observation of mutant effects. First, the mutant phenotype may be below the threshold of detection. Sometimes this difficulty can be circumvented by technical improvements; in some cases this is simply a more refined phenotypic measurement. In other cases something closer to the gene is observed, e.g., a protein product or the DNA itself. Second, the mutation may produce an effect so disastrous as to cause early death. Sometimes the death is in late fetal stages and can be studied, but there is a large residue of early lethal effects that is beyond the capability of present methods. Mutations causing sterility can also frustrate genetic studies by making it impossible to study transmission. Even here, however, there are sometimes indirect methods that can be used. For example, increased paternal age among isolated cases is an indication that the phenotype is of mutational origin, and consanguinity of the parents of affected individuals suggests autosomal recessive inheritance.

Although the range of phenotypic effects is so great and the qualitative differences so diverse as to make any generalization impossible, there is one clear observation: Mutations that produce any overt effect are almost always harmful. This, of course, is expected on the simplest of mechanistic and evolutionary considerations. The rule is considerably less certain, however, as the effects become small. Is there a large class of mutations detectable only by direct DNA or protein analysis that are totally innocuous? Clearly there are DNA changes that produce no detectable phenotypic change, but proving that they have no effect on fitness is another question. Studies of molecular evolution and polymorphism have led some (e.g., Kimura, 1968a,b, 1983; King and Jukes, 1969) to the view that most nucleotide substitutions observed in evolutionary studies and molecular polymorphisms are primarily the result of mutation and random drift with a negligible contribution from natural selection. Whether this is true or not, molecular studies have revealed a plethora of genetic variants that are at most very weakly selected.

For our purposes, the most important classification of mutation is by mode of inheritance: Is the inheritance autosomal, X-linked, or possibly Y-linked? Is it dominant or recessive? Does it depend on a chromosomal abberation? Is it multifactorial?

Almost all human biological inheritance is chromosomal. There is one well-established syndrome that is maternally inherited: mitochondrial cytopathy. It causes a variety of symptoms, and as the name suggests, involves several mitochondrial enzymes. The inheritance follows the maternal cytoplasm, as expected (Egger and Wilson, 1983).

In human genetics the word "dominant" is used in several ways. A frequent convention, and one we shall adopt, is to classify a mutation as dominant if the mutant phenotype that is usually observed is that of the heterozygote. This is more useful than the classical definition by which the allele A is regarded as dominant if the phenotypes of AA and Aa are indistinguishable. For example, achondroplasia is regularly classified as dominant; although the homozygous phenotype is considerably more severe, the phenotype usually observed is that of the heterozygote. In many other cases the homozygote is so rare that its phenotype is, in fact, unknown.

There is good evidence in experimental animals that most "recessive" mutations are actually partially dominant (i.e., have some effect on the heterzygote), and the human evidence, as far as it goes, is consistent with this observation. Furthermore, in *Drosophila,* as the effect of the mutant on viability and fitness gets smaller, the heterozygous fitness approaches the mean of the corresponding homozygotes (for reviews, see Mukai *et. al.,* 1972; Simmons and Crow, 1977; Crow, 1979). It is likely that this is true for humans as well.

Despite the virtual absence of complete dominance, there is little ambiguity if, as stated above, we define a trait as dominant or recessive according to whether the phenotype commonly observed is that of the heterozygote or the homozygote (or hemizygote for X-linked loci).

Classification by Genomic Effect

Mutation produces effects as small as a single nucleotide substitution and as great as polyploidy. Mutational changes include substitutions, additions, deletions, and rearrangements. There are also processes, such as gene conversion, that are recombinational in nature, yet produce novel effects.

It is convenient to define mutation very broadly, as encompassing all heritable changes not accounted for by normal segregation and recombination, and to place the mutation events into three classes, genomic, chromosomal, and genic. This is the vocabulary used by Vogel and Rathenberg (1975) in their review.

1. *Genome mutations* affect the number of chromosomes, but not the structure of the chomosomes themselves. Such mutations include aneuploidy and polyploidy. They are genomic in that the genome, but not its constituent chromosomes, is affected.
2. *Chromosome mutations* affect the structure of chromosomes, but not that of the individual genes. They include translocations,

inversions, deletions, deplications, and transpositions. They are chromosomal in that the chromosomes, but not the genes, are affected. For the most part, the consequences to the person are the result of chromosomal imbalance created by the meiotic irregularities to which rearranged chromosomes are subject.

3. *Gene mutations* affect the structure of the individual genes. Such changes may be substitutions, additions, deletions, or rearrangements.

The demarcation between classes 2 and 3 is ambiguous at both the causal and observational level. In *Drosophila,* chromosomal rearrangements often produce "position effects"; the human counterpart is not clear. Also, as chromosomal mutations become smaller, they become indistinguishable from genic mutations in most test systems. In the absence of molecular analysis it is often impossible to distinguish small insertions, repeat sequences, and multigene families from intragenic changes. We therefore adopt the pragmatic definition that a gene mutation is any mutation that follows Mendel's rules and is not associated with a detectable chromosomal abberation.

This review is concerned with gene mutation detected by phenotypic criteria.

Number and Incidence of Human Mendelian Traits

McKusick (1983) has provided an extensive and periodically updated list of known Mendelian phenotypes in man, classified as to their mode of inheritance. The number of known hereditary traits has increased 2.26 times since the first edition in 1966. McKusick lists traits in two categories, those that are quite certain and those that are less well established. Including both categories, the increase in known dominant, recessive, and X-linked loci has been 2.18-, 2.44-, and 2.04-fold, respectively. McKusick's numbers are reproduced in Table I.

One immediately striking fact is that autosomal recessives are only about five times as frequent as X-linked ones (almost all recessive), whereas the ratio of autosome to X-chromosome length is about 25. The comparison might be regarded as inappropriate because of X-inactivation, which suggests a different causal mechanism for X-linked and autosomal recessives. Yet, in the mouse, where there is also an X-inactivation

Table I. The Number of Loci Identified with Mendelian Phenotypes[a]

Mode of inheritance	1966	1968	1971	1975	1978	1982
Autosomal dominant	269 (568)	344 (449)	415 (528)	583 (635)	736 (753)	934 (893)
Autosomal recessive	237 (294)	280 (349)	365 (418)	466 (481)	521 (596)	588 (710)
X-linked	68 (51)	68 (55)	86 (64)	93 (78)	107 (98)	115 (128)
Total	1487	1545	1876	2336	2811	3368

[a] Data from McKusick (1983). These are the numbers in successive editions of McKusick's compendium. Numbers in parentheses refer to less well-established loci.

mechanism, there are proportionately many fewer X-linked mutants. Also, in the mouse (as well as in the much-studied *Drosophila*) autosomal recessives greatly outnumber autosomal dominants; in man there are more dominants.

These discrepancies are easily understood as being caused by the intrinsic biases of the methods of study. Dominant and X-linked mutations are strikingly apparent in pedigrees. In contrast, evidence for recessive inheritance is much more indirect and recessively inherited diseases may go undetected. On the other hand, in laboratory populations inbreeding is the rule and recessive mutants are almost as easy to discover as dominants. All this suggests that many human recessive mutations remain to be discovered. It is therefore not surprising that the number of known recessives is increasing at a faster rate than are dominant and X-linked; indeed, it is surprising that the rates are not more discrepant.

There are other reasons for the underrepresentation of recessive diseases in human data. As mentioned earlier, many and probably most recessive mutations exert some harmful effect in the heterozygous state. Therefore, they are being eliminated, undetected, before ever becoming homozygous. It is also probable that higher inbreeding levels in the past eliminated many recessive mutants, while reduced inbreeding now keeps the bulk of the remaining ones in the heterozygous state.

The incidence and prevalence of human genetic disease are hardly known at all. There are two large surveys in which an attempt was made to ascertain all cases of genetic disease in a defined region. One was in Northern Ireland (Stevenson, 1959), the other in British Columbia (Trimble and Doughty, 1974). It is disconcerting that the numbers differ so greatly, especially in the important category of Mendelian dominants.

It is still more disconcerting that there has been so little additional information since these earlier studies. There are additional data from Hungary (Czeizel, 1978; see UNSCEAR, 1982), but the emphasis is on congenital anomalies rather than Mendelian traits. The earlier data are given in Table II, along with corrections and adjustments made by the United Nations Committee (UNSCEAR, 1977).

The small number of dominants in the British Columbia survey is due to a failure to ascertain many diseases and abnormalities that are not manifest until adulthood. The large number in the Northern Ireland survey reflects the inclusion of some very mild conditions and others with more complex inheritance. The multifactorial category is heterogeneous and uncertain. Almost any number up to 100% could be defended, for there is hardly anyone without some impairment determined to some extent by genetic makeup.

We present the numbers and various adjustments in Table II mainly to emphasize the uncertainity of our current information. The estimates, however well justified for their original purpose (the assessment of radiation risks), are necessarily based on arbitrary classifications.

Carter (1982) has recently summarized the frequencies of a number of autosomal dominant, autosomal recessive, and X-linked conditions. These include monogenic hypercholesterolemia (estimated incidence of 2/1000 births), Huntington chorea (0.5), neurofibromatosis (0.4), Duchenne muscular dystrophy (0.2), hemophilia A (0.1), X-linked mental

Table II. Estimates of Incidence of Genetic Disorders[a]

Category	Stevenson (1959)	UNSCEAR (1972)	Trimble and Doughty (1974)		UNSCEAR (1982)	Carter (1982)
			Min.[c]	Adj.[c]		
Dominant	3.32	0.95	0.06	0.08	1.0[b]	0.95
Recessive	0.21	0.21	0.09	0.11	0.1	0.25
X-linked	0.04	0.04	0.03	0.04	—	0.05
Chromosomal	—	0.42	0.16	0.20	0.4	—
Malformations	1.41	2.50	3.58	4.28	4.3	—
Multifactorial	1.48	1.50	1.58	4.73	4.7	—
Total	6.46	5.62	5.50	9.44	10.5	—

[a] Frequencies are per 1000 live births.
[b] Includes X-linked.
[c] Min. = minimum; adj. = adjusted for under-ascertainment.

retardation (0.1), cystic fibrosis (0.5), phenylketonuria (0.1), and a number of less frequent conditions. The total incidences of monogenic disorders are 9.5 dominants, 0.5 X-linked, and 2.5 autosomal recessives per 1000 live births. He has also extended the method of Jones (1979a,b) to estimate the average number of years of life lost from monogenic and chromosomal conditions.

MUTATION RATE ESTIMATES

Methods

Direct Methods

Dominant Phenotypes.   The most direct and most obvious way to detect a new mutation is to find a dominant phenotype in the child of nonmutant parents (Gunther and Penrose, 1935). If the proportion of such children among all births is I, the mutation rate in females is u_f, and the rate in males is u_m, then

$$I = u_f + u_m \tag{1}$$

since the new mutation could have been transmitted by either the egg or the sperm. Alternatively, in the expression usually used, the mutation rate is given by

$$u = I/2 \tag{2}$$

where u is the unweighted mean of the rates in the two sexes.

Despite the seeming simplicity of this method, there are several pitfalls. First, the incidence I must be correctly measured. This requires that ascertainment be complete among the population of births recorded. Such a requirement limits the method to phenotypes that are conspicuous. The best data come from surveys of a defined population in which there is the opportunity to observe every child.

Second, mistaken identification of parentage can be a problem. Errors in paternity determination are frequent enough that the number of false positives may exceed the number of mutations. For this reason, most studies of mutation have concentrated on rare diseases that are disfiguring or otherwise conspicuous, and that greatly reduce survival and fertility. With the great number of alleles at the *HLA* locus and the considerable polymorphism for restriction sites, parental identification can now be quite exact. We are confident that mistaken parentage will be less of a problem in mutation rate studies of the future.

Third, difficulty arises from incomplete penetrance and phenocopies. For these not to be a serious cause of error, it is necessary for appropriate traits to be chosen. The investigator must be familiar with the phenotypes and have access to the affected individuals themselves if the study is to be trusted.

Fourth, a different kind of problem arises when "genocopies" are present. The most serious is a recessive form of the same phenotype. If the disease is only mildly harmful, the incidence of the trait from normal parents may substantially exceed the mutation rate, and hence lead to a large error. Often this can be ruled out by sufficient knowledge of the phenotypes so that the recessives can be eliminated from the study. Parental consanguinity offers grounds to suspect a recessive component. Usually, with dominant diseases there is no way to test for allelism, so there may well be several loci that produce essentially the same mutant phenotype. The mutation rate, then, is the sum of the individual rates. However, this is not likely to affect the estimates by a large factor unless a very large number of loci mimic the same phenotype.

These four sources of error are generally such as to lead to an overestimate of the mutation rate. Probably a much greater bias in the same direction comes from the choice of phenotypes. The higher the mutation rate, other things being comparable, the more likely is the trait to come to the attention of science. Thus, published mutation rates are certain to be on the high side. How large this bias is, and how important, are discussed later.

There is one biasing factor that works in the other direction, and might well be important in studies of highly deleterious traits. Those who survive to be counted may be only a fraction of the actual mutant individuals, most dying prenatally or, at least, before diagnosis. This is not likely to be nearly as large as the biasing factors mentioned above, so the general conclusion that published mutation rates are overestimates remains.

Molecular Changes. Many of the difficulties and uncertainties in the study of conspicuous phenotypes can be circumvented if there is sufficient molecular understanding of the trait. The hemoglobin alpha and beta chains are known in such detail that many mutants have been characterized at the nucleotide level. One procedure (Nute and Stamatoyannopoulos, 1981) is to identify those hemoglobin variants severe and conspicuous enough that high ascertainment can be assumed, and then determine the molecular basis of the change. This provides a mutation rate per nucleotide, and is a major step forward.

What is needed is the mutation rate per nucleotide for various classes of DNA: protein coding, unique sequence noncoding, and the various kinds of repetitive DNA. The rapid advance in molecular knowledge assures that such information will increase rapidly in the near future, provided that the requisite epidemiologic studies are undertaken.

Indirect Methods

Dominant Phenotypes. A strongly selected dominant trait has a population incidence that is directly proportional to the mutation rate and to the number of generations that the mutant gene persists in the population. The latter, in turn, is inversely proportional to the decrease in fitness of the trait. The first to call attention to this principle was Danforth (1923). Noting that the incidence of both polydactyly and syndactyly was roughly 1/1000, or one in 2000 genomes, and that each persisted for at least three generations, he concluded that the mutation rate must be less than 1/6000.

Danforth's work had little influence at first; it was essentially ignored until its resurrection by Muller (1950). The most influential worker in the early days of mutation rate estimation was Haldane. It was he who first used the indirect method to measure the rate of mutation of the hemophilia gene (Haldane, 1932, p. 188).

If not all heterozygotes are affected, we say there is "incomplete penetrance." Suppose K is the fraction of heterozygotes who manifest the disorder and $1 - K$ are normal. Then, if q is the frequency of the mutant gene, g is the selective disadvantage to those manifesting the disorder, and N the population size, there are lost through selection each generation about $2NqgK$ of the A genes. Setting this equal to $2Nu$, the input of new mutations, we find that the equilibrium gene frequency is $\hat{q} = u/Kg$. Now, $1 - Kg$ is the average fitness of all heterozygotes, that is, $K(1 - g) + 1 - K = 1 - Kg$. We might point out that in a population of stable size Danforth's mean persistence is $1/Kg$, a concept that will be discussed in more detail in section VI-D.

The considerations in the previous paragraph provide the basis for an indirect estimate of mutation rate. The incidence I of the dominant phenotype is approximately $2\hat{q}K = 2(u/Kg)K = 2u/g$. Knowing I and g, we can estimate u. This points out one advantage of the indirect method. The estimate is not affected by incomplete penetrance, provided that the unaffected heterozygotes are of normal fitness. It is also clear that mistaken paternity has no effect on the estimate, because it depends only on incidence and fitness. The method does require the assumption of equilibrium, however, which restricts its application to traits of short persistence.

Another question of interest is, what proportion of affected individuals (heterozygotes) are new mutants? We expect that the answer will depend on selection, since if the disease is lethal and the gene fully penetrant, all new cases must be mutants. The probability of a new affected mutant is approximately $2(1 - q)uK$, or roughly $2uK$; the probability of being affected is $2qK$, which is $2u/g$ at equilibrium. Thus the proportion of all affected individuals who are new mutants is approximately $2uK/(2u/g) = Kg$. As expected, for a completely penetrant, lethal gene, $K = 1$ and $g = 1$, and all cases are new mutants.

We can also ask: What proportion of cases with normal parents are new mutants? As will be shown in Section V, this proportion is $g/(g + 1 - K)$. Note that if $K = 1$, all sporadic cases are new mutants, as expected.

Let us now look at the question of mutation–selection balance more generally. We will adopt a discrete-generation, random mating model that allows for selection, mutation, and penetrance. The human population consists of individuals of all ages, which with selection will not be in Hardy–Weinberg proportions; but, as first emphasized by Haldane (1927), for rare traits near equilibrium, the simple model is a satisfactory approximation (Charlesworth, 1980, p. 142). See Nagylaki (1976) for a discussion of "quasi-Hardy–Weinberg" ratios in a continuously reproducing population.

Consider the model in Table III. Here we assume Hardy–Weinberg equilibrium and ignore back mutation, but allow for possible heterozy-

Table III. A Discrete Generation Model of Selection with Variable Penetrance

Genotype	aa	Aa	Aa	AA
Frequency before selection	p^2	$2pqK$	$2pq(1 - K)$	q^2
Fitness	w_1	w_2	w_3	w_4
Relative fitness	$1 - t$	$1 - hs$	1	$1 - s$
Mutation			$a \xrightarrow{u} A$	

gote advantage. To determine the equilibrium frequency for the A allele, we argue as follows. Only the skeleton of the argument will be shown; the algebra is not particularly interesting. Call the fitnesses of the four phenotypic classes w_1, w_2, w_3, and w_4. After selection (but before mutation) the new gene frequencies are

$$p' = p^2w_1 + pqKw_2 + pq(1 - K)w_3/W \qquad (3)$$
$$q' = pqKw_2 + pq(1 - K)w_3 + q^2w_4/W$$

where W is the average fitness. Then, after mutation, the gene frequencies are

$$q'' = q' + p'u \qquad \text{and} \qquad p'' = p'(1 - u) \qquad (4)$$

At equilibrium, we must have $q''/p'' = q/p$. If we substitute (3) into (4), we get, after some tedious algebra, the quadratic equation

$$\hat{q}^2(s + t - 2Khs) - \hat{q}(1 + u)(t - Khs) - u(1 - t) = 0 \qquad (5)$$

Although we are primarily interested in the case $t = 0$, when there is directional selection against the A gene, the model allows for heterozygote advantage, a remote possibility for some human genetic diseases. If $t > Khs$, there is heterozygote advantage and the equilibrium frequency is found to be approximately

$$\hat{q} \cong (t - Khs)(1 - u)/T \qquad (6)$$

where $T = s + t - 2Khs$. Notice that mutation in this case makes little difference, pushing q up only a small amount. Note also that if $K = 0$ and u is ignored, this is $\hat{q} = t/(s + t)$, as expected.

The case in which we are really interested, as mentioned above, is when $t = 0$. If $t = 0$, then we have

$$\hat{q}^2s(1 - 2Kh) + \hat{q}(1 + u)Khs - u = 0 \qquad (7)$$

If $u \ll sK^2h^2$,

$$\hat{q} \cong u/Khs \qquad (8)$$

approximately, as we obtained earlier for $K = 1(hs = g)$.

Under these circumstances q is small enough that q^2 may be neglected, and the incidence I of the mutant phenotype is approximately $2qK$. In much of the human genetics literature $1 - hs(= 1 - g)$ is designated by f (standing for the relative fitness of the mutant heterozygote), so (8) may be conveniently written as

$$u \cong I(1 - f)/2 \tag{9}$$

As noted earlier, the estimate is not affected by reduced penetrance.

It is of interest, although not yet practical, to separate the contribution of mutations that occur in females from those that occur in males. Letting u_f and u_m stand for the female and male rates, we have that the incidence is approximately

$$I \cong (u_f + u_m)/hs = (u_f + u_m)/(1 - f) \tag{10}$$

Therefore the rate u measured by the Haldane equation (9) measures the unweighted average of the mutation rates in the two sexes.

If the incidence is accurately measured, the only difficulty is determining $f (= 1 - hs)$. This is usually estimated by comparing survival and fertility of affected and unaffected sibs. It is clear that the larger the value of s, the more accurate is the determination of u. If $f = 0$, that is, if the mutant is lethal or sterilizing, the mutation rate is simply half the incidence. Another advantage of studying mutations that greatly reduce the fitness is that the interval between the occurrence of the mutation and its elimination is short. If it were long, it is likely that changes in environment would render fitness estimates highly uncertain.

X-Linked Recessive Phenotypes. The first to measure the mutation rate of an X-linked recessive gene was Haldane (1932, 1935). We shall use equations of Nagylaki (1977), which do not require the assumption that the heterozygous females are of normal fitness. Letting s be the selective disadvantage of homozygous females or hemizygous males and hs that of heterozygous females, the proportion of affected male newborns at equilibrium is

$$\hat{q}_m = \frac{2u_f + u_m(1 - hs)}{s(1 + 2h - hs)} \tag{11}$$

The frequency of the mutant allele in females is

$$\hat{q}_f = \frac{u_m + (2 - s)u_f}{s(1 + 2h - hs)} \tag{12}$$

The value of $\hat{q}_f$ is approximately one-half the frequency of carrier females, since for strongly selected X-linked traits female homozygotes are negligibly rare. By using Eqs. (11) and (12) one can measure the male and female mutation rates. Unfortunately, the requisite data for using these equations are not available.

When the mutant is completely recessive ($h = 0$), we have the estimating equation first used by Haldane (1935)

$$2u_f + u_m = \hat{q}_m s = \hat{q}_m(1 - f) \tag{13}$$

The quantity estimated by the familiar equation $u = \hat{q}_m(1 - f)/3$ is the weighted average rate in the two sexes, with the female rate given twice the weight of the male rate.

If s and h are known, then $\hat{q}_m s(1 + 2h - hs)$ is an estimate of $2u_f + u_m(1 - hs)$ and is an underestimate of the weighted average mutation rate. If the mutant is assumed to be completely recessive when in fact there is some selection against heterozygotes, the mutation rate obtained from (13) is an underestimate.

Equations (11) and (12) are correct even if the heterozygote is favored by selection, provided that the heterotic effect is not so large as to lead to a selectively maintained polymorphism. It is not likely that any of the X-linked traits whose mutation rate has been measured show overdominance, however. Conditions such as hemophilia and Duchenne muscular dystrophy are strongly selected against in males, while females, while possibly not of normal fitness, are superficially normal. If $|h|$ is small, the simple estimating equation (13) is a satisfactory approximation.

The same cautions are appropriate as for autosomal dominant mutations. It is important to measure X-linked recessive rates because in experimental animals the dominant phenotypes occur considerably more rarely than do the recessive. Rates for X-linked recessives are the most reliable estimates of recessive mutation rates. As for dominants, the most reliable estimates are obtained for those with very low fitness, preferably near zero. Reduced penetrance is not usually considered in the study of X-linked mutation rates. It introduces no complication, however, provided that the nonpenetrant males are of normal fitness. The equilibrium is then $3u/Ks$, of which a fraction K express the trait, leaving Eq. (13) unchanged, provided $\hat{q}_m$ is interpreted as the proportion of males expressing the trait.

Semidirect Methods

Patau and Nachtsheim (1946) and Haldane (1949) used a method that has been called semidirect (Crow, 1961). Like the indirect method, it uses the population incidence, but like the direct method, it identifies children from normal parents. For example, Nachtsheim (1954) found

Table IV. A Model of Selection with Nonrandom Mating

Genotype	AA	Aa	aa
Fitness	w	$w(1 - hs)$	$w(1 - s)$
Relative fitness	1	$1 - hs$	$1 - s$
Frequency before selection	$p^2(1 - F) + pF$	$2pq(1 - F)$	$q^2(1 - F) + qF$
Mutation		$A \xrightarrow{u} a$	

that of 56 cases of Pelger anomaly, three came from normal parents. The population incidence was taken to be 1/3000, so the mutation rate was estimated as $(1/2)(3/56)(1/3000)$, or about 10^{-5}. Note that this does not assume that the population is at equilibrium, nor is it necessary to estimate the fitness.

Another indirect estimate was obtained for an X-linked trait by Morton and Chung (1959). They used segregation analysis to determine the fraction of sporadic cases of Duchenne muscular dystrophy. This was estimated as 0.355. Then 0.355 times the proportion of affected males is an estimate of the female mutation rate, in this case 9.9×10^{-5} [compared to an estimate of 8.9×10^{-5} using Eq. (13)]. The similarity of the two estimates argues that the male and female rates are not greatly different (but see page 83).

Autosomal Recessive Phenotype

For an autosomal recessive the situation is more complicated. A realistic treatment requires that three ways of eliminating mutant alleles be considered: elimination through heterozygous effects, through consanguineous mating, and through the mutant gene's meeting a preexisting, noncomplementing mutant allele by chance. The model is given in Table IV. Here F is Wright's inbreeding coefficient, used as a measure of departure from random-mating proportions.

As with Eqs. (3) and (4), we can write the recurrence relation for gene frequency change. Letting p' be the frequency in the next generation of the normal allele A, and u be the mutation rate from A to a, we have

$$p' = w[p^2(1 - F) + pF + pq(1 - F)(1 - hs)](1 - u)/\overline{w} \quad (14)$$
$$\overline{w} = w[1 - 2pq(1 - F)hs - q^2(1 - F)s - qFs] \quad (15)$$

Setting $p' = p = \hat{p}$ for equilibrium and ignoring terms of the order of the product of three or more of F, $\hat{q}$, and h, we have

$$\hat{q} \cong u/s(\hat{q} + F + h) \tag{16}$$

as obtained by Morton *et al.* (1956).

The three terms in the parentheses correspond to the three ways in which mutant alleles are eliminated; through meeting a preexisting allele ($\hat{q}$), through inbreeding (F), and through selection against the heterozygote (h).

For a dominant or X-linked mutation it is sufficient that the incidence be known and that s be large and accurately determined. For autosomal recessives, s is usually large and can be estimated with some degree of precision. Likewise, the mutant allele frequency can be estimated, often by using data from marriages of a known degree of consanguinity. One advantage of using data from inbreeding is that the allele frequency itself is measured directly rather than its square, and therefore if more than one locus is involved, their frequencies are additive.

Yet, knowing these quantities is not sufficient. The great uncertainity arises when estimating the quantity in parentheses. For (16) to be appropriate, all three terms should be equilibrium values, and it is unlikely in the extreme that all three have remained constant during the time since the mutation occurred. Morton (1981, and references therein) has applied a number of tests of internal consistency and, by using segregation and consanguinity analysis, has estimated some of the quantities in more than one way. Nevertheless, the estimates are, at best, tentative.

We shall adopt a rather arbitrary procedure. It is very unlikely, given the stringency of natural selection and the greater amount of inbreeding in the past, that $h + F$ is less than 0.01. On the other hand, it is unlikely that it is greater than 0.10. A value of F as large as 0.085 implies an effective population number of six, or the equivalent of first cousin marriage. Persistence of lethal mutations in *Drosophila* populations is about 50 generations (Crow, 1979, and references therein), implying that the harmonic mean of h is 1/50. So we shall use the allele frequency multiplied by $0.01s$ and $0.1s$ as lower and upper estimates of the mutation rate.

Morton and his associates have also estimated the genomic rate for classes of mutants. We shall not review these studies here; this has been done by Morton (1981).

Electophoretic Variants

Neel (1983, and references therein) has summarized work done mainly by his group on mutation rates of electrophoretic variants. The direct method involves searching for rare variants in children and then looking for the absence of these in the parents, after careful inquiry into possible errors both of identification of phenotypes and of parentage. In a recent report (Neel, 1983), among 907,235 locus-person tests, two mutants had been found. This corresponds to a mutation rate of 2.2×10^{-6}. The small number of additions since the report do not materially change the estimate, which remains of the order of 10^{-6}.

On the other hand, studies of three populations, American Indians, Australian Aborigines, and New Guineans, suggest a considerably higher rate, of the order of 10^{-5}. The latter calculations are based on estimates of gene frequency and effective population number and depend on the assumption that the heterozygous variants are selectively neutral. Neel is led to "consider seriously" the possibility that the nonindustrialized, tribal populations have mutation rates an order of magnitude higher than those of large industrialized societies. The methods used in these studies are complicated (Kimura and Ohta, 1969, 1973; Nei, 1977; Rothman and Adams, 1978; Neel and Rothman, 1978; Chakraborty, 1981; Chakraborty and Roychoudhury, 1978). In our view the standard errors are so large and the assumptions too tenuous to allow any conclusion to be drawn from these studies.

Reliability and Validity of Various Methods

As we have seen, the most direct measurements of mutation rates are those for severely debilitating dominant traits. The genetic assumptions are minimal. The difficulties are the practical ones mentioned above: misidentification of parentage, incomplete penetrance, phenocopies, genocopies, and underascertainment. These can be circumvented to some extent, but never completely, by using the best epidemiologic methods and by detailed familiarity with the phenotypes.

The indirect method applied to dominant phenotypes is of comparable reliability, provided that the fitness is very low. For such traits the mean persistence of a mutant in the population is short and the equilibrium value is attained quickly. Changes in fitness in the past, or possibly changes in the mutation rate, are less influential than if the equilibrium were approached slowly. This method has the advantage that mistaken identification of parentage is not a problem, nor is incomplete penetrance. It is therefore desirable to have separate direct and indirect estimates, which add to the confidence of both when they agree.

For X-linked recessive traits with very low fitness the indirect method is almost as reliable as it is for autosomal dominants. The time to reach equilibrium is three times as long as for an autosomal dominant with the same fitness reduction. As mentioned earlier, the mutation rate estimated is the average for the two sexes, with the female rate being doubly weighted.

We conclude, as other have, that direct and indirect measurements of mutation rates of autosomal and X-linked recessives are the most valid. The extent to which these may be regarded as representatives of mutation rates in general is discussed below.

Autosomal recessive mutations may have occurred many generations in the past and their present frequency is greatly influenced by the number of consanguineous matings in the past and especially by selection in heterozygotes. Because mutant heterozygotes are so much more numerous than homozygotes, a very small selective effect—much too small to be noticed in any data—can influence the frequencies and vitiate any mutation rate estimate based on the assumption of complete recessivity. There is also uncertainty about past levels of inbreeding. Although much ingenuity has been applied to estimating recessive mutation frequencies, the necessary assumptions are tenuous.

One approach already mentioned as of possible importance is that of Nute and Stamatoyannopoulos (1981). They assembled all the data available on abnormal hemoglobins. Many of these mutants produce only minor effects on the individual, if any, and are therefore not ascertained by ordinary clinical methods. However, methemoglobins have a very conspicuous and characteristic phenotype. Likewise, unstable hemoglobins lead to chronic, hemolytic anemias that are easily detected. These are all inherited as dominants, so individuals with the trait whose parents are normal are new mutants.

Although these mutations produce a dominant phenotype, they have the same molecular basis as base-subsitution mutations that are usually inherited as recessives. By ascertaining the dominant types and multiplying their rate by the ratio of known recessive to dominant mutations in the hemoglobin molecule, one can get a direct estimate of the rate of recessive base-substitution mutations.

The hemoglobins have the great advantage that the site of the individual affected nucleotide can be determined. Nute and Stamatoyannopoulos assumed that their ascertainment was complete and so they simply divided the number of mutations by the total number of births in the relevant population during the same period. Underascertainment is balanced to some extent by noninclusion of regions where no cases were reported, but in all likelihood the estimate obtained in this manner is an underestimate.

With better epidemiology leading to complete ascertainment in a large, well-defined population this method could provide a good estimate of the mutation rate at the nucleotide level.

Results

Published Estimates

Table V gives some representative mutation rates from the reviews by Vogel and Rathenberg (1975) and Vogel and Motulsky (1979), who included the data that they thought the most valid. The average values are not appreciably changed if additional studies are included. The table includes the lowest and highest values from the earlier tables. The overall median is of the order of 10^{-5}. This value is consistent with the values reviewed 15 years earlier (Penrose, 1961; Crow, 1961).

Table V also includes values published by Childs (1982). Childs utilized various sources and arrived at his own best estimates. The details of how these conclusions were reached are given in his paper. In most cases his results are within the ranges in the first two columns of the table. The totals include additional, mostly rare, phenotypes. Two totals are given, one for which the mutation rates are reasonably well known, and a larger group including some that are more uncertain. The latter group includes, for example, hypercholesterolemia, porphyria, and otosclerosis. It is remarkable that the listed, more common types account for a large part of the total.

The study of Nute and Stamatoyannopoulos (1981), based on methemoglobin and unstable hemoglobins and assuming complete ascertainment in the areas studied, leads to an estimated mutation rate of 8.6 × 10^{-6} per thousand nucleotide pairs. This is a minimum estimate because some degree of underascertainment is almost certain. The editors of the volume in which the article appeared (Hook and Porter, 1981) suggest that the minimum value should be somewhat lower because countries with no cases were not included in the denominator. On the other hand,

Table V. Selected Mutation Rates for Human Phenotypes[a]

	Mutation rate ($\times 10^6$)		
Trait	VR upper[a]	VR lower[a]	Childs[b]
Autosomal dominants			
Achondroplasia	6	13	12
Aniridia	3	5	3
Dystrophia myotonica	8	11	28
Retinoblastoma	5	12	6
Acrocephalosyndactyly	3	4	—
Osteogenesis imperfecta	7	13	9
Tuberous sclerosis	6	11	10
Neurofibromatosis	44	100	93
Polyposis intestini	13	13	7
Marfan syndrome	4	6	5
Polycystic kidneys	65	120	76
Diaphyseal aclasis	6	9	8
Von Hippel–Lindau syndrome	0.2	0.2	—
Total: Fairly reliable	—	—	366
Including uncertain	—	—	409
X-linked recessives			
Hemophilia	22	32	—
Hemophilia A	32	57	36
Hemophilia B	2	3	3
Duchenne muscular dystrophy	43	105	60
Incontinentia pigmenti	6	20	—
Orofaciodigital syndrome	5	5	—
Total	—	—	140

[a] From Vogel and Rathenberg (1975).
[b] From Childs (1982).

if only the more recent years are included, when the ascertainment seemed to be higher, the value is raised by 50%.

We include this value not so much for its own worth, but because it is representative of the kind of information that should be more easily available in the future. Only relatively few nucleotides are involved and they may or may not be representative of DNA as a whole.

Finally, using the assumptions given earlier, we can use the data of Morton (1981) to obtain rough estimates of mutation rates for recessive diseases. Taking the allele frequency and dividing by the estimated persistence gives an estimate. The persistence, $[s(\hat{q} + F + h)]^{-1}$, probably lies between 20 and 200, which leads to estimates in the range 10^{-5}–10^{-4} with a geometric mean of 3×10^{-5}.

The Bias of Published Estimates and Possible Corrections

The most important bias in mutation rate studies arises from the fact that genes that mutate frequently are more likely to be studied than those that mutate rarely. Those that have not been observed to mutate have of course not been studied at all. This bias can enormously inflate an estimate of the typical mutation rate.

Stevenson and Kerr (1967) made the first, and so far only, serious attempt to obtain a less biased estimate. This still represents the best information available. They chose to study X-linked traits because the total number was of manageable size, the pattern of inheritance was usually clear, there was a large literature admirably summarized by McKusick [latest edition, McKusick (1983)], there had been several extensive population surveys, and Stevenson had himself "made a determined effort over a period of two and a half years to ascertain all X-linked traits in defined populations."

Table VI summarizes Stevenson and Kerr's results. Forty-nine well-established X-linked traits are included, of which 23 were rare enough not to have been encountered by Stevenson and his associates. Five traits were omitted as probably being maintained by mechanisms other than recurrent mutation. These were three types of color-blindness, glucose-6-phosphate dehydrogenase, and the Xg blood groups. Many traits for which the evidence of X-linkage was equivocal were omitted. Since these tend to be rare, to the extent that they should be included, the estimated mutation rate is biased upward.

Table VI. Distribution of 49 X-Linked Traits According to Estimated Mutation Rates[a]

Estimated mutation rate ($\times 10^6$)	Frequency of traits with this mutation rate
50	1
20–49	1
10–19	1
5–9	2
1–4	9
0.1–0.9	11
<0.1	24
Total	49

[a] From Stevenson and Kerr (1967).

The X-linked figures in Table V have a median value in the range $(10-30) \times 10^{-6}$. The median value in Table VI is not far from 0.1×10^{-6}, two orders of magnitude less. The modal mutation rate must be even smaller, because, quite generally, it is true that (mean $-$ mode) $\cong$ 3(mean $-$ median).

Cavalli-Sforza and Bodmer (1971) plotted the cumulative frequency against the log mutation rate and found the points to lie very close to a straight line, suggesting that the log-normal would be a good distribution for describing mutation rates. From the fitted line they estimated the median to be 0.16×10^{-6} and the mean about 7×10^{-6}.

The paucity of data, the tenuousness of the log-normal assumption, and still-uncorrected biases of undetermined magnitude render these estimates very uncertain. Yet, even order-of-magnitude estimates are useful. The data suggest a mean rate for X-linked phenotypes of the order 10^{-6}. The true value may be still less if there are phenotypes that are even rarer. On the other hand, these must be regarded as measures of the rate of occurrence of X-linked recessive *phenotypes,* and are not necessarily representative of the rates of mutation of the constituent genes. Many mutants may be undetected because they are lethal, because they are very mild, or because their phenotypic manifestations are deceptive.

Information from *Drosophila* is instructive. In an experimental *tour de force,* Lindsley *et al.* (1972) combined parts of different translocations to produce systematically small duplications and deletions for 85% of the autosomal chromosome complement. There was only one region where haploidy was lethal. About 50 regions produced a recognizable effect when haploid, most of them the slow-developing "minute" phenotypes. Therefore, the great majority of genes are haplosufficient. Inactivation mutations would be expected to be recessive. It is not surprising that dominants are rare, for they must represent more than the failure to reproduce a normal product.

The rate of X-linked recessive lethal mutation is 0.001–0.002 per chromosome generation. Assuming 1000 gene loci (approximately the number of salivary chromosome bands), this is a rate of $(1-2) \times 10^{-6}$ per locus. The mean rate for human X-linked recessives, uncertain though it be, is of the same order of magnitude, if the rate is per generation. The rates, of course, are enormously discrepant if measured in absolute time units. The statement by Penrose and Haldane (1935) that the human mutation rate is much less than that of *Drosophila* in absolute time units, but perhaps somewhat greater per generation, may well be true.

There is no way from present data to estimate the typical mutation rate, because of uncertainty about the frequency of loci at which mutation is very rare. There is also uncertainty about the rate of mutation in the two sexes; we know only the average. Yet, for many purposes the situation is not as bleak as the uncertainty would suggest.

In concluding this section, we should like to emphasize that, although we have commented extensively on the nonrandomness of the loci chosen for mutation study, this is not always bad. This would indeed be a serious source of error if one were, for example, to compute the total mutation rate by multiplying the average of these values by the total number of loci at risk. Yet, for many, probably most, purposes our inability to measure the rate of mutation at loci that mutate rarely does not introduce any serious problem. Nor does our ignorance about the relative mutation rates in the two sexes.

If we are interested in estimating the impact of mutation on human welfare, mutations that occur at a very low rate are of less importance than the common ones. Therefore, total rates, such as those of Childs referred to in the previous section, are what is needed. If rare traits contribute little to the total (because of their rarity, not because they are not recognized as genetic), that is how it should be.

Inability to distinguish between male and female mutation rates is not always a disadvantage. For assessing the impact of mutation on the population, it is only the average rate (unweighted for autosomal loci, females doubly weighted for X-linked) that is needed; which is precisely the information that mutation rate studies yield.

SOME SPECIAL PROBLEMS

Parental Age Effects

This topic has recently been reviewed extensively (Vogel and Rathenberg, 1975; Vogel and Motulsky, 1979), so we shall discuss it only briefly.

There are more cell divisions between the zygote and sperm than between zygote and egg. Vogel and Rathenberg estimate that there are 24 cell divisions in the female. In the male, the number is age-dependent, estimated as 380 at age 28 and 540 at age 35. There may be a large error in these estimates, especially because of uncertainty about the stem-cell divisions in the male. There is no doubt, though, that the number is substantially higher than in the female.

The first to note this was Wilhelm Weinberg over 70 years ago (Weinberg, 1912). It is one more of Weinberg's remarkable insights. He noted that achondroplastic children tended to be among the last born of a father, so that older fathers appeared to have a greater probability of having affected children. This, he suggested, argued for a mutational origin. Modern studies of paternal age effect started with Penrose (1955). Achondroplasia and Apert syndrome both show a substantial increase, the incidence of affected children of normal parents being about five times as high for the oldest age group of fathers (>40) as for those in their 20s. Other conditions with similar findings are Marfan syndrome and myositis ossificans. See also Erickson and Cohen (1974) and Friedman (1981).

Equally striking is an increase in the age of the maternal grandfather of sporadic hemophiliacs (see, for example, Hinderberger et al., 1980). The evidence for Lesch–Nyhan disease points in the same direction. On the other hand, Duchenne muscular dystrophy, which has a very high rate of mutation, seems not to show such an effect (Vogel and Rathenberg, 1975; Yasuda and Kondo, 1982).

The diseases that do not appear to have a paternal age effect are an interesting group. They include two, Duchenne muscular dystrophy and neurofibromatosis, that have unusually high mutation rates. Possibly the cause is not mutation in the usual sense, but something more like meiotic recombination that could have a high rate and not be dependent on the number of cell generations (Winter and Pembry, 1982). Another possible explanation for the absence of a paternal effect is that there is intercellular selection against early-occurring mutants; but this requires a still higher mutation rate.

Several of this group of diseases are malignancies. The best understood is retinoblastoma. Knudson (1971) suggested that inherited cases, usually bilateral, inherit one mutation and that an additional somatic mutation is required to produce the malignancy. Noninherited cases require two somatic mutations in the same cell lineage. There is good evidence that the second mutation, whether it's genic, chromosomal, or genomic, is on the homologous chromosome (Godabout et. al., 1983; Muphree and Benedict, 1984). The absence of a clear paternal effect may be due to a confounding of germinal and somatic mutations.

Sex Differences in Mutation Rates

We noted earlier that existing estimates of human mutation rates do not distinguish between mutations in males and females. Only the unweighted average rate is estimated for autosomal loci and a weighted average for X-linked loci. Despite the great interest in mutation as a subject for investigation, there is little definitive information on this matter.

As discussed earlier, it is expected that the rate in males will be higher than that in females because of the larger number of cell divisions ancestral to a mature gamete in a male. If mutation is associated with chromosome replication, as is demonstrably the case in microorganisms and as the paternal and grandpaternal age effects strongly suggest, the male mutation rate should exceed the female rate. Haldane (1947) noted that if the mutation rate is the same in both sexes and affected males have fitness zero, the proportion of affected males that are new mutations is one-third. This follows from Eq. (11). The equilibrium proportion of affected males is $\hat{q}_m$, of which u_f are new mutants; therefore, the proportion of affected males who are new mutants is

$$\frac{u_f}{\hat{q}_m} = \frac{s(1 + 2h - hs)}{2 + R(1 - hs)} \tag{17}$$

where $R = u_m/u_f$. If $h = 0$ (no selective advantage or disadvantage in the heterozygous female) and $s = 1$ (lethality or sterility in the male), then

$$u_f/\hat{q}_m = (2 + R)^{-1} \tag{18}$$

Clearly, if $R = 1$, the proportion of affected males who are new mutants is one-third. On the other hand, if the male rate is ten times the female rate, only $1/12$ of the affected males are new mutants.

Haldane thought the data argued for a greater male rate for hemophilia. This was supported by Vogel (1965, 1977) with additional data. More recently Winter (1980) and Winter and Tuddenham (1983) have presented data suggesting a tenfold or more greater rate in males. Francke et al. (1976) have reported evidence for a greater male rate in the Lesch–Nyhan syndrome. This and hemophilia both have an increase in the age of maternal grandfathers of sporadic cases. For other reports on possible differences in the mutation rates in the two sexes, see Bucher et al. (1980) and Emery (1980).

The Hawaii group (Sherman et. al., 1984) have done segregation analyses on the fragile X syndrome. This analysis suggests that the mutation rate is extremely high, estimated as 7.2×10^{-4}, and is essentially confined to males. An implication of this rate is that more than half of female carriers carry a new mutant. The analysis is complex and many assumptions are required, so these very interesting findings should be regarded as tentative until there is additional evidence.

On the other hand, for Duchenne muscular dystrophy, Cheeseman *et al.* (1958), Winter and Pembry (1982), Yasuda and Kondo (1982), and Williams *et al.* (1983) find good agreement with the figure of one-third new mutants expected if the rates were equal in the two sexes. Also, there is no grandpaternal age effect. This, together with the extraodinarily high rate, offers a strong hint that something is different about mutation for this condition. Something related to meiotic recombination suggests itself. Winter and Pembry hypothesize unequal crossing-over between the gene for muscular dystrophy and a postulated pseudogene closely linked to it. Whatever the explanation, the data point toward a substantial sex difference for hemophilia and Lesch–Nyhan disease, but not for muscular dystrophy.

It might be thought that mouse data would provide some guidance on the male–female mutation rate ratio, but the data are too scanty. The spontaneous male rate is reasonably well established for the single loci used in Russell's and Searle's radiation studies (UNSCEAR, 1977). The rate is about 8×10^{-6}. The female data are in doubt, though. There were seven mutants observed among 202,812 progeny, a face value rate of 6×10^{-6}. However, the seven include a cluster of six, so the variance is too large for any firm conclusions.

Although determining whether a particular mutation occurred in the father or mother is not possible in most cases, this situation will soon be remedied. It is already possible in many instances to distinguish between paternal and maternal origin of trisomies. There is sufficient polymorphism in the banding structure of chromosomes to make possible the identification of the source of the three components of a trisomy. At the gene level, this should also be possible soon. In amounts of DNA that are large by molecular criteria, but small relative to the length of a chromosome, there are frequent restriction polymorphisms. Thus, a restriction site, or the loss of one, could in many cases be associated with a particular parental chromosome. This should also be possible for mutants identified morphologically, provided that the gene locus is precisely mapped, i.e., mapped by molecular rather than cytological or linkage criteria.

Heterogeneity of Mutation Rates

Among the X-linked diseases reported by Stevenson and Kerr (1967), two (Duchenne muscular dystrophy and hemophilia A) accounted for more than half of the total incidence of X-linked disease. Among autosomal dominants, the mutation rates of neurofibromatosis and polycystic kidneys are far higher than the others. There is little doubt that mutation rates are enormously heterogeneous. This means, as stated earlier, that the ones that have been most studied are not typical of loci in general. The other side of this coin is that there is a grossly disproportionate contribution to the mutational burden from a few conditions.

At present, there is no information as to why certain genes are more mutable. Experimental genetics offers a number of possibilities. Mutational hot spots are well known in microbes and have a variety of explanations. Some human diseases are associated with a high degree of chromosome breakage and a susceptibility to environmental mutagens. There are a number of reports of high mutation rates, usually transient, in *Drosophila*. Usually these involve a few specific loci. Transposable elements are responsible for extremely high mutation rates in some *Drosophila* matings, and in all probability for high mutability in some natural populations (Engels, 1983). There is no information at present as to which, if any, of these mechanisms account for the extreme heterogeneity of human mutation rates.

Whatever the mechanisms, the human mutation rate is very heterogeneous. The bulk of the mutation burden, insofar as this is due to dominant and X-linked conditions, comes from a very small number of loci. If the cause could be discovered, and possibly somehow corrected, this could produce a large reduction in the mutation burden. There is no indication of any such possibility at present, but at least it seems more amenable than trying to exert some control over the mutation rate at all loci.

Population Monitoring

It is important to the public welfare to be able to detect any increase in the mutation rate, if and when it occurs. The task is not an easy one, given our uncertainty about spontaneous mutation rates and even greater uncertainty about induced rates; there is essentially no information about the induction of mutations in human germ cells by external agents. Even the enormous study of children of irradiated parents in Hiroshima and Nagasaki has yielded no significant results [for a review of radiation effects, see Denniston (1982)].

A useful system for monitoring an increase in the mutation rate would need to meet several requirements. For example, the following criteria have been suggested (Crow, 1971):

1. Relevance to the human situation.
2. Speed of detection.
3. Sensitivity to a small increase in mutation rate.
4. Sensitivity to various kinds of mutations.
5. Likelihood of determining the cause.
6. Availability now or in the near future.

In addition, the system must not be prohibitively expensive in money or human resources.

The kinds of tests suggested include: (1) direct tests for human germinal mutations (dominant sentinel phenotypes, chromosome aberrations, biochemical mutants); (2) tests for increased somatic mutation rates; somatic tests are less relevant, because the concern is for germinal mutations, although this objection is overriden by the far smaller number of individuals that need to be sampled for somatic tests; and (3) indirect tests, which include looking for sister chromatid exchange (a very sensitive system), DNA alterations, mutagens in body fluids, and sperm morphology.

A recent study (National Academy of Sciences, 1983) concluded that the technology for mutation monitoring of the human population is not yet well enough developed for wide application. However, there are systems that could be applied to selected populations, such as workers in a chemical factory. Vogel and Atland (1982) have suggested that material collected for other purposes, such as for PKU screening, could be used for mutation monitoring. For recent reviews of monitoring problems and extensive references, see Bora *et al.* (1982), Mulvihill and Czeizel, and National Academy of Sciences (1983).

Newcombe (1982) has argued that monitoring for increases in cancer is much more practical and socially useful at present than trying to monitor for mutations. In studies of exposed groups, for example, those in a specific industry, cancer followup is likely to yield the earliest evidence of something amiss: "So if exposed human populations are to be monitored, let us plan to look first for cancers in those populations, while waiting for the possible excess of genetic disease to appear in the offspring. And let us identify the exposed individuals and groups appropriately now, so that one has the option of carrying out both sorts of study eventually, using the available vital and health record systems as aids to follow-up."

Regardless of the system or endpoint chosen, monitoring poses interesting statistical problems because we do not know ahead of time when the mutation increase will occur (Denniston, 1983). The situation is as follows: The population is sampled at regular intervals (e.g., monthly, quarterly, yearly) and the spontaneous frequency of some trait with a high mutation component observed. We wish to detect a shift in this spontaneous frequency as quickly as possible so that its cause can be investigated. On the other hand, we do not want to claim an increase if none has occurred.

The statistical problem may be formulated as follows: Given observations on independent random variables $X_1, X_2, \ldots, X_n$ (taken at consecutive times), which are distributed according to some distribution function $F(X:P_i)$, $i = 1, \ldots, n$; we wish to test the hypothesis $H_0: P_1 = \cdots = P_0$ (P_0 known and no change during the time of sampling) against the composite alternative $H_1: P_1 = \cdots = P_m = P_0; P_{m+1} = \cdots = P_n = P_0 + S$ (a change during the time of sampling), where both the change point m and the magnitude of the shift S are unknown. And we want to do our testing in such a way as to minimize the average time to rejection of H_0 after a shift has occurred and maximize the average time to rejection of H_0 in the absence of any shift, subject to constraints of sample size, money, and so on.

Morton (1976), in an interesting article, has suggested using Wald's sequential probability ratio method for human population monitoring. He demonstrates the method using data on Down syndrome from Australia and Sweden. His application is essentially a two-sided sequential test, assumes an underlying Poisson distribution, and tests the simple hypothesis $P = P_0$ against the simple alternative $P = KP_0$. He discusses the relations between sample size K and the expected number of samples required for a decision with type I and type II error rates of 10%. Morton prefers the Wald scheme to the cumulative sum method (described in the next paragraph), citing greater flexibility and ease of interpretation.

Nevertheless, its seems unlikely that the Wald scheme could be optimal, because it is not specifically directed at the alternative hypothesis of interest, i.e., a shift in the parameter during the sampling process.

The other approach, advocated by Weatherall and Haskey (1976), comes from continuous inspection schemes used for quality control in industry and pioneered by Page (1954) and Barnard (1959). The cumulative sum method, as it is called, consists in recording the cumulative sums $S_r = \Sigma(X_i - K)$, where K is often the expected value of X under H_0. The value of S_r is set to zero if it becomes negative. The hypothesis H_0 is rejected when the cumulative sum reaches some predetermined value h. Again, one wants to detect a shift quickly, but not often claim a shift when none has occurred; to this end one wants the expected value of r at rejection to be small under H_1 and large under H_0. The relevant relations between h, K, sample size, and these expected run lengths are discussed, for the Poisson and normal distributions, by Ewan and Kemp (1960). For a deep discussion of the general change point problem see Kander and Zacks (1966).

The situation described above is, of course, only one of many. A slow, steady increase in the mutation rate or a sudden but temporary burst could also be looked for. Each undoubtedly requires specific statistical methods.

USE OF MUTATION RATES IN GENETIC COUNSELING

We will consider two cases in which knowledge of mutation rates is necessary to do genetic counseling.

In general, in any X-linked counseling problem, one has a pedigree containing at least one affected male or known carrier female. For convenience we will call such an individual a "root" of the pedigree. (A root may also be a proband, but that is not relevant to this discussion.) A counseling problem then always amounts to calculating the probability that some female relative of the root(s), who is not herself a root, is a carrier. There are four basic situations:

A. The female relative is a descendant of a male root.
B. The female relative is a descendant of a female root.
C. The female relative is an ancestor or collateral relative of a male root.

D. The female relative is an ancestor or collateral relative of a female root.

Simple examples of these four cases are shown in Fig. 1, in which the root is designated by an arrow and the female relative by the letter X.

Cases *a* and *b* present no particular difficulties; the risk is calculated by applying simple Mendelian arguments. Cases *c* and *d,* on the other hand, require more sophisticated calculations; in each case, the question of where the mutant gene originated arises. In particular, two population parameters are relevant: At equilibrium between selection and mutation the proportion of affected males who are new mutants is, from (17),

$$M = \frac{s + hs(2 - s)}{2 + (1 - hs)R} \tag{18}$$

where $(1 - s)$ and $(1 - hs)$ are the relative fitnesses of affected males and carrier females, respectively, and $R = u_m/u_f$, is the ratio of the male to the female mutation rates. Similarly, the proportion of carrier females who are new mutants is

$$F = \frac{(1 + R)[s + hs(2 - s)]}{2(2 + R - s)} \tag{19}$$

The risk to X in case C depends on both M and F; the risk to X in case D depends only on F. In both cases the probability that X is a carrier depends upon the selection coefficients in both males and females as well as the ratio of the two mutation rates. However, if $h = 0$, which means the carrier female is normal, then, if the trait is lethal in males ($s = 1$), we see that $F = 1/2$, i.e., F is independent of R. In general, counseling problems involving a female root are less sensitive to the (unknown) value of R than those involving a male root when the fitness of affected

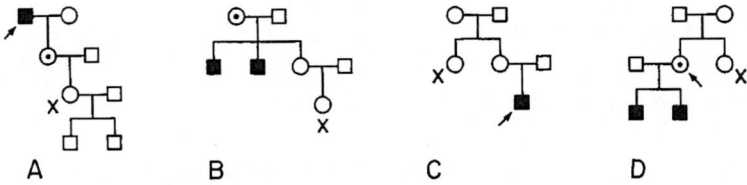

Fig. 1. Pedigrees for counseling. The root is indicated by an arrow and the female relative by an X.

Table VII. Calculation of the Posterior Probability that an Affected
Individual is a New Mutant

	One parent heterozygous	Neither parent heterozygous
Prior probability	$4q(1 - K)$	$1 - 4q(1 - K)$
Probability of affected child	$K/2$	$2u^*K$
Product	$2qK(1 - K)$	$2u^*K$
Posterior ratio	$(1 - K)$:	hsu^*/u

males is low. In any event, it is remarkable that the actual mutation rates need not be known, only their ratio. Of course, if M and F could be estimated empirically, even knowledge of the ratio would be unnecessary.

The other example of a genetic counseling problem requiring knowledge of mutation rates arises with an incompletely penetrant dominant disease. Suppose one must counsel the sibs of an isolated affected child whose parents are normal. Again, the question of whether the proband is a new mutant or not arises. Suppose, in addition, that mutation shows a paternal age affect. The probability that the affected child is a new mutant (neither of the parents is a heterozygote) can be obtained from Table VII. The last line is obtained by simplification and the substitution $q = u/Khs$. We see then that the probability that an affected child is a new mutant is

$$\frac{hsz}{hsz + 1 - K} \tag{20}$$

where $1 - sK$ is the relative fitness of heterozygotes and $z = u^*/u$; u^* is the average mutation rate of the parents (taking into account the age of the father) and u is the population average mutation rate. With a paternal age affect, z is expected to be greater than one. Again, only this ratio is required, not the individual mutation rates.

These are the only two examples that we can think of in which the mutation rate needs to be taken into account in genetic counseling. In both it turns out that the absolute mutation rates are not needed, only their ratio. This is fortunate, for the ratio can often be measured when the absolute values cannot, for example, by observing the proportion of males with an X-linked disease who come from carrier mothers.

POPULATION KINETICS OF MUTATION

In this section we consider what happens to mutant genes in the population. We shall consider three cases, autosomal dominant, X-linked recessive, and autosomal recessive. In each instance, the mutant gene is deleterious and we assume that the selective disadvantage of the mutation is large relative to the mutation rate.

Equilibrium between Mutation and Selection

Consider first an autosomal dominant mutation with complete penetrance, using the model given in the section, Mutation Rate Estimates. From Eq. (8) if penetrance is complete ($K = 1$), we have the approximate equilibrium allele frequency

$$\hat{q} \cong u/hs \tag{21}$$

where u is the average mutation rate in the two sexes and hs is the selective disadvantage of mutant heterozygotes. This assumes that $h^2s \gg u$, where, as before, s is the selective disadvantage of the mutant homozygote.

To determine the rate of approach to equilibrium, let $x_t = q_t - \hat{q}$. We use the subscript t to designate time, measured in generations, and assume that $x_t \ll 1$. Substituting this into (3) and (4) and neglecting all terms involving $\hat{q}^2$, x^2, or $x\hat{q}$, we have the approximate relation

$$x_{t+1} \cong x_t(1 - hs) \tag{22}$$

or

$$x_t \cong x_0(1 - hs)^t \tag{23}$$

This linearized approximation is most accurate near the equilibrium.

The approach to equilibrium is exponential and the rate is dependent on the value of hs. Strongly selected genes approach their equilibrium values very rapidly. A convenient way to express the rate of approach is the number of generations required to go halfway to equilibrium. Designating this as $t_{1/2}$, we let $x_t = x_0/2$, leading to

$$t_{1/2} = \ln(1/2)/\ln(1 - hs) = -0.693/\ln(1 - hs) \tag{24}$$

Table VIII. Equilibrium Mutant Gene Frequency and Time to Go Halfway to Equilibrium[a]

Mutant inheritance	s	z	z'	u/z	$t_{1/2}$ Discrete	$t_{1/2}$ Continuous
Autosomal dominant	0.5	0.5	0.5	2.0×10^{-5}	1	1.39
$z = z' = s$	0.2	0.2	0.2	5.0×10^{-5}	3	3.46
	0.1	0.1	0.2	1.0×10^{-4}	6	6.93
X-linked recessive	1.0	0.333	0.333	3.0×10^{-5}	2	2.08
$z = z' = s/3$	0.5	0.167	0.167	6.0×10^{-5}	4	4.15
	0.2	0.067	0.067	1.5×10^{-4}	10	10.34
Autosomal recessive	1.0	0.05	0.05	2.0×10^{-4}	14	13.86
$z = s(\hat{q} + h + F)$	1.0	0.02	0.02	5.0×10^{-4}	34	34.65
$z' = s(2\hat{q} + h + F$	0.5	0.01	0.01	1.0×10^{-3}	69	68.31
	1.0	0.0031	0.0062	3.1×10^{-3}	111	111.8
	0.1	0.001	0.002	1.0×10^{-2}	346	346.5

[a] The mutation rate u is taken as 10^{-5}; s is the selective disadvantage of the mutant heterozygote for autosomal dominants, of mutant males for X-linked recessives, and of mutant homozygotes for autosomal recessives; the mutant gene frequency is u/z; the number of generation to go halfway to equilibrium is $t_{1/2}$. The time to reach equilibrium is $-0.693/\ln(1 - z')$ with discrete generations (nearest whole number) and $0.693/z'$ for a continuous model.

The human population consists of individuals of all ages. A simple continuous model, although ignoring the realities of departure from age-structure equilibrium, is still probably more realistic than a discrete generation model. Instead of (22) we can write

$$x_{t+1} - x_t = -hsx_t \tag{25}$$

for which the continuous analog is

$$dx/dt = -hsx \tag{26}$$

which integrates to

$$x(t) = x(0)e^{-hst} \tag{27}$$

The time required to go halfway to equilibrium, obtained by setting $x(t) = x(0)/2$, is

$$t_{1/2} = (\ln 2)/hs = 0.693/hs \tag{28}$$

Some numerical examples are given in Table VIII.

For an X-linked recessive mutant the result is similar. The equilibrium allele frequency in males from (12) is

$$\hat{q}_m = 3u/s \tag{29}$$

where u is the weighted average of the mutation rates in the two sexes, $(u_m + 2u_f)/3$, and s is the selective disadvantage of mutant males. The rate of approach to equilibrium is complicated and may even be oscillatory if the male and female gene frequencies are on opposite sides of their equilibrium values. To a first approximation, not too far from the equilibrium we can treat x as an absolute deviation from the equilibrium, leading to

$$x_t = x_0(1 - z)^t \tag{30}$$

where $z = s/3$. The time to halve the absolute deviation is

$$t_{1/2} = -0.693/\ln(1 - z) \tag{31}$$

or, for a continuous model,

$$t_{1/2} = 0.693/z \tag{32}$$

For an autosomal recessive, we use the equilibrium equation (16), which is

$$\hat{q} = u/s(\hat{q} + F + h) = u/z \tag{33}$$

and where the letters have the same meanings as in the section, Mutation Rate Estimates.

Using Eq. (14) and (15) and writing $x = q - \hat{q}$, we obtain

$$x_t = x_0(1 - z')^t \tag{34}$$

where

$$z' = s(2\hat{q} + F + h) \tag{35}$$

As before, the time to go halfway to equilibrium is

$$t_{1/2} = \ln(1/2)/\ln(1 - z') \tag{36}$$

or, for the continuous model,

$$t_{1/2} = (\ln 2)/z' = 0.693/z' \tag{37}$$

The numbers in Table VIII illustrate the main features. A dominant mutation that causes a large reduction in fitness equilibrates at a low frequency, of the same order as the mutation rate, and attains this frequency in a small number of generations, inversely related to s. The closer s

approaches one, the more likely the population is to be near an equilibrium. The shorter the time to reach equilibrium, the more reasonable is the assumption that the value of s has remained constant during this period. Hence strongly selected dominant mutants are best for mutation rate estimates, or for predicting the future consequences of mutations.

X-linked recessive mutants are similar, but for a corresponding value of s the equilibrium frequency in males is three times as high and the rate of approach to equilibrium is one-third as fast.

The situation with autosomal recessives is quite different. The kinetics depends strongly on how the mutant alleles are eliminated from the population. If $F \to 0$, the mutant gene is incompletely recessive, and $h^2 s \gg u$; most eliminations are through heterozygous effects and the kinetics are the same as for a dominant mutation with heterozygous fitness $1 - hs$. If there is enough inbreeding that most elimination is through homozygotes produced by inbreeding, the equilibrium mutant gene frequency is u/sF.

If the mutant gene is completely recessive and mating is at random, the equilibrium mutant gene frequency is $(u/s)^{1/2}$ In this case the rate of approach to equilibrium is $2\hat{q}s$ and it requires $0.693/2\hat{q}s$ to go halfway to equilibrium, usually a very long time.

In Table VIII, under "autosomal recessive" the first three items illustrate typical cases where eliminations are through heterozygous selection or inbreeding. The time to go halfway to equilibrium is typically tens of generations. The last two illustrate the situation for complete recessivity and random mating, where the time to go a significant fraction of the way to equilibrium is hundreds of generations. In any of these cases the rate of approach is so slow that it is unrealistic to rely on equilibrium assumptions.

The Rarity of Complete Recessivity

As we have already indicated, there are many reasons for believing that the great majority of recessive mutant genes are partially dominant. We now give some evidence, the strongest of which comes from *Drosophila*.

One line of evidence comes from heterozygous deletions. Despite the fact that almost all loci in *Drosophila* are haplosufficient, as discussed earlier, it has been known for many years that all sizable deletions are lethal when heterozygous. This must be caused by the cumulative effect of many heterozygous effects, each too small to be noticed alone (Muller, 1950; Lindsley *et. al.,* 1972).

More direct evidence comes from the study of lethal mutations. New "recessive" lethal mutations reduce heterozygous viability by 4–5%. Recessive lethals extracted from natural populations cause a 1–2% reduction. The difference is expected, because those mutants that are found in natural populations are present in proportion to the number of generations that they persist after mutation, and this is greatest for those causing the least heterozygous disadvantage. When total fitness is measured rather then viability alone, the heterozygous effect is some three times as large (Simmons and Crow, 1977; Lee and Watanabe, 1977). Stated another way, the average recessive lethal mutation persists in the population some 50 generations before being eliminated by natural selection. This is much too short a time to be consistent with elimination through homozygote lethality, either because of inbreeding or because the lethal mutant meets up with a preexisting allelic mutant.

The conclusion regarding partial dominance is also true for mutant genes with less than a lethal effect. In fact the data taken at face value suggest that the persistence of mildly deleterious mutants is no greater than that of lethals (Crow, 1979, and references therein). Thus, the heterozygous effect on fitness, relative to the homozygous effect, appears to approach one-half as s approaches zero.

Human data are less convincing, but the evidence points in the same direction. One line of evidence comes from the aforementioned low frequency of individual recessive phenotypes, often less than their probable mutation rates. Another line of evidence comes from consanguineous matings. If $s = 0.5$ and $u = 5 \times 10^{-5}$, the equilibrium frequency of the mutant gene is $\hat{q} = 0.01$. The number of human gene loci is not known, but the number of loci capable of producing a lethal mutation in *Drosophila* is about 5000. The human is not likely to be simpler, so we assume 10,000. With this number the average gamete carries 100 serious or disease-causing recessive mutations. The average child of a cousin marriage ($F = 1/16$) would have 100/16, or about six highly deleterious mutations. If the number of loci is greater, the number of lethal equivalents would be larger. Even if the mutation rate were 5×10^{-6}, there would be two recessive mutants per child of a cousin marriage. Clearly, no such thing happens; mutant genes are far below the frequency expected at equilibrium with complete recessivity. It is probable that inbreeding was much more common in the past, but considering all the evidence, partial dominance is a much more likely explanation.

This discussion concerns average values only. The value of hs is expected to vary from locus to locus and at the same locus over time. In particular, improvements in hygiene and living standard would be expected to make the value less than in the past. Selection against recessive heterozygotes is probably much less effective than in the past, with the implication that their frequency is slowly increasing.

Effects of a Change of Mutation Rate and of Environment

If there is a permanent change in the mutation rate, the new equilibrium and the rate of approach can be obtained from Eqs. (21–37), using the new mutation rate. For any particular mutant the approach to the new equilibrium is exponential (when the new equilibrium is not too far from the old). However, the rates of different mutants will differ greatly, the rate being greatest for the most strongly selected dominant mutants and smallest for weakly selected or nearly recessive mutants. For the whole genome, then, the approach to a new equilibrium will be the average of a family of exponentials, illustrated in Fig. 2.

The effect of an improved environment lowering the s value is very similar (Fig. 2). Since all the equilibrium frequencies (except for complete recessives) are proportional to u/s, multiplying the mutation rate by a certain factor has about the same consequence as dividing the value of s by the same factor. Table IX, taken from Morton (1982), gives formulas for a number of common situations.

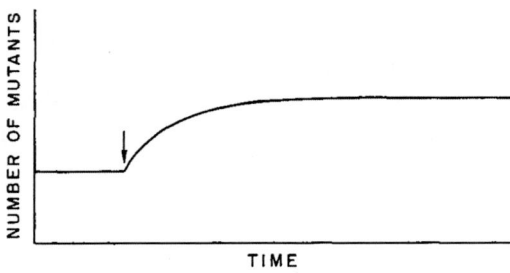

Fig. 2. Effect of a changed mutation rate or selection intensity on mutant allele frequency. The arrow indicates the time when either the mutation rate is doubled or the decrease in fitness caused by the mutation is halved.

Table IX. Consequences of Changes in Parameters[a]

Nature of inheritance and initial condition	Initial gene frequency q_0	New condition	Equilibrium gene frequency Q	Generations to go halfway to the new equilibrium
Autosomal dominant				
Mutation–selection balance	u/s	$u \to cu$	cu/s	$0.693/s$
Mutation–selection balance	u/s	$s \to s/c$	cu/s	$0.693c/s$
X-linked recessive				
Mutation–selection balance	$3u/s$	$u \to cu$	$3cu/s$	$0.693(3/s)$
Mutation–selection balance	$3u/s$	$s \to s/c$	$3cu/s$	$0.693(3c/s)$
Autosomal recessive				
Mutation–inbreeding balance	u/Fs	$F \to 0, h = 0$	$(u/s)^{1/2}$	$0.693/2Qs$
Mutation–inbreeding balance	u/Fs	$F \to 0, h > 0$	u/hs	$0.693/hs$
Mutation–selection balance	u/hs	$h \to 0$	$(u/s)^{1/2}$	$0.693/2Qs$
Mutation–selection balance	$u/s(h + q + F)$	$F \to F, F > F'$	u/Fs	$0.693/Fs$
Mutation–selection balance	$u/s(h + q + F)$	$u \to cu, h + F \to 0$	$(cu/s)^{1/2}$	$0.693/2Qs$
Mutation–selection balance	$u/s(h + q + F)$	$s \to s/c, h + F \to 0$	$(cu/s)^{1/2}$	$0.693/2Qs$
Heterozygote advantage				
Mutation–selection balance	$u/(h + v + F)s$	$h + F \to 0, v > q_0$	$v/(s + v)$	$0.693/(2Qs + v)$
Selection–selection balance	$v/(s + v)$	$v \to 0, h + F \to 0$	$(u/s)^{1/2}$	$0.693/2Qs$
Selection–selection balance	$v/(s + v)$	$s \to s/c$	$cv/(s + cv)$	$0.693c/(2Qs + cv)$
Selection–selection balance	$v/(s + v)$	$v \to cv$	$cv/(s + cv)$	$0.693/(2Qs + cv)$

[a] From Morton (1982). u, Mutation rate; s, selection coefficient against disease, h, dominance in carriers, v, selection coefficient against normal homozygote.

Although in terms of the number of mutant genes in the population an increased mutation rate and a relaxation of selection have the same consequence, from the standpoint of human welfare they are greatly different. In most cases a reduction of s means not only a reduction in the mutant's effect on fitness, but also a reduction in its effect on human welfare. The effects are not likely to be strictly proportional, however. The least desirable environmental improvement is one that reduces the effect of a mutant on fitness while not decreasing the amount of suffering or anguish that it causes. See ICRP (1977) for a discussion of some of the problems involved in devising an index of harm, and Jones (1979a,b) for attempts to assess years of life lost.

Childs (1981) has made systematic, disease by disease, estimates of the increased disease incidence following a doubling of the mutation rate. The incidence data come largely from Carter (1977), with some modifications by Childs. The mutation rates are from the literature and the effects on reproductive fitness are estimated by the author. From this information, he calculated the increase in successive generations after the doubling of the mutation rate. The curve for each disease is shaped like that in Fig. 2. The curve for the total rises rapidly at first, but the rate diminishes as the more severe diseases reach their equilibrium frequencies.

Childs estimates that, altogether, six per 1000 liveborn individuals have a monogenic disorder, of which one per 1000 are new mutations. If the mutation rate were doubled permanently, the frequency would increase by 15% the first generation, by 24% in the second, and would reach 50% of the final equilibrium value in nine generations.

The Effect of a Single Burst of Mutations

A single-generation increase in the mutation rate will cause an increase in the proportion of mutant genes in the population, but the number will gradually decay back to the old equilibrium value. The approach to the original equilibrium value is given by the same equations we have been discussing; the approach is exponential, with the rate determined by z', as before. This is illustrated in Fig. 3.

One relationship is of particular interest. The *per generation* excess of mutant individuals at equilibrium produced by a permanent increase of X percent is equal to the *total* number of mutant individuals resulting

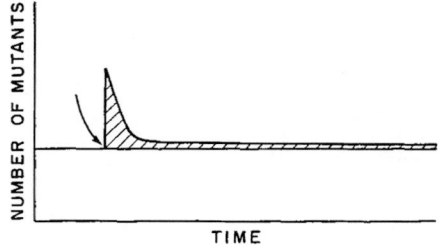

Fig. 3. Distribution of mutant alleles in a population after a single-generation burst of mutations. The arrow indicates the time when the increase occurred.

from a single-generation increase of X percent. (This assumes a constant population size and no change in s values; if the population number is changing, the mutant frequency should be expressed as a proportion of the total rather than as an absolute number.) This conclusion is easily seen by recalling that at equilibrium the number of additional mutants each generation is $2Nu/z$, where N is the population number, u is the increase in gametic mutation rate, z is the inverse of the persistence, and the 2 comes from diploidy. The additional number from a burst of mutations is multiplied each generation by a factor $(1 - z)$. Thus the total excess mutant individuals for all time is

$$2Nu[1 + (1 - z) + (1 - z)^2 + (1 - z)^3 + \cdots] = 2Nu/z \quad (38)$$

the same as the increase per generation at equilibrium.

It is noteworthy that the expected number affected by a mutant gene is unchanged when the problem is treated stochastically, provided the mutant gene is rare enough that homozygotes can be ignored (Li and Nei, 1972).

ASSESSING THE POPULATION MUTATION BURDEN

The Mutation Load and Mutation Impact

The earliest attempt to assess the total impact of mutation on the fitness of a population was made by Haldane (1937). In a widely influential article entitled, "The effect of variation on fitness," Haldane stated that the effect of recurrent mutation on fitness is to reduce the mean fitness by a value somewhere between one and two times the total mutation rate per gamete. Essentially the same idea was put forth by Muller (1950) in his address as first president of the American Society of Human Genetics, entitled "Our load of mutations." Both Haldane and Muller realized that the effect of mutation on the population does not depend on the magnitude of the effect of the mutations, but only on the mutation rate, provided that the effect is measured as reduced fitness.

The Haldane–Muller concept is appealing in its simplicity and elegance and was used by the First National Academy Committee on Biological Effects of Atomic Radiation (National Academy of Sciences, 1956) as one way of attempting to assess the total impact of mutation on the population. The method has fallen from favor in recent years. The principal reasons are: (1) Nonindependence of gene effects upsets the linearity on which the principle depends; in particular, truncate or rank order selection may greatly decrease the load. (2) More important, most geneticists are not willing to accept fitness reduction as a realistic measure of the impact of mutation on future human well-being. Later we develop a concept that uses some of the theory of the mutation load, but measures the impact of the mutation in terms of human welfare. First, we review genetic load theory. For a more thorough treatment, see Crow (1970).

Calculating the Mutation Load

The mutation load is defined (Crow, 1958) as

$$L = (w - \overline{w})/w \tag{39}$$

where w is the fitness of a mutant-free individual and $\overline{w}$ is the mean fitness of the population at equilibrium under mutation and selection. Applying this to a semidominant mutation ($h = 1/2$), we have from Eqs. (14) and (15) (setting $p = p'$ and $F = 0$),

$$\overline{w} = w(1 - sq) \tag{40}$$
$$\hat{q} = 2u/s(1 + u) \tag{41}$$

and substituting these into (39) gives

$$L = 2u/(1 + u) \tag{42}$$

or approximately

$$L \cong 2u \tag{43}$$

This value is almost independent of h as long as $h^2s \gg u$.

For completely recessive mutations we use (15) and (16) for $h = F = 0$, obtaining

$$q^2 = u/s \qquad (44)$$
$$\overline{w} = w(1 - sq^2) \qquad (45)$$

and

$$L = u \qquad (46)$$

The general statement is: The mutation load is twice the average mutation rate per gamete divided by the number of mutant genes eliminated by each genetic death. This number is one for partial dominants and X-linked recessives, and two for autosomal recessives. Twice the gametic rate is of course the zygotic rate. If $h^2s \gg u$, near-recessives behave like dominants.

This statement is correct for multiple loci with dominance and epistasis. For a derivation, see Crow and Denniston (1981).

For an X-linked recessive mutation

$$L = (sq_m + 2hsq_f)/2 \qquad (47)$$

and substituting from the equilibrium equations (9) and (10), we have

$$L = (2u_f + u_m)/2 \qquad (48)$$

as might have been expected.

Equation (48) illustrates a nice property of genetic load theory and mutation rate estimation. The standard methods of measuring mutation rates do not measure the rates separately for each sex, as we noted earlier. However, the mutation rates measured are the unweighted average for autosomal loci and the weighted average for X-linked loci. The mutation rates required for estimating the mutation load are weighted exactly the same way—equally for autosomal loci and twice as heavily for females at X-linked loci. In this case there is no necessity for separate measurements in the two sexes, which is fortunate, since it cannot now be done.

We can illustrate the mutation load principle in another way, more akin to the way Muller (1950) used it. Muller stated that each new mutant required one extinction, or "genetic death," unless two (as with recessives) or more (with some forms of epistasis) were eliminated at once. There is an implicit assumption of constant population size (unless the load is expressed as a fraction of the total population rather than as an absolute value). We can compute the load immediately from Eq. (38). For a dominant mutant, $z = hs$. The load is the total number of mutants multiplied by the fitness reduction caused by each, so

$$\text{absolute load} = (2Nu/z)z = 2Nu \tag{49}$$

where N is the population number. The load per individual is then $2u$, as we obtained before.

It should be mentioned that this principle does not depend on z being constant. Letting primes stand for successive generations, we can write the load as

$$2Nu[z + (1 - z)z' + (1 - z)(1 - z')z'' + \cdots]$$

or letting $x = 1 - z$, we have

$$2Nu[1 - x + x - xx' + xx' - xx'x'' + xx'x'' \cdots] = 2Nu \tag{50}$$

Thus, the value of z can vary from generation to generation without affecting the conclusion (Crow, 1957). It can even take occasional negative values; a sufficiently variable environment might convert a mutant gene whose long-time average effect is deleterious into one that is sometimes beneficial.

Distinction between Mutation Load and Mutation Impact

The mutation load, as we have seen, measures the effect of mutation on the population in terms of reduced fitness or genetic extinctions. For evolutionary considerations this is the appropriate measure. For most human considerations, though, we are interested in the effect of the mutations on human welfare. We designate this as the impact I.

The frequency of the gene is determined by its mutation rate and the rate of elimination by natural selection, which is related to its effect on fitness. The impact is the effect of the condition on fitness multiplied by a quality factor to adjust for the amount of the burden. The quality factor measures the severity of the impairment or its effect on the welfare of the individual. It might, in principle, include effects on the welfare of other individuals, such as family members who are indirectly affected or even all of society. It adjusts for the fact that different mutants with the same effect on fitness need not cause the same amount of suffering or other burden.

The Mutation Component of Genetic Disease

Estimating the Mutation Component from Load Theory

For traits maintained by balance between mutation and selection, the mutation load is proportional to the mutation rate, where the proportionality constant depends on dominance and epistasis. We can then write the impact I of the trait as

$$I = a + bu \tag{51}$$

where a and b are constants. The mutation component M is

$$M = bu/(a + bu) \tag{52}$$

One can interpret M as the proportion of the total impact of the disease that is attributable to recurrent mutation, while $a/(a + bu)$ is the proportion that is due to other causes. If the mutation rate is increased from u to $u(1 + k)$, the impact will increase to a value $a + bu(1 + k)$ at equilibrium; that is, it will have increased from I to $I(1 + Mk)$. So, M represents the proportion of an increased mutation rate that is directly reflected in an increased impact. If there is an increment du in the mutation rate, the increment in the impact dI is given by

$$dI/I = M \, du/u \tag{53}$$

$$M = \frac{u}{I} \frac{dI}{du} \tag{54}$$

Since I and L are proportional, we can replace I by L in these equations and make use of genetic load theory.

Traits that are maintained by mutation–selection balance and with no environmental component have an incidence and impact proportional to the mutation rate. Thus, $I = bU$, where U is the total mutation rate of relevant loci. From (54) the mutation component is one.

Now consider that the trait has two components, a genetic part that is maintained by mutation–selection balance, $bu/(a + bu)$, and an independent environmental part, $a/(a + bu)$. The genetic part has a mutation component of one; the environmental part is independent of the mutation rate. The mutation component is analogous to heritability in the broad sense, so the techniques used to measure heritability give an estimate of the mutation component. This extends the analysis to quantitative traits.

Still assuming that the genetic part of the trait is determined by mutation–selection balance, we can consider a quantitative measurement for which the optimum value is intermediate. For such a trait the mean and the optimum will roughly coincide and the effect of mutation is mainly to increase the genetic variance. For such a trait, if the mutation rate is high and the individual mutant effects small, the mutation load is proportional to the square root of the mutation rate if the mean and optimum coincide (Crow and Kimura, 1964; Kimura, 1965; Lande, 1975; Fleming, 1979). This implies a mutation component of one-half. To the extent that the mean and optimum do not coincide, the situation is comparable to directional selection and the mutation component is one. Thus the value is somewhere between one-half and one, this to be multiplied by the heritability if there is an environmental component to the variance (Crow and Denniston, 1981).

The problem is more complicated, however. Latter (1960) and Bulmer (1972, 1980) have presented a two-allele, multilocus model that leads to a mutation load proportional to the mutation rate, rather than its square root, and therefore with a mutation component of one. This troublesome dilemma has recently been resolved by Turelli (1984), who showed that they represent opposite extremes of a mathematical continuum (see also Nagylaki, 1983). As the mutation rate increases and individual mutant effects decrease, the Kimura–Lande model is approached. At lower mutation rates the Latter–Bulmer model is approached. The truth undoubtedly lies somewhere between, and it is not clear where. Fortunately, our earlier conclusion that the mutation component for traits with an intermediate optimum has a value between one-half and one times the heritability still stands.

Using Heritability to Estimate the Mutation Component

So far, we have assumed that the genetic part of the trait is maintained by mutation–selection balance. Alternatively, the trait may be maintained by some sort of balanced selective forces, of which the most obvious example is heterozygote advantage. Such a trait may have a high heritability, so our heritability criterion is not sufficient.

We can get more information by considering heritability in two

Table X. Relationship of Heritabilities to the Mutation Component[a]

Broad-sense heritability h_B^2	Narrow-sense heritability h_N^2	Mutation component M	Example
High	High	High	Rare dominant
High	Low	High	Rare recessive
High	Low	Low	Overdominant
Low	Low	Low	Environmental

[a] From Crow and Denniston (1981).

senses (see, for example, Falconer 1981). Heritability in the broad sense h_B^2 is the proportion of the total variance that is genetically determined. It can be measured by correlations between identical twins, preferably reared in independent environments.

Heritability in the narrow sense h_N^2 is the proportion of the total variance that is additively genetic. It is measured by the correlation between parent and child or other unilineal relatives. Table X gives some examples of heritabilities and mutation components.

As the table shows, classes 2 and 3 are ambiguous in that heritability measurements are insufficient to distinguish between high and low mutation components. A rare recessive has a high value. This could be mimicked by a trait in which the homozygote is affected but the heterozygote is favored by selection. It is not possible on present information to say whether cystic fibrosis owes its high incidence to a high mutation rate, multiple loci, or to selection of heterozygotes.

There is one clear conclusion, however. A trait for which the broad-sense heritability is high and the narrow-sense heritability low is not quickly responsive to a change in mutation rate. A change in mutation rate either has no effect or the new equilibrium will be approached very slowly.

This is of practical value in assessment of the possible impact of environmental mutagens on fugure generations. Figure 4 is taken from the National Academy of Sciences (1983, p. 186). This shows the long-time consequences of a single-generation doubling of the mutation rate. The mutation component is taken to be 0.1 for congenital malformations and other multifactorial conditions and one for other categories. The mean persistence times are taken as 4 for dominant and X-linked, 100 for recessives, 1.25 for chromosomal effects, and 10 for congenital anom-

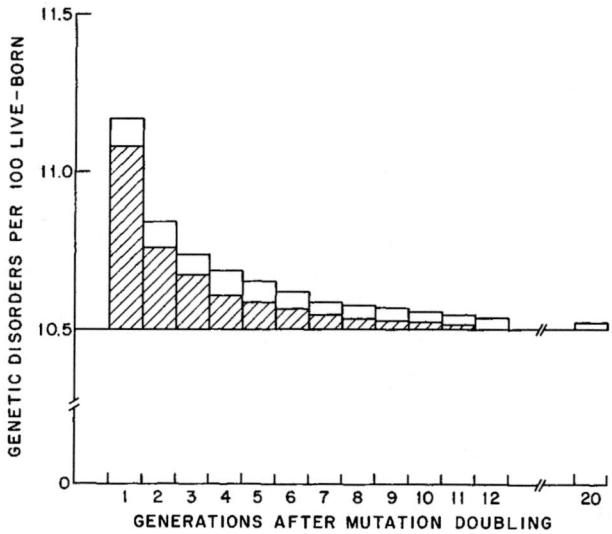

Fig. 4. An example of the increase in genetic disorders when the mutation rate is doubled for a single generation. The contribution of dominant, X-linked, and cytogenetic disorders is hatched. The white area is caused by congenital malformations, multifactorial conditions, and a very small contribution from autosomal recessives. (From National Academy of Sciences, 1983.)

alies and multifactorial conditions. The normal incidences are taken from UNSCEAR (1977, 1982) (see Table II).

Traditionally, studies of heritability have not been done to determine the mutation component, but this provides another reason for such research. For traits with a high parent–child correlation, a higher regression of child on parent than of parent on child indicates a contribution from *new* mutations to the incidence of the trait. For a more extensive discussion of the mutation component, see Crow and Denniston (1981).

MUTATION AND EVOLUTION

The Importance of Mutation Rate in Evolution

Mutation as a factor in evolution was first emphasized by DeVries (1901) almost immediately after the rediscovery of Mendel's laws at the turn of the century. Actually, the "mutations" that DeVries saw in *Oen-*

othera lamarckiana were segregants from complex translocation heterozygotes. These were both much more frequent and much more conspicuous than typical gene mutations. True gene mutations would probably
not have been noticed. Important as the discovery of mutation was in the
history of genetics, it was in fact based on a misinterpretation.

In the first quarter of the twentieth century there was considerable
controversy, especially in Britain, between those who regarded Darwinian natural selection as the guiding force in evolution and those who
argued for mutation. The latter usually assumed an adaptive direction to
mutation leading to steady improvement. The contrast between these and
Darwinian views was accentuated by the conflict between the Mendelists
and the biometricians (Provine, 1971). The resolution of the conflict
came from the demonstration by Fisher (1918) that the observed correlations for human measurements were consistent with Mendelian polygenic inheritance. In the United States, in contrast, it seems to have been
assumed by many geneticists from the beginning that quantitative inheritance is also Mendelian, differing from the inheritance of conspicuous
monogenic differences only in the number of loci involved and by the
fact that the individual Mendelian factors produced effects too small to
be noticed individually. Yet, there were still differences of opinion as to
whether natural selection, acting on small variations, or individual
mutants of larger magnitude were more important in accounting for
major advances in evolution.

By now most geneticists have accepted the neo-Darwinian view.
Because of the work of Fisher (1930), Haldane (1932), and Wright (1931)
there is now the widely held assumption that, although mutation is the
ultimate source of variability, natural selection is the guiding force of
evolution. The most influential opponent of this view in the 1930s was
Goldschmidt (1940), who did not accept the idea that major changes in
evolution are the result of the accumulation of many small differences,
but postulated major, "systemic" mutations. He did not win many adher-
ents, however, and the Haldane–Fisher–Wright view prevailed.

Recently there has been a resurrection of some of the older views.
Gould and Eldridge (1977) have argued from the paleontological record
that evolution is characterized by long periods of stasis interspersed with
sudden, large changes ("punctuated equilibria"). That evolutionary rates
are highly variable has been recognized all along (e.g., Simpson, 1953),
but whether the jumps are as instantaneous as claimed by "punctualists"
is far from established. Exactly what the mechanisms might be, both to

maintain the long periods of constancy and the saltations, is not clear. Some have suggested that the jumps are due to systemic ("regulatory") mutations, somewhat like those of Goldschmidt. It is not clear that any special mechanisms need be postulated. A well-adapted species in a constant environment need not change, while a changed environment could easily lead by natural selection to changes rapid enough to appear as a jump in the incomplete fossil record. Our own preference is to wait for more convincing evidence of "punctuated equilibria" before postulating any new mechanisms [for a critique of the Gould–Eldridge view, see Charlesworth *et al.* (1982)].

Renewed emphasis on mutation has also arisen in connection with the discovery of mutable and mutator genes (Green, 1977; Engels, 1983). Episodes of high mutability have been reported in many species, especially *Drosophila* and maize, and doubtless many more have gone unreported. Typically a high mutation rate, often involving a few specific mutant phenotypes, is observed, but the property is lost before it can be fully analyzed. It is now clear that at least some of these, and perhaps the great majority, are due to transposable elements.

Whether such systems exist primarily as parasites or "selfish DNA" or whether their hosts have used them to further their own evolutionary progress is an open question. Bacterial transposons, such as those that carry drug resistance factors, are clearly advantageous both to themselves and to their hosts. But whether the great number of newly discovered examples of transposable DNA play a useful evolutionary role for their hosts is unknown. The null hypothesis, we believe, should be that these are parasites. However, we should fully expect that, as with other kinds of parasites, some would evolve into a symbiotic or mutually beneficial liaison.

For the purpose of this review, we want to inquire: Under what circumstances is mutation the rate-limiting process and in what circumstances is it not? How do these apply to human evolution?

Circumstances in Which Mutation Is Rate-Determining

When a new gene mutation occurs, usually it will be lost by random processes within a few generations. This is true even if the mutation is favorable. Occasionally a mutation will be lucky and sweep through the population to ultimate fixation. This is much more probable if the gene is favorable, but this can also happen if the gene is neutral or even slightly detrimental. The differences in individual nucleotides that characterize different species give every appearance of having arisen in this way, since populations are monomorphic at most nucleotide sites.

The rate of nucleotide substitution is given by

$$R = 2NuP \tag{55}$$

where N is the population number, u the mutation rate per nucleotide per generation, and P is the probability that the mutation is eventually fixed. The accuracy of this formula depends on the time scale of observation being long relative to the time required for the mutant gene to go to fixation. For a selectively neutral mutation this time is $4N_e$ (Crow and Kimura, 1970, pp. 430–432), where N_e is the effective population number (Wright, 1931); the effective number is roughly the number of reproducing adults, somewhat less if there is non-Poisson variation in fertility. A selectively favored mutant takes less time on the average and, somewhat surprisingly, so does one that is fixed despite being unfavorable (Maruyama and Kimura, 1974). Comparative species studies involve divergence times measured in hundreds of millions of years, so these conditions are met. The relative rarity of nucleotide polymorphisms argues that not many are caught in the process of substitution.

The value of P, the probability of fixation, is

$$P = \frac{1 - \exp(-2sN_e/N)}{1 - \exp(-4sN_e)} \tag{56}$$

(Crow and Kimura, 1970, p. 426). Here, s is the selective advantage of the mutant heterozygote and, as before, N and N_e are the actual and effective population numbers. The fitness of the mutant homozygote does not matter much, as long as it is equal to or larger than s, since the ultimate fate is determined largely by random processes in the early generations while the mutation is almost entirely in heterozygotes.

Notice that when $N = N_e$, $s \ll 1$, $Ns \gg 1$, the probability of fixation is approximately $2s$. As s approaches zero, P approaches $1/2N$, as expected. Finally, it should be noted that (56) is correct even for negative values of s, although the probability of random fixation of a deleterious gene becomes extremely small unless $|s|$ is very minute.

Note that if evolution depends on incorporating favorable mutations ($s > 0$), then R is approximately $(2Nu)(2s) = 4Nus$. The rate of evolution is then proportional to the selective advantage and to the population number, but from the standpoint of our present interest, also proportional to the mutation rate. So we can say that, to the extent that evolution depends on the successive substitution of favorable mutations, the rate is proportional to the mutation rate.

There has been no chance to test this prediction against actual observations in nature, but there have been chemostat experiments where this prediction is verified. Cox and Gibson (1974) were the first to show that under such circumstances a mutable strain adapted more rapidly to life in the chemostat than did one with a normal mutation rate. Presumably the ratio of favorable to unfavorable mutants was high enough in this new environment for an increased mutation rate to be advantageous. Chao and Cox (1983) have verified another prediction of the Kimura formula, namely the proportionality to population size. In two competing populations with the same mutation rate, the eventual winner was the one with the larger initial population size. A sufficient size discrepancy could offset a difference in mutation rates.

This shows that, at least in some circumstances, in particular when bacteria are grown in a chemostat, the simple kinetics of Eqs. (55) and (56) holds. Evolution does indeed appear to be a succession of substitutions of favorable mutants.

Thus, when evolution is dependent on successive substitution of mutations that were favorable from the beginning, the rate of evolution is proportional to the mutation rate. The only difficulty would arise if the ratio of deleterious to favorable mutations is high enough that the former cannot be eliminated rapidly enough to prevent the population from deteriorating faster than the favorable mutants cause improvement.

The important question is: To what extent do clonally propagated strains of bacteria in a chemostat mimic the evolution of sexually reproducing eukaryotes, including man? One opportunity to check the prediction of this kinetics is by observations on the rate of molecular evolution. There is now an abundance of data on evolutionary substitution of nucleotides or amino acids in many lineages. The prediction that evolutionary rates are proportional to species population size is not met at all. Large populations do not in general change more rapidly than small ones. Insects evolve no faster than mammals; herbivores evolve no more rapidly than carnivores.

Thus the observations of molecular evolution argue strongly against these being mainly the result of the substitution of favorable mutations. In fact the rates of amino acid substitution are, to a first approximation, constant for a given protein. Notice that when the gene substitutions are neutral, $P = 1/2N$ [from (56)] and the evolution rate R is simply proportional to the mutation rate, as first emphasized by Kimura (1968a,b). However, the observed rate is roughly constant per year, whereas the prediction of the theory is for constancy per generation. Thus the organisms with longer reproductive life cycles appear to evolve more rapidly per generation than those with shorter cycles. In broad generality, organisms that are the largest have longer life cycles and smaller populations than those that are smaller. Note from Eqs. (55) and (56) that if s is negative, the evolution rate R is negatively correlated with population size. Thus, as improbable as it would seem *a priori,* the data are more consistent with a majority of molecular substitutions being slightly deleterious than with their being neutral or favorable (Kimura, 1979). We should emphasize that the predicted downward trend in fitness caused by such a mechanism is very, very slow and easily offset by a few favorable mutations or alterations of gene frequencies.

Regardless of whether the steady downhill drift in fitness predicted from random fixation of very slightly deleterious mutations stands up under further research, molecular evidence offers no support to the hypothesis that most nucleotide substitutions occur because the mutations are favorable.

Circumstances in Which Mutation Is Not Rate-Determining

One of the most important properties of particulate Mendelian inheritance is its capacity to conserve genetic variance. The rate of random decay of variance in a randomly mating population of effective size N_e is $1/2N_e$ per generation, an amount that is very slight in all but the smallest populations. Selection, unless it is balancing, reduces variance at a somewhat more rapid rate, but in general a very small mutational input is sufficient to maintain a great deal of genetic variance.

The relationship between the amount of standing variability in a population and the per generation input to this by mutation has been investigated mainly in *Drosophila.* Clayton and Robertson (1955) showed that for some bristle characters the amount of variance created by a single generation of mutation is only of the order of 1/1000 that of the standing variance. For mutants with minor effects on viability and fertility the ratio is about 1/50 (Crow, 1979), about the same as that for "recessive" lethal mutations. The existing variability in a population is more promising as raw material for future evolution, for the most grossly deleterious mutations have already been weeded out by purifying selection.

A second property of Mendelian segregation and recombination is that the potential variability is enormously greater than the standing variability. By combining existing genes, phenotypes far beyond the range of the current population can be produced in a few generations of selection. Complete dominance is ordinarily not found in genes that contribute to polygenic variability; the heterozygote is typically not far from the average of the two corresponding homozygotes (e.g., Mukai *et al.* 1972). Thus, the phenotype, insofar as it is genetically determined, responds rapidly to directional selection. For most quantitative traits an intermediate level is optimum for fitness and the curve relating fitness (as ordinate) to phenotypic value is humped. Small changes in phenotype cause even smaller changes in fitness. Thus a great deal of phenotypic variance is conserved with relatively little cost in fitness.

For such reasons a system of Mendelian inheritance determined by multiple, independent factors, each lacking in dominance, is in many ways optimum for rapid response to environmental changes. The response is very much faster than if it were dependent on new mutations. There is no reason to expect any correlation between mutation and rapidity of response to environmental change, except for the minimum requirement of sufficient mutations to offset a slow decay of genetic variability.

So we conclude that to the extent that evolution is dependent mainly on shifts of frequencies of existing genes, its rate is largely independent of the mutation rate. To the extent that it is dependent on substitution of new mutations that were favorable from the beginning, the evolution rate is directly proportional to the mutation rate.

Evolution theorists, largely following the influential writings of Fisher and Wright, have emphasized changes of gene frequencies in response to changes in the environment as the major mechanism of microevolution. By extension, the evolution of higher categories has been assumed to be due to the same processes acting over greater time periods. Contemporary speciation is regarded as being the same essential process, accompanied by some isolating process. However much they differed on the importance of epistasis in creating evolutionary novelty and on the importance of a structured population, Fisher and Wright agreed on the more basic principles. The weight of authority of these two, to which the names of Haldane and Muller could be added, has been such as to silence those who argued for mutational determination of evolutionary rate and direction. However, recent research in transposable genes has brought out latent Goldschmidtian tendencies in some molecular biologists.

We suspect that the conventional wisdom derived from Fisher and Wright is correct and that this is not changed by the recent discoveries of transposable and mutable genes, but the case certainly cannot be regarded as closed.

Evolutionary Adjustment of Mutation Rates

Asexual Populations

Adjustment of the mutation rate in an asexual species is easily understood. A clone with a higher or lower mutation rate will propagate this mutation rate to all the descendants, provided of course that the mutation rate is genetically determined. Whether an increase or decrease in the mutation rate will be favored depends on such factors as the existing rate, the ratio of beneficial to deleterious mutations, and the stability of the environment. A mutation that affects the rate of mutation at all loci can be subject to quite strong selection, and especially in rapidly reproducing species the average mutation rate can be changed rapidly. The distinction between individual and group selection is blurred, and unless the population is broken up into partially isolated groups, the entire population will eventually be descended from a single individual. There is a tradeoff between the pressure to lower the mutation rate in order to decrease the incidence of harmful mutant phenotypes and the need for greater variability to keep up with a changing environment. It is quite likely that at any given time the mutation rate is not optimum. One reason is that changes in the environment are not predictable. Another is that there is a cost to the organism of reducing the mutation rate to lower levels; for example, more accurate polymerases may be slower or more energy-demanding than less accurate ones.

Experimental verification of this principle has been provided by the chemostat experiments mentioned above, in which a highly mutable strain replaced its slowly mutating competitor (Cox and Gibson, 1974). Presumably the chemostat environment was enough different from that of the usual environment to make the ratio of beneficial to harmful mutants high enough to make an increased mutation rate advantageous.

Similar results have been reported when transposon-carrying strains have replaced competitors without the transposon in chemostat experiments (Chao *et al.,* 1983). We must be cautious in interpreting such experiments as evidence for the adaptive value of a high mutation rate, because of such results as those of Biel and Hartl (1983). They, as had others, found that the transposable element Tn5 in *E. coli* produced a selective advantage in strains carrying it. However, this was not due to an increased mutation rate, because the winning strain retained the same number and positions of the transposon. The transposon in this case must have a beneficial function other than an effect on the mutation rate. The transposon carries a kanamycin-resistance gene, but this was shown not to be the cause.

Sexual Populations

Evolutionary adjustment of the mutation rate in a Mendelian population is quite a different matter. One possibility is locus-by-locus adjustment by selection among alleles with different mutation rates. It is likely to be of limited applicability, however, because such alleles may not exist and because the process of selection at any particular locus would be extremely slow.

A gene that increases the general mutation rate might be thought to provide a way for the species to adapt to a continually changing environment. Yet, such changes occur over many generations and the effect of a single generation of mutant genes is not very significant. At the same time, the mutator gene is separated from most of the rest of its genome at a rate of 50% each sexual generation, so it could influence effectively only those loci closely linked to it.

Selection for a lowered mutation rate to decrease the mutation load is somewhat more direct, for the load due to dominant mutations exerts its major impact within the first few generations of their occurrence. Selection against the rate of occurrence of highly deleterious dominant mutations is quite direct in affecting the number of descendants of individuals with different mutation rates. Yet, the selection is still less direct than that on genes having an immediate effect on fitness. The question has been discussed by several authors (e.g., Leigh, 1973).

In view of the inefficiency of the adjustment of the mutation rate toward whatever rate would be optimal for evolutionary advance, it may be that the existing mutation rate is not determined to any significant extent by evolutionary considerations. Although selection to reduce the rate must surely be occurring all the time, such selection is weak. At the same time, lowering the mutation rate has its own cost to the organism, as mentioned before. It seems likely, then, that the mutation rate in sexual species is determined largely by the tradeoff between a high mutation load and the energetic expense of lowering it. The evolutionary functions of mutation are then a byproduct of this selection. The ability of a Mendelian population to maintain a great deal of genetic variability (and especially, potential genetic variability) with a wide range of mutation rates means that the actual mutation rate is not determined mainly by evolutionary considerations. If these arguments are correct, the existing mutation rate does not prevail because it approximates some evolutionary optimum, but simply because it costs too much to reduce it further.

It is possible that the major selective force to reduce the mutation rate is not acting on germinal rates but on somatic mutation rates; and, because both rates are to some extent responsive to the same mechanisms, selection affects germinal rates indirectly. Selection on somatic mutation rates acts directly on the survival and fertility of the individual in which the mutations occur, and hence the problems of adjusting germinal rates are not a handicap. It has been suggested that protection against recessive or partially dominant mutants may be a reason for the evolution of diploidy (Crow and Kimura, 1965). Keeping the somatic mutation rate low is obviously of survival value. Somatic mutations may damage crucial cells or tissues or might lead to malignancy. We therefore suggest that it is reasonable that the germinal mutation rate is a byproduct of evolutionary adjustments of the somatic mutation rate, which natural selection tends to lower until the price becomes too great.

A Possible Role of Transposons

Chao *et al.* (1983) have suggested that transposons may have an evolutionary effect by partially compensating for the inability of sexual populations to adjust the mutation rate effectively. They note that a transposon can convert a normal locus into a mutable one. If there is an evolutionary advantage to this locus being mutable, a transposon can help the species to this extent. The mutability property follows the transmission of this locus, and others closely linked to it, even in a population with segregation and free recombination. Whether such a process in fact ever plays a useful evolutionary role is yet to be demonstrated.

Although there were foreshadowings in both *Drosophila* (Demerec, 1941; Neel, 1942; Mampell, 1943) and maize (McClintock, 1956), and possibly even man (Auerbach, 1949), detailed molecular understanding of transposable elements came from bacterial studies (Kleckner, 1981; Calos and Miller, 1980). Recently this knowledge is being extended at a very rapid rate in various organisms, especially *Drosophila* (Shapiro, 1983). With the discovery of the ubiquity and frequency of elements that move DNA around the genome, it is all the more remarkable that the gene order has remained as stable as it has.

The Human Population

The considerations just discussed apply to the human population, as to all large, sexually reproducing populations. There is not way to know how well the human mutation rate is adjusted toward an evolutionary optimum. There is every reason, though, to think that if it ever was adjusted, it is now badly out of date. For one thing, the human reproductive life span is longer than that of our distant ancestors and the slowness of any mutational adjustment may mean that the rate per generation (to the extent that this is time-dependent rather than cell division-dependent) is now too high. For another, the environment has changed very rapidly. Finally, there are many new chemicals in our present environment, some of which are almost certain to be mutagenic. Increased amounts of radiation may also play a role, although in all likelihood a very minor one. The changes in the environment (better food storage, for example) may have decreased the number of chemical mutagens, but it is also likely that new chemicals more than offset this. Finally, in long-lived organisms the immediate disadvantages of mutation reduction, such as metabolic costs of more accurate polymerases and repair enzymes, may be such that a higher than optimum mutation rate is tolerated.

For all these reasons it is doubtful that the human mutation rate is near the optimum value for future evolution, if it ever was. We suspect that it is more likely to err on the high side, but this is not a question that can be answered with present information.

Although we are curious about long-time human evolutionary trends, our far greater concern is for the welfare of the population in the next few generations. Our interest in a descendant in the future diminishes perhaps at a rate not very different from the 50% decay rate of the fraction of shared genes. From the standpoint of the immediate future *any* mutations are solely a debit. If our germinal mutation rate would suddenly drop to zero, we should recognize this only by the reduced incidence of the most debilitating dominant diseases. The store of genetic variability is sufficient to satisfy the desires of even the most enthusiastic eugenicist. Clearly anything that keeps the mutation rate from increasing or that reduces "spontaneous" mutation would be of social benefit.

REFERENCES

Auerbach, C., 1949, A possible case of delayed mutation in man, *Ann. Hum. Genet.* **20**:266–269.

Barnard, G. A., 1959, Control charts and stochastic processes, *J. R. Stat. Soc. (B)* **21**:239–257.

Biel, S. W., and Hartl, D. L., 1983, Evolution of transposons: Natural selection for Tn5 in *Escherichia coli, Genetics* **103**:581–592.

Bora, K. C., Douglas, G. R., and Nestmann, E. R., eds., 1982, *Chemical Mutagenesis, Human Population Monitoring and Genetic Risk Assessment. Progress in Medical Research,* Vol. 3, Elsevier Biomedical Press, Amsterdam.

Bucher, K., Ionasescu, V., and Hanson, J., 1980, Frequency of new mutants among boys with Duchenne muscular dystrophy, *Am. J. Med. Genet.* **7**:27–34.

Bulmer, M. G., 1972, The genetic variability of polygenic characters under optimizing selection, mutation and drift, *Genet. Res.* **19**:17–25.

Bulmer, M. G., 1980, *The Mathematical Theory of Quantitative Genetics,* Clarendon Press, Oxford.

Calos, M. P., and Miller, J. H., 1980, Transposable elements, *Cell* **20**:579–596.

Carter, C. O., 1977, Monogenic disorders, *J. Med. Genet.* **14**:316–320.

Carter, C. O., 1982, Contribution of gene mutations to genetic disease in humans, in: *Progress in Mutation Research,* Vol. 3, pp. 1–8, Elsevier/North-Holland Biomedical Press, Amsterdam.

Cavalli-Sforza, L. L., and Bodmer, W. F., 1971, *The Genetics of Human Populations,* Freeman, San Francisco.

Chakraborty, R., 1981, Estimation of mutation rates from the number of rare alleles in a sample, *Ann. Hum. Biol.* **8**:221–230.

Chakraborty, R., and Roychoudhury, A. K., 1978, Mutation rates from rare variants of proteins in Indian tribes, *Hum. Genet.* **43**:179–183.

Chao, L., and Cox, E. C., 1983, Competition between high and low mutating strains of *Escherichia coli, Evolution* **37**:123–134.

Chao, L., Vargas, C., Spear, B. B., and Cox, E. C., 1983, Transposable elements as mutator genes in evolution, *Nature* **303**:633–635.

Charlesworth, B., 1980, *Evolution in Age-Structured Populations,* Cambridge University Press, Cambridge.

Charlesworth, B., Lande, R., and Slatkin, M., 1982, A neo-Darwinian commentary on macroevolution, *Evolution* **36**:474–498.

Cheeseman, E. A. S., Kilpatrick, J., Stevenson, A. C., and Smith, C. A. B., 1958, The sex ratio of mutation rates of the sex-linked recessive genes in man with particular reference to Duchenne type muscular dystrophy, *Ann. Hum. Genet.* **22**:235–263.

Childs, J. D., 1981, The effect of a change of mutation rate on the incidence of dominant and X-linked recessive disorders in man, *Mutat. Res.* **83**:145–158.

Childs, J. D., 1982, Dominant and X-linked recessive mutation rates in man, in: *Progress in Medical Research,* Vol. 3, pp. 163–167, Elsevier Biomedical Press, Amsterdam.

Clayton, G. A., and Robertson, A., 1955, Mutation and quantitative variation, *Am. Nat.* **89**:151–158.

Cox, E. C., and Gibson, T. C., 1974, Selection for high mutation rates in chemostats, *Genetics* **77**:169–184.

Crow, J. F., 1957, Possible consequences of an increased mutation rate, *Eugen. Q.* **4**:67–80.

Crow, J. F., 1958, Some possibilities for measuring selection intensities in man, *Hum. Biol.* **30**:1–13.

Crow, J. F., 1961, Mutation in man, *Prog. Med. Genet* **1**:1–26.

Crow, J. F., 1970, Genetic loads and the cost of natural selection, in: *Mathematical Topics in Population Genetics* (I. Kojima, ed.), pp. 128–177, Springer-Verlag, Berlin.

Crow, J. F., 1971, Human population monitoring, in: *Chemical Mutagens. Principles and Methods for Their Detection* (A. Hollaender, ed.), pp. 591–605, Plenum Press, New York.

Crow, J. F., 1979, Minor viability mutants in *Drosophila, Genetics* **92s**:165–172.

Crow, J. F., and Denniston, C., 1981, The mutation component of genetic damage, *Science* **212**:888–893.

Crow, J. F., and Kimura, M., 1964, The theory of genetic loads in: *Proceedings XI International Congress of Genetics,* Vol. 3, pp. 495–505.

Crow, J. J., and Kimura, M., 1965, Evolution in sexual and asexual populations, *Am. Nat.* **99**:439–450.

Crow, J. F., and Kimura, M., 1970, *An Introduction to Population Genetics Theory,* Harper and Row, New York.

Czeizel, A., 1978, The baseline data of the Hungarian congenital Malformation Register, 1970–1976, *Acata Acad. Sci. Hung.* **19**:149–156.

Danforth, C. H., 1923, The frequency of mutation and the incidence of hereditary traits in man, in: *2nd International Congress Eugenics,* Vol. I, pp. 120–128.

Demerec, M., 1941, Unstable genes, *Cold Spring Harbor Symp. Quant. Biol.* **9**:145–149.

Denniston, C., 1982, Low level radiation and genetic risk estimation in man, *Ann. Rev. Genet.* **16**:329–355.

Denniston, C., 1983, Are human studies possible? some thoughts on the mutation component and population monitoring, *Env. Health Persp.* **52**:41–44.

DeVries, H., 1901, *Die Mutation Theorie,* Viet, Leipzig [*The Mutation Theory,* Open Court, Chicago, 1909].

Egger, J., and Wilson, J., 1983, Mitochondrial inheritance in a mitochondrically mediated disease, *N. Engl. J. Med.* **309**:142–146.

Emery, A. E. H., 1980, Duchenne muscular dystrophy: Genetic aspects, carrier detection and antenatal diagnosis, *Br. Med. Bull.* **3**(2):117–122.

Engels, W. R., 1983, The P family of transposable elements in *Drosophila, Annu. Rev. Genet.,* **17**:315–344.

Erickson, J. D., and Cohen, M. M., 1974, a study of paternal age effects on the occurence of fresh mutations for the Apert syndrome, *Ann. Hum. Genet.* **38**:89–96.

Ewan, W. D., and Kemp, K. W., 1960, Sampling inspection of continuous processes with no autocorrelation between successive results, *Biometrika* **47**:363–380.

Falconer, D., 1981, *Quantitative Genetics,* Longmans, New York.

Fisher, R. A., 1918, The correlation between relatives on the supposition of Mendelian inheritance, *Trans. R. Soc. Edinb.* **52**:321–341.

Fisher, R. A., 1930, *The Genetical Theory of Natural Selection,* Clarendon Press, Oxford.

Fleming, W. H., 1979, Equilibrium distributions of continuous polygenic traits, *SIAM J. Appl. Math.* **36**:148–168.

Francke, U., Felsenstein, J., Gartler, S. J., Migeon, B. R., Dancis, J., Seegmiller, J. E., Bakay, F., and Nyhan, W. L., 1976, The occurrence of new mutants in the X-linked recessive Lesch–Nyhan disease, *Am. J. Hum. Genet.* **38**:123–137.

Friedman, J. M., 1981, Genetic disease in the offspring of older fathers, *Obstet. Gynecol.* **57**:745–749.

Godabout, R., Dryja, T. P., Squire, J., Gallie, B. L., and Phillips, R. A., 1983, Somatic inactivation of genes on chromosome 13 is a common event in retinoblastoma, *Nature* **304**:451–453.

Goldschmidt, R., 1940, *The Material Basis of Evolution,* Yale University Press, New Haven.

Gould, S. J., and Eldredge, N., 1977, Punctuated equilibria: The tempo and mode of evolution reconsidered, *Paleobiology* **3**:115–151.

Green, M. M., 1976, Mutable and mutator loci, in: *The Genetics and Biology of Drosophila* (M. Ashburner and E. Novitski, eds.), pp. 929–946, Academic Press, New York.

Gunther, M., and Penrose, L. S., 1935, The genetics of epiloia, *J. Genet.* **31**:413–430.

Haldane, J. B. S., 1927, A mathematical theory of natural and artificial selection. Part V. Selection and mutation, *Proc. Camb. Philos. Soc.* **23**:838–844.

Haldane, J. B. S., 1932, *The Causes of Evolution,* Harper & Brothers, New York.

Haldane, J. B. S., 1935, The rate of spontaneous mutation of a human gene, *J. Genet* **31**:317–326.

Haldane, J. B. S., 1937, The effect of variation on fitness, *Am. Nat.* **71**:337–349.

Haldane, J. B. S., 1947, The mutation rate of the gene for hemophilia and its segregation ratios in males and females, *Ann. Eugen.* **13**:262–271.

Haldane, J. B. S., 1949, The rate of mutation of human genes, *Hereditas (Suppl.)* **1949**:267–273.

Hinderberger, P., Moser, H., Beck, E. A., and Pflugshaupt, R., 1980, Heterozygotenerfassung bei der Hämophilie A—Genealogische und biochemische Resultate einer Feldstudie an 25 Bluterfamiliern, *Schweiz. Rundschau Med.* **69**:1349–1360.

Hollaender, A., ed., 1971, *Chemical Mutagens. Principles and Methods for Their Detection,* Plenum Press, New York.

Hook, E. B., and Porter, I. H., eds., 1981, *Population and Biological Aspects of Human Mutation,* Academic Press, New York.

ICRP, 1977, *Problems Involved in Developing an Index of Harm,* International Commission on Radiological Protection, Publication 27, Pergamon Press, Oxford.

Jones, M. B., 1979a, Years of life lost due to Down's syndrome, *J. Med. Genet.* **16**:379–383.

Jones, M. B., 1979b, Years of life lost due to Huntington's disease, *Am. J. Hum. Genet.* **31**:711–717.

Kander, Z., and Zacks, S., 1966, Test procedures for possible changes in parameters of statistical distributions occurring at known time points, *Ann. Math. Stat.* **37**:1196–1210.

Kimura, M., 1965, A stochastic model concerning the maintenance of genetic variability in quantitative characters, *Proc. Natl. Acad. Sci. USA* **54**:731–736.

Kimura, M., 1968*a*, Evolutionary rate at the molecular level, *Nature* **217**:624–626.

Kimura, M., 1968*b*, Genetic variability maintained in a finite population due to mutational production of neutral and nearly neutral isoalleles, *Genet. Res.* **11**:247–269.

Kimura, M., 1979, Model of effectively neutral mutations in which selective constraint is incorporated, *Proc. Natl. Acad. Sci. USA* **76**:3440–3444.

Kimura, M., 1981, Possibility of extensive neutral evolution under stabilizing selection with special reference to non-random usage of synonymous codons, *Proc. Natl. Acad. Sci. USA* **78**:5773–5777.

Kimura, M., 1983, *The Neutral Theory of Molecular Evolution: Fundamental Random Processes in Evolution,* Cambridge University Press, Cambridge.

Kimura, M., and Ohta, T., 1969, The average number of generations until extinction of an individual mutant gene in a finite population, *Genetics* **63**:701–709.

Kimura, M., and Ohta, T., 1973, Mutation and evolution at the molecular level, *Genetics (Suppl.)* **73**:19–35.

King, J. L., and Jukes, T. H., 1969, Non-Darwinian evolution, *Science* **164**:788–798.

Kleckner, N., 1981, Transposable elements in prokaryotes, *Annu. Rev. Genet.* **15**:341–404.

Knudson, A. G., 1971, Mutation and cancer: Statistical study of retinoblastoma, *Proc. Natl. Acad. Sci. USA* **68**:820–823.

Lande, R., 1975, The maintenance of genetic variability by mutation in a polygenic character with linked loci, *Genet. Res.* **26**:221–235.

Latter, B. D. H., 1960, Natural selection for an intermediate optimum, *Austr. J. Biol. Sci.* **13**:30–35.

Lee, W. H., and Watanabe, T. K., 1977, Accumulation of deleterious genes in a cage population of *Drosophila melanogaster, Genetics* **86**:657–664.

Leigh, E., 1973, The evolution of mutation rates, *Genetics (Suppl)* **73**:1–18.

Li, W. H., and Nei, M., 1972, Total number of individuals affected by a single deleterious mutation in a finite population, *Am. J. Hum. Genet.* **24**:667–679.

Lindsley, D. L., Sandler, L., Baker, B. S., Carpenter, A. T. C., Denell, R. E., Hall, J. C., Jacobs, P. A., Miklos, G. L. G., Davis, B. K., Gethmann, R. C., Hardy, R. W., Hessler, A., Miller, S. M., Nozawa, H., Parry, D. M., and Gould-Somero, M., 1972, Segmental aneuploidy and the genetic gross structure of the *Drosophila* genome, *Genetics* **71**:157–184.

Mampell, K., 1943, High mutation frequency in *Drosophila pseaudoobscura* race B, *Proc. Natl. Acad. Sci. USA* **29**:137–144.

Maruyama, T., and Kimura, M., 1974, A note on the speed of gene frequency changes in reverse directions in a finite population, *Evolution* **28**:161–163.

McClintock, B., 1956, Controlling elements and the gene, *Cold Spring Harbor Symp. Quant. Biol.* **21**:197–216.

McKusick, V. A., 1983, *Mendelian Inheritance in Man: Catalogs of Autosomal Dominant, Autosomal Recessive, and X-Linked Phenotypes,* 6th ed., Johns Hopkins University Press, Baltimore.

Morton, N. E., 1976, Surveillance of Down's syndrome as a paradigm of population monitoring, *Hum. Hered.* **26**:360–371.

Morton, N. E., 1981, Mutation rates for human autosomal recessives, in: *Population and Biological Aspects of Human Mutation* (E. B. Hook and I. H. Porter, eds.), pp. 361–375, Academic Press, New York.

Morton, N. E., 1982, *Outline of Genetic Epidemiology,* S. Karger, Basel.

Morton, N. E., and Chung, C. S., 1959, The formal genetics of muscular dystrophy, *Am. J. Hum. Genet.* **11**:360–379.

Morton, N. E., and Chung, C. S., eds., 1978, *Genetic Epidemiology,* Academic Press, New York.

Morton, N. E., Crow, J. F., and Muller, H. J., 1956, An estimate of the mutational damage in man from data on consanguineous marriages, *Proc. Natl. Acad. Sci.* **42**:855–863.

Mukai, T., Chigusa, S. I., Mettler, L. E., and Crow, J. F., 1972, Mutation rate and dominance of genes affecting viability in *Drosophila melanogaster, Genetics* **72**:335–355.

Mulvihill, J. J., and Czeizel, A., 1983, A 1983 view of sentinel phenotypes, *Mutat. Res.* **123**:345–361.

Muller, H. J. 1950, Our load of mutations, *Am. J. Hum. Genet.* **2**:111–176.

Murphree, A. L., and Benedict, W. F., 1984, Retinoblasoma: clues to human oncogenesis, *Science* **223**:1028–1033.

Nachtscheim, H., 1954, Die Mutations rate menschlicher Gene, *Naturwissenschaften* **41**:358–392.

Nagylaki, T., 1976, The evolution of one- and two-locus systems, *Genetics* **83**:583–600.

Nagylaki, T., 1977, Selection and mutation at an X-linked locus, *Ann. Hum. Genet.* **41**:241–248.

Nagylaki, T., 1983, Selection on a quantitative character, in: *Human Population Genetics: The Pittsburgh Symposium* (A. Chakravarti, ed.), Hutchinson Ross, Stroudsburg, Pennsylvania.

National Academy of Sciences, 1956, *The Biological Effects of Atomic Radiation,* National Research Council, Washington, D.C.

National Academy of Sciences, 1972, *The Effects on Populations of Exposure to Low Levels of Ionizing Radiation,* National Academy of Sciences–National Research Council, Washington, D.C.

National Academy of Sciences, 1980, *The Effects on Populations of Exposure to Low Levels of Ionizing Radiation,* National Academy of Sciences, Washington, D.C.

National Academy of Sciences, 1983, *Identifying and Estimating the Genetic Impact of Chemical Mutagens,* Report of the Committee on Chemical Environmental Mutagens, National Academy of Sciences, Washington, D.C.

Neel, J. V., 1942, A study of a case of high mutation rate in *Drosophila melanogaster, Genetics* **27**:519–536.

Neel, J. V., 1983, Frequency of spontaneous and induced "point" mutations in higher eukaryotes, *J. Hered.* **74**:2–15.

Neel, J. V., and Rothman, E. D., 1978, Some indirect estimates of mutation rates in tribal Amerindians, *Proc. Natl. Acad. Sci. USA* **75**:5585–5588.

Nei, M., 1977, Estimation of mutation rates from rare protein variants, *Am. J. Hum. Genet.* **29**:225–232.

Newcombe, H. B., 1982, Quantitative assessment of induced genetic ill-health in humans as a model for assessing genetic risks from chemicals, in: *Chemical Mutagenesis, Human Population Monitoring, and Genetic Risk Assessment* (K. C. Bora, G. R. Douglas, and E. R. Nestmann, eds.), pp. 53–62, Elsevier Biomedical Press, Amsterdam.

Nute, P. E., and Stamatoyannopoulos, G., 1981, Estimates of mutation rates of *de novo* hemoglobin mutants, in: *Population and Biological Aspects of Human Mutation* (E. B. Hook and I. H. Porter, eds.), pp. 337–350, Academic Press, New York.

Page, E. S., 1954, Continuous inspection schemes, *Biometrika* **41**:100–116.

Patau, K., and Nachtscheim, H., 1946, Mutations- und Selectionsdruck beim Pelger gen des Menschen, *Z. Naturforsch.* **1**:345–348.

Penrose, L. S., 1955, Parental age and mutation, *Lancet* **2**:312–313.

Penrose, L. S., 1961, Mutation, in: *Recent Advances in Human Genetics* (L. S. Penrose, ed.), pp. 1–18, Churchill, London.

Provine, W. B., 1971, *The Origins of Theoretical Population Genetics,* University of Chicago Press, Chicago.

Rothman, E. D., and Adams, J., 1978, Estimation of expected number of rare alleles of a locus and calculation of mutation rate, *Proc. Natl. Acad. Sci. USA* **75**:5094–5098.

Shapiro, J. A., 1983, *Mobile Genetic Elements,* Academic Press, New York.

Sherman, S. L., Morton, N. E., Jacobs, P. A., and Turner, G., 1984, The marker (X) syndrome: a cytogenetic and genetic analysis, *Ann. Hum. Genet.* **48**:21–37.

Simmons, M. J., and Crow, J. F., 1977, Mutations affecting fitness in *Drosophila* populations, *Annu. Rev. Genet.* **11**:49–78.

Simpson, G. G., 1953, *The Major Features of Evolution,* Columbia University Press, New York.

Stevenson, A. C., 1959, The load of hereditary defects in human population, *Rad. Res. Suppl.* **1**:306–325.

Stevenson, A. C., and Kerr, C. B., 1967, One the distributions of frequencies of mutation to genes determining harmful traits in man, *Mutat. Res.* **4**:339–352.

Trimble, B. K., and Doughty, J. H., 1974, The amount of hereditary disease in human populations, *Ann. Hum. Genet.* **38**:199–223.

Turelli, M., 1984, Heritable genetic variation via mutation–selection balance: Lerch's zeta meets the abdominal bristle, *Theor. Popul. Biol.,* **25**:138–193.

UNSCEAR, 1972, Genetic effects of radiation, in: *Ionizing Radiation: Levels and Effects,* United Nations Scientific Committee on the Effects of Ionizing Radiation, United Nations, Twenty-Seventh Session, Supplement No. 25 (A/8725), pp. 199–302.

UNSCEAR, 1977, Genetic effects of radiation, in: *Sources and Effects of Ionizing Radiation,* United Nations Scientific Committee on the Effects of Ionizing Radiation, United Nations, Thirty Second Session, Supplement No. 40 (A/32/40), pp. 425–564.

UNSCEAR, 1982, Genetic effects of radiation, in: *Ionizing Radiation: Sources and Biological Effects,* United Nations Scientific Committee on the Effects of Atomic Radiation, United Nations, Thirty Seventh Session, Supplement No. 45 (A/37/45), pp. 425–569.

Vogel, F., 1965, Sind de Mutationstrate für die X-chromosomal recessive Hamophilieformen in Keimzellen von Frauen neidriger als in Keimzellen von Männern? *Humangenetik* **1**:253–363.

Vogel, F., 1977, A probable sex difference in some mutation rates, *Amer. J. Hum. Genet.* **29**:312–319.

Vogel, F., 1983, Mutation in man, in: Principles and Practice of Medical Genetics (A. E. Emergy and D. L. Rimoin, eds.) pp. 26–48, Longman, Edinburgh.

Vogel, F., and Altland, K., 1982, Utilization of material from PKU-screening programs for mutation screening, *Prog. Mut. Res.* **3**:143–157.

Vogel, F., and Motulsky, A. G., 1979, *Human Genetics,* Springer-Verlag, Berlin.

Vogel, F., and Rathenberg, R., 1975, Spontaneous mutation in man, in: *Advances in Human Genetics,* Vol. 5 (H. Harris and K. Hirschhorn, eds.), pp. 223–318, Plenum Press, New York.

Vogel, F., and Röhrborn, G., eds., *Chemical Mutagenesis in Mammals and Man,* Springer-Verlag, New York.

Weatherall, J. A. C., and Haskey, J. C., 1976, Surveillance of malformations, *Br. Med. Bull.* **32**:39–44.

Weinberg, W., 1912, Zur Vererbung des Zwergwuches, *Arch. Rass. Ges. Biol.* **9**:710–717.

Williams, W. R., Thompson, M. W., and Morton, N. E., 1983, Complex segregation analysis and computer-assisted risk assessment for Duchenne muscular dystrophy, *Am. J. Med. Genet.* **14**:315–333.

Winter, R. M., 1980, Estimation of male to female ratio of mutation rates from carrier-detection tests in X-linked disorders, *Am. J. Hum. Genet.* **32**:582–588.

Winter, R. M., and Pembry, M. E., 1982, Does unequal crossing over contribute to the mutation rate in Duchenne muscular dystrophy? *Am. J. Med. Genet.* **12**:437–441.

Winter, R. M., and Tuddenham, E. G. D. 1983, A maximum likelihood estimate of the sex ratio of mutation rates in hemophilia A, *Hum. Genet.,* **64**:156–159.

Wright, S., 1931, Evolution in Mendelian populations, *Genetics* **16**:97–159.

Yasuda, N., and Kondo, K., 1980, No sex difference in mutation rates of Duchenne muscular dystrophy, *J. Med. Genet.* **17**:106–111.

Yasuda, N., and Kondo, K., 1982, The effect of parental age on rate of mutation for Duchenne muscular dystrophy, *Am. J. Med. Genet.* **13**:91–99.

Chapter 3

Genetic Mutations Affecting Human Lipoprotein Metabolism

Vassilis I. Zannis and Jan L. Breslow

Children's Hospital Corporation and Harvard Medical School
Boston, Massachusetts 02115

GENERAL REVIEW

Introduction

Lipoproteins are macromolecular complexes of lipids and proteins that are synthesized mainly by the liver and intestine and catabolized by hepatic and extrahepatic tissues. Their main well-defined physiological function is to transport dietary and/or endogenously synthesized lipids (cholesterol, triglycerides, and phospholipids) from one organ to another,[1] although they may also be involved in the regulation of other important physiological processes. In normal plasma, there are traditionally considered to be four lipoprotein classes: (1) chylomicrons, (2) very low-density lipoproteins (VLDL), (3) low-density lipoproteins (LDL), and (4) high-density lipoproteins (HDL) (Table I). Several subfractions of VLDL, LDL, and HDL and a lipoprotein class of density intermediate between VLDL and LDL (IDL) have also been described. The plasma lipoproteins are spherical particles with cores of nonpolar neutral lipid consisting of cholesteryl ester and triglycerides and coats of relatively polar materials consisting of phospholipid, free cholesterol, and proteins[2,3] (Table I; for reviews see Refs. 4–6). The protein components of lipoproteins are called apoproteins and have been designated apo A-I, apo A-II, apo A-IV, apo B, apo CI, apo CII, apo CIII, apo D, and apo E.[7]

It has become increasingly apparent that single-gene mutations in

Table I. Properties and Composition of Human Plasma Lipoproteins[a]

Lipoprotein class	Size, Å	Density range, g/ml	Triglycerides, % wt	Phospholipids, % wt	Free cholesterol, % wt	Esterified cholesterol, % wt	S_f, [b]S	Electrophoretic mobility	Proteins, % wt	Major apoproteins	Minor apoproteins
Chylomicrons	750–12,000	0.94	80–95	3–6	1–3	2–4	400	Origin (cathode)	1–2	A-I, A-IV, B, CI, CIII, E	A-II, CII
VLDL	300–700	0.94–1.006	45–65	15–20	4–8	16–22	20–400	Prebeta	6–10	B, E, CI, CII, CIII	A-I, A-II, A-IV
LDL	180–300	1.019–1.063	4–8	18–24	6–8	45–50	0–12	Beta	18–22	B	CI, CII, CIII, E
HDL	50–120	1.063–1.21	2–7	26–32	3–5	15–20	0–9[c]	Alpha	45–55	A-I, A-II, E	CI, CII, CIII, D, F

[a] Modified from Herbert et al.[5]
[b] Corrected flotation rate at $d = 1.063$, expressed in svedbergs [10^{-13} cm/(sec dyne g)].
[c] Corrected flotation rate at $d = 1.20$.

apoproteins, lipoprotein receptors, or various activities involved in lipo-protein metabolism may underlie lipoprotein disorders characterized by hyper- or hypolipoproteinemia, some of which lead to premature athero-sclerosis. In this chapter we will review current knowledge about lipopro-tein and apoprotein metabolic pathways. These pathways are complex and encompass several steps. Special emphasis will be given to genetic mutations in the apoprotein moieties of lipoproteins that affect these pathways.

Recent findings suggest that variability exists in the human popula-tion in the structural genes specifying apo A-I, apo B, apo CII, and apo E. In addition, post-translational modification of apoproteins has recently been identified and may be yet another important factor in lipo-protein metabolism. In the future, we expect that current progress in pro-tein and recombinant DNA technologies will permit the description of the majority of hereditary disorders of lipoprotein metabolism in terms of changes that occurred at specific sites in protein and DNA molecules.

Pathway of Lipoprotein Metabolism

Although only partially understood at the present time, lipoprotein metabolism is complex and includes the following steps: (1) apopro-tein synthesis, (2) intracellular apoprotein modification, (3) lipoprotein assembly, (4) lipoprotein secretion, (5) extracellular apoprotein modifi-cation, (6) hydrolysis of lipoprotein triglycerides by lipoprotein lipase and hepatic lipase, (7) esterification of lipoprotein cholesterol by lecithin cho-lesterol acyltransferase, (8) enzyme-catalyzed exchange and/or transfer of cholesteryl esters and phospholipids, (9) exchange and/or transfer of apo-proteins, (10) reverse transport of cholesterol from cells to lipoproteins, (11) receptor-mediated catabolism of lipoproteins.

Synthesis and Intracellular Modification of Apoproteins*

In mammalian species, two organs in the body, liver and intestine, are thought to produce most of the apoproteins synthesized.[8-20] In stud-ies with rats, hepatic synthesis of all the major lipoprotein apoproteins has been demonstrated.[11,18-20] Similar studies have shown that rat small intestine synthesizes large amounts of the apoproteins apo A-I, apo A-IV,

---

* See addendum, p. 383ff, for additional information.

and apo B,[12-16,19,20] but only small amounts of the apo C peptides and little or no apo E.[13,14,16,19,20] A quantitative study in rat indicated that the liver contributes 81% and the intestine 19% to the total apoprotein pool. The percent contribution of the intestine to individual apoproteins was apo A-IV 59%, apo A-I 56%, apo B 16%, apo C's 5%, and apo E <1%.[19] Apoprotein synthesis has also been demonstrated by human liver cell cultures[21-25] and by organ cultures of human intestine and liver.[26-28] Recent evidence suggests that, besides liver and intestine, other tissues may also contribute to apoprotein synthesis. In avian species apo B synthesis has been reported in kidney[29] and apo A-I synthesis in a variety of peripheral tissues.[30] Finally, in mammalian species, apo E synthesis has been shown to occur in kidney, adrenal gland, and reticuloendothelial cells.[31-33] Varying amounts of apo E mRNA have been found in all major human and monkey tissues.[33a]

Most secreted proteins synthesized in cell-free translation systems have been shown to contain a 16 to 25-amino acid-long (usually) NH_2-terminal signal peptide sequence.[34,35] Blobel and Dobberstein proposed that these leader sequences direct the cotranslational translocation of secreted proteins across the membrane of the rough endoplasmic reticulum. In most[34,36] but not all[37] cases the signal peptide is cleaved cotranslationally by a membrane-bound enzyme (signal peptidase) of the rough endoplasmic reticulum.[34,36] An 18-amino acid-long signal peptide sequence has been demonstrated for human and rat apo A-I[38-40] and apo E[41,42] and human apo A-II.[42a] A 20-amino acid-long signal peptide has also been demonstrated for rat apo A-IV[43] and human apo CIII[43a] In preliminary experiments, a signal peptide has been identified for human apo CII.[44] Figure 1A, 1B, 1E and 1F show the primary translational products of human apo A-I and apo E mRNA, respectively, and their conversion to different forms by treatment with dog pancreatic membranes that cleave the signal peptide.

Four of the plasma apoproteins, apo B, apo CIII, apo D, and apo E, are glycoproteins that contain carbohydrate chains that terminate in sialic acid.[44-50] Early experiments showed carbohydrate incorporation into apoproteins synthesized by membrane fractions of rat liver[51-53] and suggested that the post-translational glycosylation of apoproteins occurs in the Golgi apparatus. Pulse-chase experiments utilizing primary cultures of chicken hepatocytes showed that carbohydrate was added to apo B cotranslationally in two stages corresponding to the times at which the native polypeptide has acquired approximately 34 and 80% of its length.[54] Inhibition of apo B glycosylation with tunicamycin did not affect its secretion.[55] Figure 1C shows that apo A-I is secreted after cleavage of the signal peptide without further modification, whereas apo E, as shown in Figures 1G and 1H, is further modified prior to secretion with carbohydrate chains containing sialic acid.

Assembly and Secretion of Lipoproteins

Earlier studies have shown that lipoproteins are secreted by the intestine and liver. The intestine secretes triglyceride-rich chylomicrons (and VLDL) and nascent HDL.[8,13,15] Chylomicrons are formed from dietary lipids and intestinal apoproteins, mainly apo B-48, apo A-I, and apo A-IV,[17,56,57] and are released into the mesenteric lymph. The sequence of steps involved in assembly and secretion of chylomicrons and other lipoproteins has not been completely worked out. It is known that the products of digestion of dietary fat (mainly free fatty acids, 2-monoglycerides, and lysolecithin) are absorbed by the brush border membrane of the intestinal epithelial cell[58] and reesterified in the smooth endoplasmic reticulum (SER) of these cells.[13,14,59,60] Dietary or endogenously synthesized cholesterol is similarly absorbed and a portion of this is reesterified. Association of lipids and apoproteins is believed to occur between the rough endoplasmic reticulum (RER) and the Golgi apparatus.[61,62] Inhibition of apoprotein synthesis[63] inhibits secretion of chylomicrons. The importance of apo B for chylomicron (and VLDL) secretion has been underscored by the complete absence of chylomicrons and VLDL from the plasma of patients with abetalipoproteinemia, who are believed to have a defect in apo B synthesis.[5] Intestinal HDL is also formed from lipid and apoproteins and is secreted into the mesenteric lymph as well as the plasma compartment. Intestinal HDL contains spherical as well as disc-shaped particles enriched in phospholipid and cholesterol and contains apo A-I as its main apoprotein.[15]

The liver secretes triglyceride-rich VLDL and nascent HDL,[8,11,18] and, under certain conditions, LDL.[64-68] Hepatic lipoproteins are secreted into both the plasma and lymph compartments. Hepatic VLDL is formed from triglycerides and phospholipids, which are synthesized from precursor molecules in the endoplasmic reticulum of the hepatocytes. The cholesterol moiety of these particles apparently originates from *de novo* synthesis or from intracellular degradation of lipoproteins. Tri-

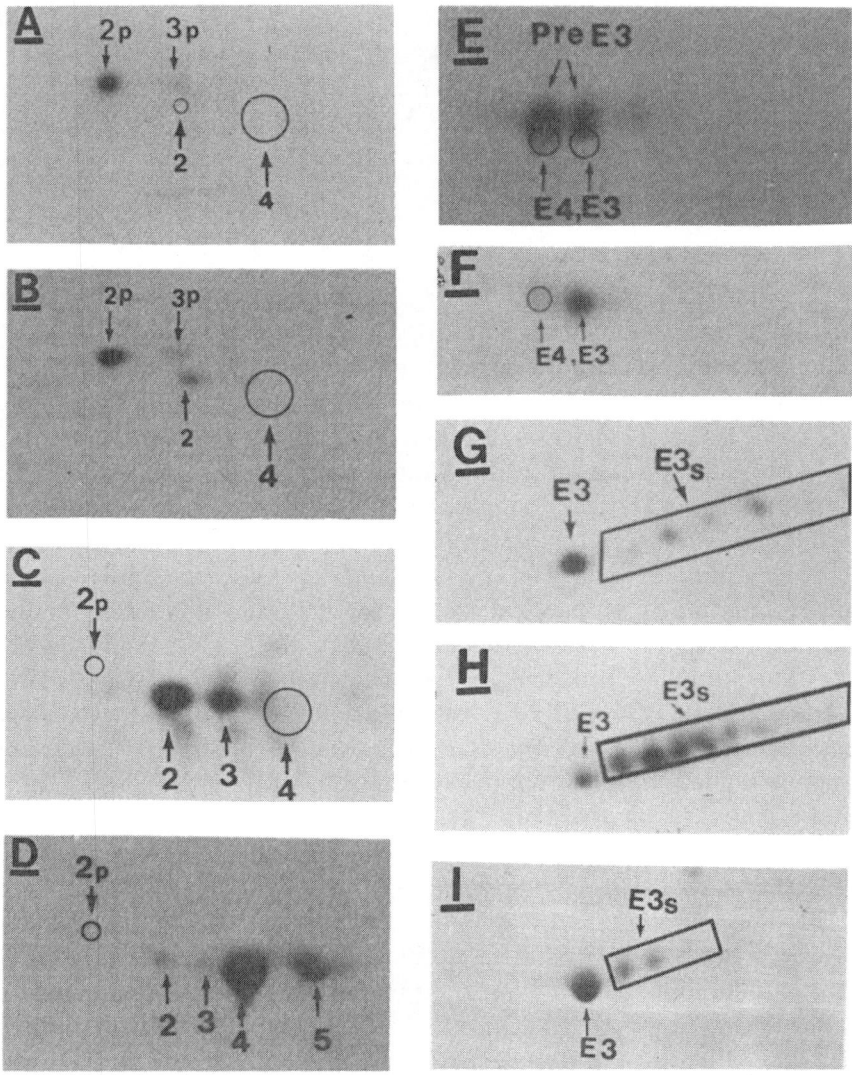

Fig. 1. Comparison of intra- and extracellular forms of human apo A-I and apo E. (A) Analysis by 2D-PAGE and autoradiography of proteins synthesized by cell-free translation of apo A-I mRNA after precipitation with specific anti-apo A-I antibodies. An aliquot of 50 μ l of the translation cocktail of human liver mRNA was mixed with 15 μg of human HDL and immunoprecipitated with anti-human apo A-I and IgGsorb as explained in Ref. 39. The immunoprecipitate was dissolved in lysis buffer, and analyzed by 2D-PAGE and autoradiography. Shown is the autoradioagram obtained from this analysis. The position of plasma apo A-I$_4$, indicated by open circles, was established by superimposing the autora-

glyceride-rich particles first accumulate in the region between the smooth and rough endoplasmic reticulum.[69] Association of these particles with apoproteins, mainly apo B and apo E,[70-73] occurs in the region between RER and the Golgi apparatus.[61] The VLDL secretion is stimulated by free fatty acids[22,74] and hormones and is diminished by inhibitors of both protein synthesis[22,74,75] and microtubule chain formation.[76] Similar to intestinal HDL, hepatic HDL synthesized in the presence of LCAT inhibitors has a discoidal shape, and is enriched in phospholipid and cholesterol. These particles have apo E as their major apoprotein.[10,18] Discoidal shape HDL particles are found in the plasma of patients with LCAT deficiency[77,78] and may represent the nascent form of HDL. The major portion of plasma IDL and LDL is derived from catabolism of VLDL, as will be discussed later[67,79]; however, direct secretion of LDL has been demonstrated in patients with hypercholesterolemia and type III hyperlipidemia[64,67,68] and by perfused livers of cholesterol-fed animals.[65,66]

---

diogram of this figure on the corresponding two-dimensional slab gel that was stained for protein as explained in Refs. 25 and 28. (B) An autoradiogram obtained after similar analysis of the translation products of human liver mRNA was processed cotranslationally with dog pancreatic membranes as explained in Ref. 39. Note the partial conversions of apo A-I$_{2p}$ to apo A-I$_2$. (C) An autoradiogram obtained after 2D-PAGE analysis of apo A-I secreted from hepatic organ cultures grown in ^{35}S-methionine. The proteins were precipitated from the cell extract or culture medium as explained in Ref. 28. (D) The 2D-PAGE of plasma apo A-I (20 μg) obtained from normal human subjects. (E) The analysis by 2D-PAGE and autoradiography of proteins immunoprecipitated from the cell-free translation cocktail with specific anti-apo E antibodies. An aliquot of 50 μl of the translation cocktail containing HepG2 mRNA was mixed with 100 μg of human VLDL and immunoprecipitated with anti-human apo E as explained in Refs. 25 and 42. The immunoprecipitate was dissolved in lysis buffer, and analyzed by 2D-PAGE and autoradiography. Shown is the autoradiogram obtained from this analysis. The position of plasma apo E4 and apo E3, indicated by open circles, was established by superimposing the autoradiogram of this figure on the corresponding two-dimensional slab gel that was stained for protein as explained in Refs. 25 and 28. (F) An autoradiogram obtained after similar analysis of the translation products of HepG2 mRNA processed cotranslationally with dog pancreatic membranes as explained in Ref. 42. Note the conversion of preapo E3 to apo E3. (G,H) Autoradiograms obtained after 2D-PAGE analysis of intracellular and secreted apo E synthesized by HepG2 cells grown in ^{35}S-methionine. The proteins were precipitated from the cell extract or culture medium as explained in Ref. 25. (I) The 2D-PAGE of plasma apo E (25 μg) obtained from normal human subjects. Note the decreased sialation of the plasma apo E (compare H with I). In all panels only the area of the gel or autoradiogram in the vicinity of apo E is shown. The cathode is on the left and anode is on the right.

Extracellular Apoprotein Modification*

Recent studies have shown that the secreted forms of apo A-I and apo E undergo additional post-translational alterations in plasma.[25,28,39,40,50] As will be discussed later, the secreted form of apo A-I contains a six-amino acid-long N-terminal extension.[39,40] Cleavage of the N-terminal hexapeptide in plasma and/or lymph converts the secreted to the plasma apo A-I form[39,40] (Figs. 1C and 1D). This post-translational conversion of apo A-I may be important for the stability of HDL.[80] The same studies have also shown synthesis of a low-molecular weight protein, designated X, by human hepatic tissues or cells.[25,28] This protein has been shown recently to be a proapo A-II form containing either a five[42a] or six[80a] amino acid long prosegment and is converted to the plasma form by a similar extracellular apoprotein modification. Finally, these studies suggest strongly that apo E is secreted as sialo apo E and is subsequently desialated in plasma (Figs. 1G–1I).[25,28] A schematic representation of the intra- and extracellular post-translational modifications of human apo A-I and apo E are shown in Figs. 2A and 2B. Besides desialation, another form of alteration has been observed for monkey apo E *in vitro*.[81] The physiological significance of sialation of apo E and apo B in lipoprotein catabolism requires further clarification.[82,83]

Alterations of Lipoproteins in Plasma

Following secretion, lipoproteins undergo a series of alterations in plasma, prior to their uptake and catabolism by lipoprotein receptors. These alterations include (1) hydrolysis of chylomicron and VLDL triglycerides by lipoprotein lipase, (2) hydrolysis of lipoprotein triglycerides by hepatic lipase (3) esterification of HDL cholesterol by lecithin cholesterol acyltransferase, (4) enzyme-catalyzed exchange or transfer of cholesteryl ester and phospholipids, (5) exchange and transfer of apoproteins, (6) reverse transport of cholesterol from cells to lipoproteins.

Lipoprotein Lipase (LPL). LPL hydrolyzes preferentially the 1,3 ester bonds of chylomicrons and VLDL triglycerides, generating free fatty acids and mainly 2-monoglycerides.[84,85] The enzyme is activated by apoprotein CII (apo CII)[88–91] and inhibited by 1 M NaCl.[85,91] LPL is present on the luminal surface of the vascular endothelium attached to a mem-

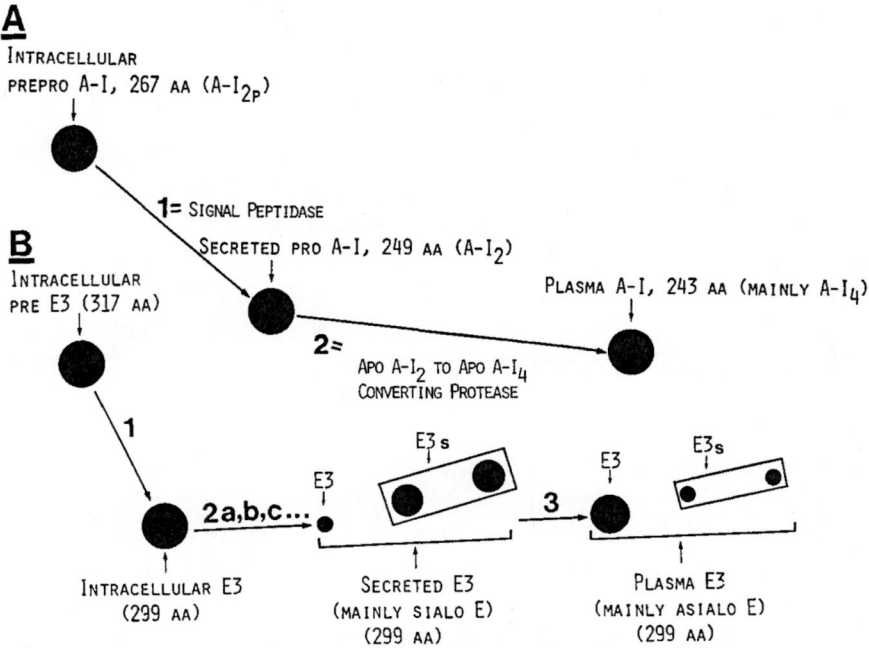

A

INTRACELLULAR
PREPRO A-I, 267 AA (A-I$_{2P}$)

1= SIGNAL PEPTIDASE

SECRETED PRO A-I, 249 AA (A-I$_2$)

PLASMA A-I, 243 AA (MAINLY A-I$_4$)

B

INTRACELLULAR
PRE E3 (317 AA)

2= APO A-I$_2$ TO APO A-I$_4$
CONVERTING PROTEASE

1

E3

E3s

E3

E3s

2a,b,c...

3

INTRACELLULAR E3
(299 AA)

SECRETED E3
(MAINLY SIALO E)
(299 AA)

PLASMA E3
(MAINLY ASIALO E)
(299 AA)

Fig. 2. Schematic presentation of the intra- and extracellular modification of (A) human apo A-I and (B) apo E. The numbers indicate: (A)1, signal peptidase; 2, apo A-I$_2$ to apo A-I$_4$ converting protease present in plasma, lymph, and/or on cell surfaces; (B) 1, signal peptidase; 2a,b,c, . . . , putative glycosyl transferases; 3, desialating enzyme present in plasma and/or on cell surfaces.

brane-bound glycosaminoglycan and can be released into plasma by injection of heparin.[92,93] LPL activity has been demonstrated in postheparin plasma, skeletal muscle, heart, lung, mammary gland, and adipose tissue.[92,94–98] LPL synthesis and secretion have also been observed in the murine macrophage cell line J774.[99] Two forms of rat LPL with high (heart enzyme) and low (adipose tissue enzyme) substrate affinity, respectively, have been described.[100] Subunit molecular weight values of 60,000–70,000[85] and 34,000–37,000[91,101] and carbohydrate content of 3–10% have been reported for LPL.[91,92,101] The activity of LPL is regulated by nutrients[102–104] and hormones.[105–107] Inhibition of LPL by antibodies[96] or genetic defects of LPL[108] and/or apo CII[109,110] cause excessive accumulation of VLDL and chylomicrons in plasma.[108–110] This indicates that the initial hydrolysis of VLDL and/or phospholipids by lipoprotein lipase is a necessary step for the subsequent catabolism of these particles.

Hepatic Triglyceride Lipase (HTL). HTL has been localized by immunofluorescent studies on the surface of hepatic endothelial cells[111] and can be released by injection of heparin.[111-114] Biochemical and genetic evidence[108,115-119] suggests that HTL is a lipolytic activity distinct from LPL. The purified enzyme has a glycoprotein with subunit molecular weight of 62,500.[120] HTL is not activated by apo CII,[85] is not affected by protamine and high salt,[92,115] but is inhibited by SDS.[118] Human patients and animal models have been described with deficiencies either of HTL or LPL or both enzymes.[107,117,121] HTL hydrolyzes VLDL and chylomicron triglycerides and phospholipids *in vitro*.[6,85,112,120,122] Decreased activity of HTL in several diseases[123-125] or inhibition of the enzyme with antibodies[120,126,127] causes accumulation of certain lipoprotein species (HDL_2, LDL_2) that are enriched in phospholipids, mainly phosphatidylethanolamine.[123-127] These data suggest that these lipoproteins may be the natural substrates of HTL and that HTL may play some role in phospholipid catabolism.

Lecithin Cholesterol Acyltransferase (LCAT). LCAT is the enzyme responsible for the formation of cholesteryl esters in plasma.[128] It has been proposed that LCAT forms a complex in plasma with components of HDL[129] and catalyzes the esterification of HDL cholesterol using HDL lecithin as the acyl donor. The C-2 fatty acyl group of lecithin is preferentially transferred and the specific fatty acyl groups at the C-1 and C-2 positions of lecithin affect the rate of the reaction.[130,131] The products of the reaction are 2-lysolecithin and cholesteryl ester. The prefered substrates of LCAT are nascent HDL cholesterol,[6,15,18] HDL_3 cholesterol, and, to a lesser extent, HDL_2 cholesterol.[132] LDL cholesterol and VLDL cholesterol are poor substrates. The enzyme is activated by apo A-I and to a lesser extent by apo CI.[133-135] LCAT also catalyzes the reverse reaction (esterification of lysolecithin), and this process is activated by LDL,[136] as well as the hydrolysis of lecithin to lysolecithin and free fatty acids.[137] LCAT is synthesized mainly by the liver and is subsequently secreted into palsma.[138,139] Plasma LCAT has been purified and is a monomer of molecular weight 59,000–70,000 which contains 24% carbohydrate by weight.[85,137,140,141] Fielding and Fielding have shown that the rate of HDL cholesterol esterification depends on the cholesteryl ester content of acceptor VLDL and LDL particles.[142] This finding suggests that the synthesis and transfer of cholesteryl esters in plasma may be functionally linked.

Exchange and Transfer of Lipid and Protein Moieties among Lipoprotein Classes. Several investigators have observed that the lipid and protein moieties are not statically fixed on the lipoprotein molecules but rather that they exchange readily among lipoprotein classes. The specific enzymatic activities and the other factors that regulate the change of composition of the lipoprotein molecules are only partially understood and are the subject of extensive investigations.[143] Several activities have been identified in plasma that catalyze the exchange and/or transfer of lipid moieties between lipoproteins. These include the cholesteryl ester transfer-exchange protein, the phospholipid transfer protein, and the triglyceride transfer protein. The cholesteryl ester transfer (CET) protein has been identified in the lipoprotein-free plasma of all species studied[144-150] except the rat[146] and the pig.[150] The CET activity of different species correlates with the concentration of VLDL cholesterol.[151] Most studies indicate that this protein promotes the bidirectional transfer of cholesteryl ester among all lipoprotein classes.[143-149] Other studies indicate that there is a net cholesteryl ester transfer from HDL to VLDL and LDL.[152-155] The suggestion that apo D might be involved directly in cholesteryl ester transfer[152] was not supported by subsequent experiments.[49,155] Several studies suggest that cholesteryl ester transfer from one lipoprotein particle to another is associated with equimolar reciprocal transfer of triglycerides.[152,154,156-158] Present evidence indicates that cholesteryl ester and triglyceride transfer may be mediated by the same protein[159-161] However, triglyceride transfer activity can be inhibited preferentially with mercurial compounds.[154,159,162] Earlier studies indicated that CET is a glycoprotein molecular weight 78,000 and isoelectric point of 5,[145] which binds to HDL.[163] Morton and Zilversmit have shown, with additional purification, that the transfer protein has two components on SDS gels of apparent molecular weight 66,400 and 58,300.[159] Both components have CET and triglyceride transfer activity. The relative rate of the two activities is maintained through the various purification steps.[159] Albers, et al. have recently purified two distinct lipid transfer proteins (LTP) designated LTP-1 (MW 64K, PI5) and LTP-2. The two activities have different lipid transfer specificities and thermal stability, and may have similarities with the various lipid transfer activities described by others.[159a] A protein complex of 150,000 molecular weight, purified from human plasma, has been shown to catalyze the bidirectional exchange of cholesteryl ester and phospholipid at a 1:1 ratio between HDL and LDL.[164,165] This protein complex is absent from rat plasma, which contains only a phospholipid exchange protein.[164] Finally, a protein of 35,000 molecular weight and isoelectric point of ≥ 4 has been purified from plasma and inhibits the transfer or exchange of cholesteryl ester and triglycerides between lipoproteins.[66] The physiological significance and the specificity of these transfer and/or exchange activities in lipoprotein metabolism require further investigation.

Several studies have established that exchange and/or transfer of all apoproteins (with the exception of apo B) occurs during various stages of lipoprotein metabolism. As mentioned above, lymph chylomicrons are composed primarily of apo B-48, apo A-I and apo A-IV.[12,15−17,56,57] Chylomicrons as they enter the plasma compartment receive apo C and apo E from HDL. Following hydrolysis of chylomicrons by LPL, they transfer their apo A-I to HDL[167,168] and their apo A-IV either to HDL or to the $d > 1.21$ g/ml fraction.[169,170] Apo A-I and apo A-II in plasma are found in HDL and exchange readily between the HDL_2 and HDL_3 subclasses.[171,172] Other studies have shown that hepatic Golgi VLDL contain mainly apo B and apo E but only small amounts of apo C's.[73] This implies that when nascent VLDL enters the plasma compartment, it acquires apo C's from other plasma lipoproteins, possibly HDL_2.[167] In addition, nascent VLDL may acquire additional apo E from nascent HDL.[173] When VLDL triglycerides are hydrolyzed by lipoprotein lipase, apo CII, apo CIII, and some apo E are transferred back to HDL.[6,167,173−175]

The enzyme-catalyzed lipolysis of chylomicron and VLDL triglycerides and esterification of HDL cholesterol and the ensuing exchange and transfer of lipid and protein moieties result in the conversion of one lipoprotein class into another. Plasma chylomicrons, when acted upon by LPL,[84,85] lose the bulk of their triglycerides, transfer their phospholopids and apoproteins to HDL,[168,176−178] and become chylomicron remnants. Chylomicron remnants are then cleared from plasma by the liver with a half-life of less than 10 min by a saturable high-affinity process.[179,180] Similarly, sequential hydrolysis of VLDL by LPL and the ensuing loss of apo C's and apo E result in the generation of plasma IDL ($d = 1.006–1.019$ g/ml) and LDL,[67,79] which are catabolized by extrahepatic as well as by hepatic tissues. The discoidal HDL of patients with LCAT deficiency[77,78] can be converted to a spherical particle by the action of LCAT.[181] This conversion is associated with transfer of the nascent HDL apo E to VLDL,[173] transfer of VLDL apo C to the spherical plasma HDL,[173] and possible altered affinity of the spherical HDL for apo A-I.[182] As will be discussed later, HDL may either be catabolized directly by some tissues or, as already discussed, it may transfer its cholesteryl ester content to

VLDL and LDL for further catabolism.[143-159] The VLDL and LDL$_2$ particles of unusual size and composition found in the plasma of patients with LCAT deficiency[78,173] could represent intermediates of lipoprotein metabolism that may be converted rapidly to other lipoproteins in normal plasma.[183] A schematic presentation of various steps of lipoprotein metabolism outlined in this section is shown in Fig. 3.

Reverse Cholesterol Transport. Glomset and colleagues have proposed that HDL may be involved in the reverse transport of cholesterol from the peripheral tissues to the liver and other organs.[128,181] According to this hypothesis, HDL attracts the excess of cholesterol from plasma membranes of tissues or red blood cells. The free cholesterol is esterified by LCAT[128] and is either catabolized by some tissues[184-189] or transferred as cholesteryl esters to VLDL and LDL,[143-159] which are subsequently removed from the circulation by various tissues. A portion of the cholesteryl esters delivered to the liver is secreted into the bile either as free cholesterol or in the form of bile acids.[190] Several subsequent studies are consistent with the proposed role of HDL in the reverse transport of cholesterol.[191-194] Oram et al.[193] and Biesbroeck et al.[194] have shown that HDL$_3$ (d = 1.1-1.21) promotes cholesterol efflux from cells and regulates intracellular sterol synthesis and esterification. In other studies, it has been shown that mouse peritoneal macrophages catabolize modified LDL through a receptor-mediated pathway.[195,196] This process results in a dramatic increase of the intracellular cholesteryl ester content of these cells.[196] However, in the presence of HDL in the culture medium, the modified LDL cholesteryl esters are hydrolyzed intracellularly and secreted into the medium.[197,198] At the same time, macrophages secrete apo E through a pathway that is independent of that of cholesterol secretion.[199] It has been proposed that the apo E and cholesterol secreted by macrophages are incorporated into HDL$_3$ to form HDL$_2$, HDL$_1$, and HDL$_c$ particles, which transfer the cellular cholesterol back to the liver.[199] A role for HDL in the reverse transport of cholesterol could explain the inverse correlation between HDL cholesterol levels and the risk of developing coronary artery disease.[200,201]

Receptor-Mediated Catabolism of Lipoproteins

Our current understanding of the molecular events involved in lipoprotein catabolism has been shaped mainly by the pioneering work of

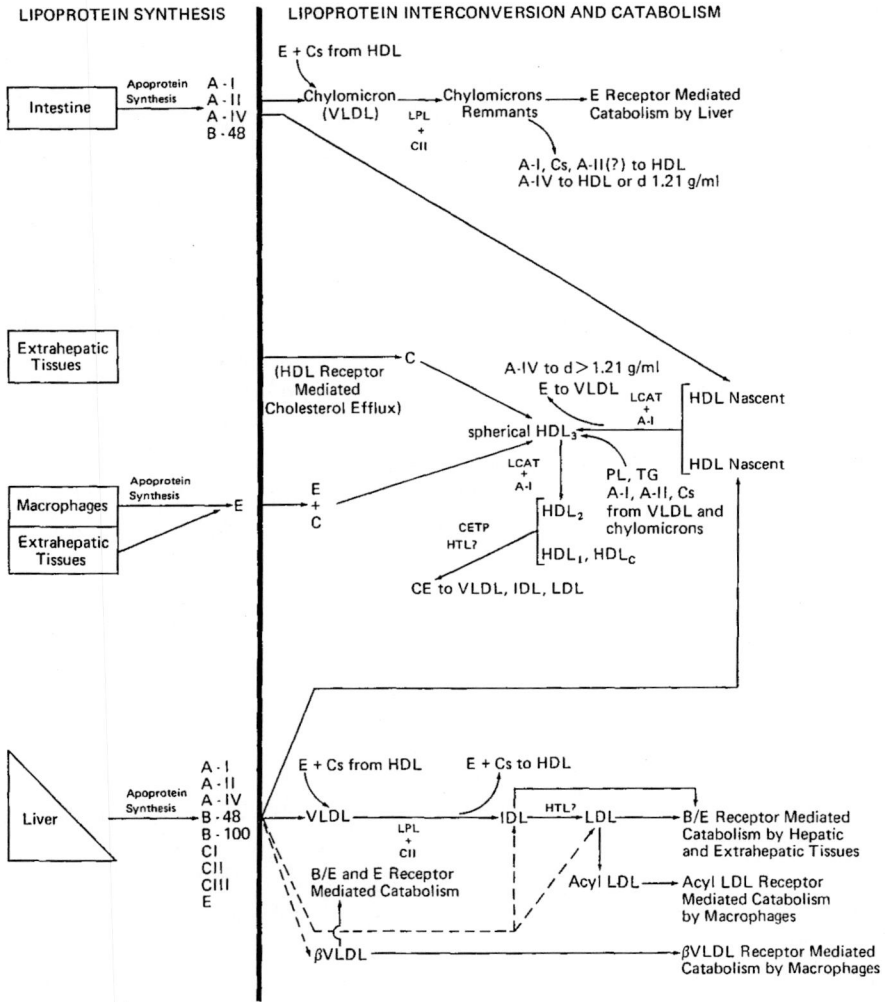

Fig. 3. Schematic representation of the pathway of lipoprotein metabolism. The pathway is based on the information presented in the text. LCAT, Lecithin:cholesterol acyltransferase; CETP, cholesteryl ester transfer protein; LPL, lipoprotein lipase; HTL, hepatic triglyceride lipase; C, cholesterol; TG, triglyceride; PL phospholipid; A-I, E, . . . , apo A-I, apo E, . . .

Goldstein and Brown and colleagues, who first demonstrated the presence of specific LDL receptors on cell surfaces. Since then, several other distinct lipoprotein receptors have been described. The basic properties of the different lipoprotein receptors are shown in Table II and are also reviewed briefly in this section.

LDL (B/E) Receptor.* Biochemical and genetic studies have demonstrated that the cell surface of cultured human fibroblasts contains high-affinity receptors for LDL, the major cholesterol transport protein in human plasma.[202-206] It has been estimated that each fibroblast cell contains 50,000–100,000 receptors.[203,207,208] Electron microscopy studies have shown that 50–80% of the receptors are clustered in regions of the plasma membrane called coated pits.[209-212] The binding of LDL is Ca^{2+}-dependent and pronase-sensitive.[204,206,208] The LDL receptor binds LDL by interacting with apo B.[204,206,213-215] Modification of apo B lysine[215] or arginine[214] residues destroys its ability to bind to the receptor. The development of an assay for LDL receptor activity in cell membrane preparations[216] has allowed the purification of the LDL receptor from bovine adrenal cortex.[217,218] The mature receptor is a glycoprotein of apparent molecular weight 160,000, and isoelectric point 4.3,[219,220] and contains both N-linked and O-linked oligosaccharides.[221] The purified receptor retains all of the properties of the LDL receptor.[217,218] Following synthesis, the LDL receptor undergoes post-translational modification, presumably in the Golgi apparatus, which increases its apparent molecular weight (120,000 to 160,000).[219] The molecular nature of this modification is not clear.[222] Polyclonal[223] and monoclonal[224] antibodies against the LDL receptor have been raised and immunologic cross-reactivity of LDL receptors from bovine adrenal cortex, canine liver and adrenal gland, rat liver, and human fibroblasts has been demonstrated.[223] One of the monoclonal antibodies has been shown to bind in stoichiometric amounts to the LDL receptor.[220,224] LDL binds to the LDL receptor at 4°C but is not internalized.[204,206] The dissociation constant of the LDL–LDL receptor complex is 2.8 nM.[208] When cell cultures are incubated at 37°C, the coated pits with the LDL receptor complex invaginate into the cell and pinch off to form endocytic vesicles called endosomes that carry LDL to lysosomes.[225] The process of receptor internalization and movement to the lysosomes requires 10–15 min.[204,206] During this time, the endosome developes an acidic pH that is believed to mediate the dissociation of the lipoprotein receptor complex.[221] The free receptor recycles to the cell surface prior to the fusion of endosomes with primary

Table II. Lipoprotein Receptors[a]

Name of receptor	Cell or tissue origin	Ligand	Affinity K_d, nM	Binding characteristics
LDL (B/E) receptor	Skin fibroblasts (various extrahepatic tissues and cells)	LDL	2.8	Binds one LDL molecule/ receptor
LDL (B/E) receptor	Skin fibroblasts	HDL with apo E	0.12	Binds one HDL with apo E molecule/ four receptors
LDL (B/E) receptor	Skin fibroblasts	DMPC apo E	0.1	Binds one HDL with apo E molecule/ four receptors
LDL (B/E) receptor	Liver	LDL	11.0	—
E Receptor (chylomicron remnant receptor)	Liver	HDL with apo E, DMPC apo E	0.23	—
HDL	Liver	HDL (apo E free)	82.0	Nonspecific
HDL	Skin fibroblasts	HDL (apo E free)	~200	Nonspecific
HDL	Adrenal ovary gonads	HDL	—	—
βVLDL Receptor	Monocyte– macrophage	βVLDL	—	—
Modified LDL receptor	Monocyte– macrophage	Modified LDL	—	—

[a] The references on which this table is based are given in the text.
[b] With the exception of HDL receptor, "receptor regulation" is manifested by (1) decrease of intracellular cholesterol synthesis, (2) increase in intracellular cholesterol esterification,

Other features	Receptor–ligand internalization	Receptor regulation[b]	Function
Ca^{2+}-Dependent, pronase-sensitive	Yes	Yes	Regulation of body and cellular cholesterol homeostasis (steroid hormone synthesis by adrenal gland, ovaries, and gonads)
Ca^{2+}-Dependent, pronase-sensitive	Yes	Yes	
Ca^{2+}-Dependent, pronase-sensitive	—	—	
Ca^{2+}-Dependent, pronase-sensitive, age-dependent, inducible by hypocholesterolemic agents (cholestyramine)	Yes	Yes	Clearance of IDL and LDL cholesterol by the liver for excretion, regulation of body and cellular cholesterol homeostasis
Ca^{2+}-Dependent, pronase-sensitive, age-independent, noninducible	Yes	Yes	Clearance of chylomicron remnant cholesterol by the liver for excretion, regulation of body and cellular cholesterol homeostasis
Ca^{2+}-independent, pronase-insensitive	No	—	Reverse transport of cholesterol
Ca^{2+}-independent, pronase-insensitive	No	Yes	Reverse transport of cholesterol
—	—	—	Provision of cholesterol for steroid hormone synthesis
Ca^{2+}-Dependent	Yes	Yes (at higher ligand concentrations than LDL receptor)	Scavenging diet-induced lipoprotein particles; role in foam cell formation
Ca^{2+}-Independent, pronase-sensitive	Yes	No	Scavenging modified particles; role in foam cell formation

and (3) decrease in number of surface receptors. Receptor regulation following HDL (apo E free) is manifested by (1) increase in number of LDL receptors, (2) increase in cellular sterol synthesis, and (3) decrease in cellular cholesterol esterification.

lysosomes.[221,226] Recycling of the receptors is inhibited by the carboxylic ionophore monensin.[226] Fusion of endosomes with primary lysosomes results in the hydrolytic degradation of apo B to amino acids and hydrolysis of cholesteryl esters by the lysosomal enzyme, acid lipase.[202,227] Liberated cholesterol is used by cells for membrane synthesis.[228] It also triggers three regulatory responses that assure cellular cholesterol homeostasis: (1) suppression of HMG CoA reductase, the rate-limiting enzyme of cholesterol biosynthesis,[229] turning off cellular cholesterol synthesis, (2) activation of acyl-CoA:cholesterol acyltransferase (ACAT), which reesterifies excess cholesterol preferentially with oleic acid, resulting in cytoplasmic storage of cholesteryl ester droplets,[230] and (3) decrease in the number of surface LDL receptors, which prevents additional cholesterol influx into the cell.[203,204,206] In addition to fibroblasts, many other animal and human cells, including lymphoid cells,[231,232] arterial smooth muscle cells,[233,234] endothelial cells,[235] and adrenocortical cells, have LDL receptors.[188,189] The LDL receptors are particularly important in adrenocortical cells, where the cholesterol derived from LDL provides one source of substrate for steroid hormone synthesis.[188,189]

LDL receptors could not be demonstrated in perfused rat liver and rat and adult canine liver membrane preparations.[236,237] In the rat system, treatment with pharmacological doses of 17 α-ethinyl estradiol lowers plasma lipoprotein levels[236] and induces Ca^{2+}-dependent LDL binding to hepatic membranes.[186,236,238] In similar experiments, adult dogs who have ingested cholestyramine have liver membranes that bind LDL specifically with high affinity ($K_d = 1.5 \times 10^8$ M). High-affinity binding of LDL ($K_d = 1.1 \times 10^8$ M) is also exhibited by liver membranes from young, rapidly growing puppies. In all three cases binding of ^{125}I-LDL to liver membranes appeared to be mediated by LDL receptors similar to the extrahepatic LDL receptors. The ^{125}I-LDL binding is pronase-sensitive and is competitively inhibited by unlabeled LDL or lipoproteins containing apo E.[237] These observations are in agreement with reports of increased receptor-mediated clearance of LDL in man[239] and rabbits[240] after cholestyramine treatment, and of increased LDL binding to rat livers after estradiol treatment. These observations also suggest a relationship between an increase in hepatic LDL receptors and decreased plasma cholesterol levels.[186] The Watanabe hereditary hyperlipidemic (WHHL) rabbit has been proposed as a model for familial hypercholesterolemia. This animal shows LDL receptor deficiency in cultured fibroblasts[241] as well as adrenal and hepatic tissues and cells,[242,243] which suggests that the hepatic and extrahepatic LDL receptors are the products of the same gene.[242,243]

Experiments by Mahley and colleagues[244–249] have demonstrated that the LDL receptor specifically binds apo E-containing lipoproteins in addition to apo B-containing lipoproteins, and is thus more accurately described as an apo B/E receptor. It was shown that a subfraction of HDL induced in dogs by cholesterol feeding, which has apo E as the only apoprotein (HDL with apo E or previously designated HDL_c),[244] binds to the LDL receptor.[245] Cultured fibroblasts from patients with receptor-negative, homozygous familial hypercholesterolemia cannot bind HDL with apo E.[245] The binding of HDL with apo E was competitively inhibited by LDL. The binding of LDL was competitively inhibited by HDL with apo E.[208,246] It was also shown that chemical modification of apo E arginine (by cyclohexanedione[214]) or lysine residues (by acetylation or reductive methylation[247]) inhibited binding of HDL with apo E to the LDL receptor. The metabolic fate of HDL with apo E bound by the LDL receptor is similar to that of LDL itself.[204,245] Bound HDL with apo E is internalized and transferred to lysosomes, where the apoprotein is degraded and cholesteryl esters are hydrolyzed. This is followed by inhibition of cellular cholesterol biosynthesis and stimulation of cholesterol esterification.[245] The affinity of HDL with apo E for the LDL receptor was over 20 times greater than that for LDL itself. The dissociation constant K_d of the lipoprotein–receptor complex was 1.2×10^{-10} for HDL with apo E and 2.8×10^{-9} for LDL. Furthermore, four times as many HDL particles as HDL with apo E particles were required for saturation of the receptors at maximal binding.[208] Since HDL with apo E and LDL bind the same receptor, these data indicate that one HDL with apo E particle binds to four LDL receptors.[248,249] In other studies, it has been shown that, besides HDL with apo E, other apo E-containing lipoproteins, such as chylomicron remnants, βVLDL, and HDL_1 show apo E-mediated binding to cultured fibroblasts.[250–253] Liver membranes from normal rabbits have been shown to have high-affinity binding sites ($K_d \approx 0.5$ μg/ml) for βVLDL. The receptor that binds βVLDL resembles the extrahepatic LDL receptor in having high affinity for B- and/or E-containing lipoproteins, requiring Ca^{2+}, and being sensitive to pronase. This receptor appears to mediate the rapid hepatic clearance of βVLDL in normal rabbits. After cholesterol feeding, saturation of these receptors by the high concentration of endogenous βVLDL and a down regulation of the number of hepatic receptors appeared to be responsible for the accumulation of βVLDL in plasma and profound hypercholesterolemia.[253] Finally, metabolic studies have shown faster catabolic rates for apo E in VLDL as compared to apo E in HDL particles.[254,255] This indicates that in addition to the apoproteins, the lipid composition and the overall configuration of the lipoprotein particles play an important role in their recognition by the LDL receptor.

   Chylomicron Remnant (Apo E) Receptor.* As discussed earlier, chylomicron remnants result from the hydrolysis of chylomicron triglycerides by LPL.[84,85] A specific, high-affinity chylomicron remnant receptor has been identified on rat liver plasma membranes from animals not treated with estradiol that do not exhibit the apo B/E receptor. The dissociation constant of the remnant–receptor complex is 27 μM cholesterol. This receptor did not bind LDL or VLDL, and only weakly bound HDL and chylomicrons.[256] Chylomicron remnants contain both apo B and apo E.[257] In perfused rat liver, transport kinetics for chylomicron remnants resemble those observed for canine HDL with apo E, the particles induced by cholesterol feeding, that contain no other apoproteins. Competitive binding studies also indicate that chylomicron remnants and HDL with apo E bind to identical receptor sites.[258] Furthermore, *in vivo* studies in rats and dogs demonstrate that arginine or lysine modification of HDL with apo E results in the retarded hepatic clearance of these lipoproteins from plasma, and suggests the importance of apo E in hepatic uptake of these lipoproteins.[259,260] In addition, when apo E is added to small chylomicrons obtained from estrogen-treated rats, which contained very little apo E, or to rat lymph chylomicrons, or to triglyceride emulsions, this results in rapid hepatic uptake of all these particles by the perfused rat liver similar to that observed for chylomicron remnants. Of interest was the finding that the addition of apo C's to apo E-enriched chylomicrons or triglyceride emulsions inhibited their hepatic uptake.[257,261–263] These observations suggest that apo E is one of the protein determinants for hepatic uptake of chylomicron remnants, with the apo C's (mainly apo CIII) having a regulatory role.[257,261–263] Other studies with hepatic membranes from adult dogs that do not exhibit the apo B/E receptor have shown high-affinity receptors specific for apo E-containing lipoproteins (HDL with apo E). These receptors have been designated apo E receptors.[237] Scatchard analysis of the binding of ^{125}I-HDL with apo E to adult canine hepatic membranes suggests the presence of two binding sites: a higher affinity ($K_d = 2.3 \times 10^{-10}$ M), calcium-dependent, pronase-sensitive site, and a lower affinity ($K_d = 2 \times 10^{-8}$ M), calcium-independent, pronase-resistant site. Arginine or lysine modification of HDL with apo E abolished binding to the higher but not to the lower affinity site. The specificity of the high-affinity receptor for apo E was established by competition experiments. Iodine-125-labeled HDL with apo E, which can bind either to LDL (apo B/E) or apo E receptors, is only partially displaced by excess unlabeled LDL that contains apo B and not apo E, but is totally displaced by excess unlabeled HDL with apo E.[237] Earlier *in vivo* experiments in rats suggested that the low-molecular weight or intestinal form of apo B (designated apo Bl) may play some role in the catabolism of at least a subpopulation of chylomicron remnants.[57,264-268] The same experiments showed that the higher molecular weight form of apo B (designated apo Bh) was taken up less efficiently by the liver.[57,264-268] Variants of apo B corresponding to the Bl and Bh forms seen in rats have also been observed in human lymph chylomicrons and have been designated B-48 and B-100, respectively.[269] Recent studies have shown that apo E, but not apo B-48, is important for the binding of βVLDL and chylomicron remnants to extrahepatic lipoprotein receptors.[269a] Further experiments are needed to clarify the role of the two forms of apo B in lipoprotein catabolism. The current data do not allow a distinction between the chylomicron remnant receptor and the apo E receptor. However, the difference between the LDL receptor and the chylomicron remnant receptor is suggested by the observation of normal hepatic chylomicron remnant catabolism in patients with homozygous familial hypercholesterolemia, who are LDL receptor-negative,[206,270] as well as in the WHHL rabbit.[271-273] For instance, as a result of the LDL receptor defect,[241] the WHHL rabbit accumulates in its plasma apo B-containing lipoproteins (VLDL, IDL, and LDL), but not apo B-48-containing chylomicron remnants.[271-273] The metabolic block in the hepatic clearance of IDL that exists in the WHHL rabbit causes an increase in the conversion of IDL to LDL and results in elevated plasma LDL levels in this animal model as well as in patients with familial hypercholesterolemia.[271,273]

βVLDL Receptor. Animals fed cholesterol accumulate β-migrating, very low density lipoprotein particles, designated βVLDL, in plasma, which are rich in cholesterol and contain apo B and apo E.[274-276] Similar lipoprotein particles are found in the plasma of patients with type III hyperlipoproteinemia.[276-279] The βVLDL obtained from various animals causes cholesteryl ester accumulation in cultures of mouse peritoneal macrophages.[274,275] VLDL, LDL, and HDL cholesterol are substantially less effective in causing cholesteryl ester accumulation in macrophage cultures when compared to βVLDL.[274] In these cultures, the increase in cellular cholesteryl ester content is associated with down regulation of βVLDL receptor activity, similar to the phenomenon observed for the LDL receptor.[274] However, down regulation is mediated at high concentrations of βVLDL or modified LDL in the culture medium and occurs only after extensive cellular cholesteryl ester accumulation.[274] Cholesteryl ester accumulation in macrophages *in vivo* may result in foam cell formation, which is thought to be a precursor of atherosclerotic lesions.[280-283] Chemical modification of lysine residues of the apoprotein moieties blocks binding of βVLDL to macrophage receptors. However, other factors, such as cholesterol content and conformation of βVLDL may be important for its recognition and catabolism by the βVLDL receptor.[276,284] Lipoprotein binding studies and the kinetics of cholesteryl ester accumulation caused by βVLDL indicate that the βVLDL receptor is distinct from the LDL receptor.[274,275] This notion is further supported by the observation that monocyte-macrophage cultures from patients with homozygous familial hypercholesterolemia have near-normal βVLDL receptor activity.[285] The βVLDL activity of freshly isolated human monocyte-macrophages is threefold higher than LDL receptor activity. However, the activity of both receptors decreases approximately to the same level with time in culture.[285] Beside macrophages, βVLDL receptors have also been demonstrated on endothelial cells.[285a]

Acyl LDL (or Modified LDL) Receptor. It has been estimated that in normal humans two-thirds of LDL is catabolized through the LDL receptor pathway and one-third by a receptor-independent pathway which may reside in scavenger cells.[206,286,287] The molecular basis of LDL degradation by scavenger cells has been investigated using mouse peritoneal macrophages and cultures of human monocyte-macrophages. Mouse peritoneal macrophages contain a receptor that binds specifically and with high affinity to acyl LDL, but not to native LDL.[195,196] The human monocyte-macrophage system contains specific, high-affinity receptors for both LDL and acyl LDL.[288] The bound, modified LDL is internalized and the protein moiety degraded to amino acids.[195,196] The regulation of cellular cholesterol homeostasis following acyl LDL degradation is fundamentally different from that following LDL degradation by reticuloendothelial cells.[206] The cholesteryl ester moiety of modified LDL is hydrolyzed presumably by a nonlysosomal cholesteryl esterase.[198] When the cells are grown in serum-containing medium, half of the free cholesterol is secreted and the remainder is reesterified by ACAT and stored in the cytoplasm as cholesteryl ester droplets.[196] In the continuous presence of acyl LDL in the culture medium, the macrophages apparently fail to down regulate their receptor activity and this results in a dramatic increase in cellular cholesteryl ester content.[196] Such cholesteryl ester accumulation in the monocyte-macrophages may lead to the formation of foam cells that are found in atherosclerotic lesions.[280-283] This hypothesis is further supported by the observation that aortic foam cells have receptors for both βVLDL as well as modified LDL.[283] The acyl LDL receptor has been partially purified from membranes of the murine macrophage cell line p388D1 after solubilization with octylglucoside.[289] The purified receptor has a molecular weight of 200,000 to 283,000, and an isoelectric point of 5.9, and maintains its specificity for acyl LDL.[289] A molecular weight of 200,000 has been reported for the acyl LDL receptor isolated from rabbit alveolar macrophages.[289a] Other recent experiments have shown that similar to the LDL receptor, the acyl LDL receptor recycles from the cytoplasm to the cell surface every 18 minutes[289b] and this process is inhibited by monensin.

The physiological importance of this receptor and the manner in which acyl LDL may be actively produced *in vivo* are not completely understood. Fogelman *et al.*[287] have proposed that one form of modified LDL may be produced *in vivo* by malonyldialdehyde that is released by platelets or is produced during lipid peroxidation. Recent studies also have shown that incubation of LDL with cultured vascular endothelial cells apparently modifies LDL in a still unknown way. This putative modification results in the recognition and uptake of modified LDL by the modified LDL receptor.[284,290]

HDL Receptor. HDL binding to primary cultures of hepatocytes,[155,291,292] nonparenchymal cells,[291,293] cultured human fibroblasts,[294,295] and adrenal gland[188,189] as well as to membrane preparations of rat and dog liver[186,237] and rat testis[187] has been demonstrated. The number of HDL binding sites per hepatocyte and nonparenchymal cell has been estimated to be 10^5–10^6.[185,292,293] The dissociation constant of the HDL–receptor complex is in the range of 10^{-6}–10^{-7} M.[186,292,293] The binding is Ca^{2+} independent[186,237,292] and is not affected by acetylation or reductive methylation of HDL.[237,292,293] However, nitrosylation severely inhibited the binding of HDL, or the apo A-I liposomes to the HDL receptor.[293a] This finding suggests that tyrosine(s) in apo A-I may be involved in the binding of HDL to the HDL receptor. Pronase treatment of the membrane preparations or of cell cultures does not significantly affect HDL binding.[186,237,292,294] Various lipoproteins including HDL_3,

HDL$_2$,[293a] HDL with apo E,[237], LDL, and VLDL,[185,293] as well as lipo-somes containing apo A-I or apo A-II[293a] compete to varying degrees for the HDL-receptor binding site. Recent studies showed an induction of HDL binding sites in cultured human fibroblasts by increasing the cho-lesterol concentration of the culture medium. This induction was inhib-ited by cycloheximide, suggesting a requirement for protein synthesis in the production of new HDL receptors.[296] The same studies also showed that human fibroblasts and arterial smooth muscle cells contain specific, high-affinity receptors for HDL free of apo E (maximum saturation 20 μg HDL/ml).[194] Bound HDL was not internalized or degraded by these cells; instead it caused an increase in LDL receptor activity, sterol syn-thesis, and cholesterol efflux. These processes were saturated at HDL con-centrations of 20 μg/ml, as was the specific, high-affinity HDL binding, suggesting they were also mediated by the HDL receptor.[194] In addition to the role of HDL in promoting cholesterol efflux from peripheral tissues through the HDL receptors, some studies suggest that HDL may directly or indirectly deliver cholesterol to steroid-hormone-producing cells.[187-189] This process may be mediated by a specific HDL receptor.

Apoprotein Structure and Function

Following the nomenclature system proposed by Alaupovic,[7] the protein components of lipoproteins, known as apoproteins, have been designated by the letters A, B, C, etc. Apoproteins after exposure to lipid increase their α-helical character. Primary sequence analysis of apopro-teins indicates that these α-helices are amphipathic. The nonpolar surface of the helix is presumed to interact with nonpolar lipids, such as choles-teryl ester and triglycerides, and the polar surface with the polar head group of the phospholipid as well as with the aqueous phase.[297] This is consistent with the role of apoproteins in lipoprotein structure and/or lipid transport. In addition, research of the last decade has provided ample evidence that some apoproteins are not merely structural compo-nents of lipoproteins, but can be cofactors in enzymatic reactions that affect lipoprotein metabolism[85-91,133-135] or can be involved in receptor-mediated catabolism of lipoproteins.[204,237,245,246,258] The apoprotein com-position of the lipoproteins is summarized in Table I. Our current knowl-edge of apoprotein structure and function is summarized in Table III[298-301] and reviewed in detail in this section as well as in section II, 2.

Table III. Apoproteins and Their Association with Human Diseases[a]

Apoprotein	Plasma concentration, mg/ml	Isoelectric point	Molecular weight	Primary amino acid sequence of mature proteins	Function	Association with clinical disorders
A-I	1.0–1.2	5.85–5.40[b]	28K	243 A.A.	Activates LCAT	Tangier disease, apo A-I–apo C-III deficiency
A-II	0.3–0.5	5.0	8.5K	77 A.A.	—	—
A-IV	0.16	5.45	46K	Unknown	—	—
B-100	0.7–1.0	—	549K	Unknown	Receptor-mediated catabolism of LDL	Abetalipoproteinemia, normotriglyceridemic abetalipoproteinemia (B-100 deficiency)
B-48	—	—	246K	Unknown	Chylomicron remnant catabolism	—
CI	0.04–0.06	7.5	6.5K	57 A.A.	Activates (moderately) LCAT	—
CII	0.03–0.05	4.9	9K	79 A.A.	Activates lipoprotein lipase	Familial type I hyperlipoproteinemia
CIII	0.12–0.14	4.7–5.0[c]	9K	79 A.A.	Inhibits catabolism of apo E-containing lipoproteins	Apo A-I–apo CIII deficiency
D	0.06–0.07	5.0–5.2[d]	32.5K	Unknown	—	—
E	0.025–0.050	5.7–6.0[e]	34.2K	299 A.A.	Receptor-mediated catabolism of apo E-containing lipoproteins	Familial type III hyperlipoproteinemia

[a] The references regarding molecular weight and function of individual apoproteins are given in the text. The isoelectric point values are those obtained in our laboratory and Ref. 49. The plasma concentrations of apoproteins are based on Refs. 49, 169, 298–301.
[b] The isoelectric points of individual normal apo A-I isoproteins are: A-I_2 = 5.85, A-I_3 = 5.74, A-I_4 = 5.64, A-I_5 = 5.52, A-I_6 = 5.40.
[c] The isoelectric points of individual apo C-III isoproteins are: apo CIII-0 = 5.0, apo CIII-1 = 4.85, apo CIII-2 = 4.65.
[d] The isoelectric points of individual apo D isoproteins are: apo D_1 = 5.2, apo D_2 = 5.08, apo D_3 = 5.0.
[e] The isoelectric points of individual apo E3 isoproteins are: apo E3 = 6.02, apo $E3_{s-1}$ = 5.89, apo $E3_{s-2}$ = 5.78, apo $E3_{s-3}$ = 5.68. The isoelectric points of the major apo E variatns are: apo E2 = 5.89, apo E4 = 6.18.

Apo A-I

Apo A-I is the major apoprotein of high-density lipoproteins (HDL) and is a relatively abundant plasma protein, with a concentration of 1.0–1.2 mg/dl.[300] Plasma apo A-I is a single polypeptide chain composed of 243 amino acid residues of known primary amino acid sequence.[302] Apo A-I serves as a cofactor for the plasma enzyme lecithin:cholesterol acyltransferase (LCAT), which is responsible for the formation of most cholesteryl esters in plasma.[133-135] A synthetic peptide containing apo A-I residues 121–164 is 30% as effective in activating LCAT as is apo A-I itself.[135] The activation of LCAT by apo A-I and a variety of synthetic peptides correlates with their α-helix content in 50% trifluoroethanol.[135] Association of A-I with phospholipid increases α-helical content from 55% to 75%. Apo A-I in lipoprotein particles of $d > 1.1$ g/ml promotes cholesterol efflux from cells and through this mechanism might be important in maintaining cellular cholesterol homeostasis.[191-194] Earlier work showed that apo A-I could be resolved by DEAE chromatography into several fractions with similar amino acid compostions.[303,304] Two-dimensional polyacrylamide gel electrophoresis (2D-PAGE) of apo A-I has shown that plasma apo A-I is composed of several isoproteins with the same apparent molecular weight (28,000) but different isoelectric points (Fig. 1D and Table I). In mammalian systems, apo A-I synthesis is thought to occur exclusively in liver and small intestine.[10-20,25-28] Synthesis of apo A-I by other tissues besides liver and intestine has also been demonstrated in avian species.[30] In all systems studied, the major newly secreted apo A-I isoprotein differs from the major plasma apo A-I isoprotein.[25,27,28,30,305] In humans, newly secreted apo A-I (apo A-I$_2$) is two charge units more basic than the major plasma apo A-I isoprotein (apo A-I$_4$) (Figs. 1C and 1D). Sequence analysis of the newly synthesized apo A-I$_2$ revealed that it contains a six-amino acid-long N-terminal extension with a sequence of ArgHisPheTrpGlnGln.[39,40] The N-terminal hexapeptide has two additional positively charged amino acids at the isoelectric point of apo A-I (pH $<$ 6). This finding explains the observed isoelectric point differences between apo A-I$_2$ and apo A-I$_4$ (Figs. 1C and 1D). In addition, it suggests that the apo A-I$_2$ to apo A-I$_4$ conversion is performed by a plasma and/or lymph protease (tentatively designated apo A-I$_2$:apo A-I$_4$ converting protease), which recognizes and cleaves the Gln $-$ 1 to Asp $+$ 1 peptide bond.[39] The importance of the converting protease for the pathogenesis of Tangier disease is discussed in section II, 2A. Recent studies have also shown that the 249-amino acid-long apo A-I$_2$ originates from a 267-amino acid-long precursor (designated apo A-I$_{2p}$ or preproapo A-I), which is the primary translation product of human apo A-I mRNA.[39,40,306,307] The first 18 N-terminal amino acids of this longer precursor are cleaved intracellularly by the signal peptidase of the rough endoplasmic reticulum,[34,36,39,40,308] resulting in the formation of apo A-I$_2$, which, as explained above, is the secreted form of apo A-I (25, 27, 28) (Figs. 1 and 2). The gene coding for human apo A-I has recently been isolated and characterized.[306,307] This gene is approximately 2.0 kb in length and is interrupted by three intervening sequences (IVS). The IVS-1 (197 bp) occurs in the region corresponding to the 5′ noncoding region of apo A-I mRNA. The IVS-2 (185 bp) interrupts the codon specifying amino acid 10 of the preprosegment of apo A-I. Finally, IVS-3 (588 bp) interrupts the codon specifying amino acid 43 of mature apo A-I (Fig. 4A). Recent findings indicate that human apo A-I is located approximately 2.6 kb upstream of the apo CIII gene[309] and that both genes are on human chromosome 11.[309a] The apo A-I DNA sequence contains six tandemly repeated 66-bp regions corresponding to codons 99–230. These are highly homologous to each other, and may have originated by internal gene duplications.[306] Based on the amino acid sequence analyses then available for the apoproteins, which included the sequences of apo A-I, apo A-II, apo CI, and apo CIII, it was proposed that the apo A-I gene has been elongated by internal gene duplications[310,311] and that all of the apoproteins were derived from a common ancestral precursor.

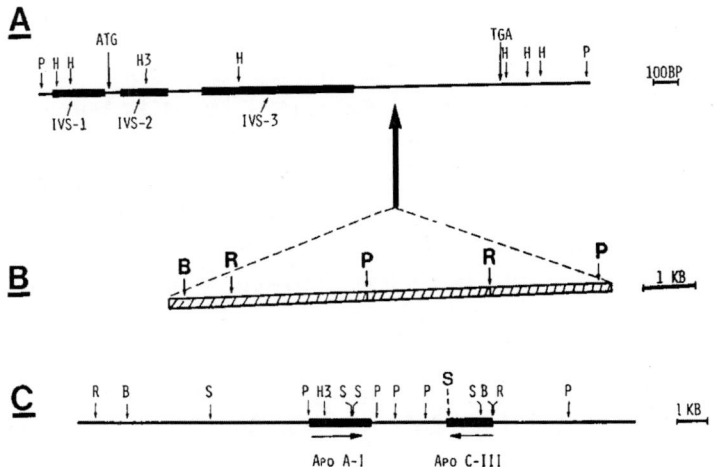

Fig. 4. (A) Restriction map of human apo A-I gene.[306] Thick lines indicate the intervening sequences. (B) Restriction map and position of the DNA element that was inserted in the gene of the patients with apo A-I–apo CIII deficiency.[417,418] (C) Linkage map of human apo A-I and apo CIII genes.[309] Thick lines represent the apo A-I and apo CIII genes. Horizontal arrows beneath the thick lines indicate the direction of transcription of each gene. The dashed line arrow shows the location of the SacI restriction fragment length polymorphism observed in the hypertriglyceridemic patients.[309,479] Restriction sites are: EcoRI (R), BamHI (B), PstI (P), HindIII (H3), HpaII (H).

Apo A-II

Apo A-II contains two identical polypeptide chains of 77 amino acid residues of known sequence,[312] which are linked by a disulfide bond at residue 6. Complexes of apo A-II and apo E arising from mixed disulfide bridges have been observed in plasma[315] and probably involve amino acids 50–55.[316] Apo A-II is synthesized by the liver and to a lesser extent by the small intestine.[19,26] Recent studies have shown that the primary translation product of human apo A-II mRNA consists of 100 amino acids and contains a preprosegment. The presegment (signal peptide) consists of either 17 or 18 amino acids and the prosegment of either 6 or 5 amino acids.[42a,80a] The proposed roles of apo A-II in the activation of hepatic lipase[317,318] and the inhibition of LCAT[6,133,134] are uncertain. The finding that human apo A-II displaces apo A-I from HDL indicates that both proteins occupy overlapping domains on the HDL surface.[319] The physiological significance of this apoprotein requires further investigation.

Apo A-IV

Apo A-IV is a major component of rat HDL and chylomicrons.[320] Human apo A-IV (molecular weight 46,000) has recently been found in lymph, chylomicrons, VLDL, and the $d > 1.21$ g/ml plasma fraction.[168,321–323] In rats, apo A-IV is synthesized by liver and small intestine.[19] Intestinal synthesis of apo A-IV has also been demonstrated in humans.[169] Rat apo A-IV has a 20-amino-acid long signal peptide (43). Human apo A-IV binds to triglyceride emulsions with a Kd of 2.3 μM and can be displaced from these particles by apo CIII or HDL$_2$. The data are consistent with the displacement of apo A-IV from triglyceride rich particles by apo CIII (323a). Nevertheless, the physiological role of apo A-IV requires further clarification.

Apo B

Apo B is the main apoprotein of LDL, comprising approximately 25% of the weight of this particle.[204] The delipidated apoprotein is sensitive to oxidation, and without proper precautions it forms insoluble aggregates of large molecular weight.[324] Apo B is a glycoprotein containing 8–10% carbohydrate terminating in sialic acid. Recent experiments have shown that the carbohydrate is added to apo B cotranslationally in two stages corresponding to the times the native polypeptide has acquired approximately 34% and 80% of its length.[54] Earlier reports suggested that the protein is composed of subunits of 10,000–30,000 molecular weight.[325,326] However, recent studies have shown that human plasma apo B exists in two primary forms, designated B-100 (molecular weight 549,000) and B-48 (246,000).[269] Two other apo B forms designated B-74 (molecular weight 409,000) and B-26 (126,000) may represent degradation products of the B-100 form. Biochemical[264–269] and genetic[327] evidence indicates that the two apo B forms are the products of different genes. Apo B of high (335,000) and low (240,000) molecular weight have been identified in the rat.[57,264–268,328] The 335,000 form is synthesized predominantly by the liver and has a slower catabolic rate, whereas the 240,000 form is synthesized by both liver and intestine and has a faster catabolic rate.[57,2640268] As discussed in section I, 2E, apo B (B-100) is the protein determinant for the cellular recognition and catabolism of LDL by the LDL receptor.[204,206] The structure and function of apo B, as well as the specific roles of apo B forms in lipoprotein metabolism, remain the subject of active investigation.

Apo CI

Apo CI is a single polypeptide chain of 57 amino acid residues of known sequence.[329,330] It is the most basic of the apoproteins and contains nine lysines and three arginines.[329,330] After association with phospholipid vesicles, apo CI increases its α-helical content to 73%.[331] Apo CI activates LCAT, but with 25% of the activity of apo A-I.[134] There are conflicting reports on the role of apo CI in the activation of lipoprotein lipase.[91,332] There is no definitive information on the site of synthesis or the physiological role of this apoprotein.

Apo CII

Apo CII is a polypeptide chain of 78 amino acid residues of known sequence.[333] Newly synthesized apo CII contains an N-terminal signal peptide.[44] Most individuals have one isoprotein form of apo CII; how-ever, variants have been reported,[334] which may represent structural gene mutations. Apo CII synthesis occurs almost exclusively in the liver.[19,25,28] Association of apo CII with phospholipid increases α-helical content from 30% to 45%.[335,336] Apo CII is a potent activator of LPL but not HTL.[85-91] Maximal stimulation of LPL is achieved at a molar ratio of apo CII to enzyme of 1:1. The domain of apo CII that activates LPL has been localized to the 23 COOH-terminal amino acid residues.[337-339] The physiological importance of apo CII in activating LPL has been estab-lished by the finding of individuals with inherited apo CII deficiency who have great difficulty in clearing triglyceride-rich lipoprotein particles from their plasma.[109] Human apo CII has been mapped on chromosome 19.[44]

Apo CIII

Apo CIII is a glycopeptide composed of 79 amino acids of known sequence.[45,340] Newly synthesized apo CIII contains an N-terminal signal peptide (S. K. Karathanasis et al., unpublished data). The polysaccharide moiety contains 1 mole each of galactose and galactosamine and either 0, 1, or 2 moles of sialic acid, which results in three isoproteins, designated CIII-0, CIII-1, and CIII-2, respectively.[44,341] In normal plasma, apo CIII-1, apo CIII-2, and apo CIII-0 comprise approximately 59%, 27%, and 14% of apo CIII, respectively.[342] Recent studies have shown that apo CIII-0 and apo CIII-1 are composed of more than one isoprotein with different molecular weight but the same isoelectric point (Fig. 5).[50] The molecular basis of these isoproteins is not known. Association of apo CIII with phospholipid increases its α-helical content from 22% to 54%.[343] The phospholipid-binding domain of apo CIII is located in the 39 COOH-minal amino acid residues.[344] It has been reported that in rats synthesis of apo CIII occurs in the liver and to a much lesser extent in the small intestine.[19,25,28] However, in recent experiments we have found approxi-mately equal concentrations of apo CIII mRNA in both human liver and intestine.[33a] It has been shown that apo CIII inhibits lipoprotein lipase.[91,345,346] However, the physiological significance of this in vitro inac-tivation is not clear. Recent work has shown that the receptor-mediated hepatic catabolism of lipoproteins that is enhanced by apo E is inhibited by apo CIII.[257,261-263] Finally, recent findings indicate that the apo CIII

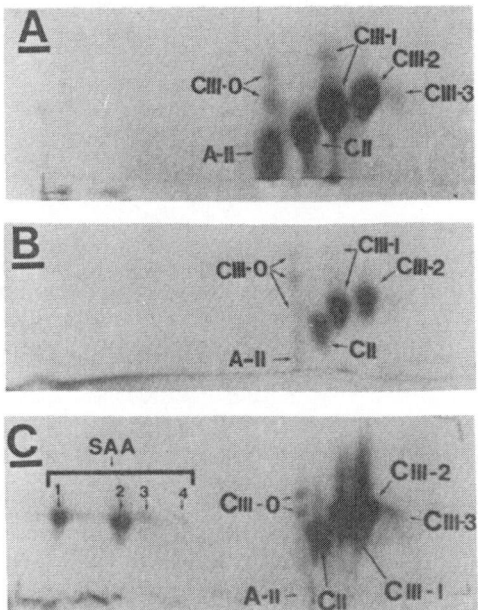

Fig. 5. Two-dimensional PAGE analysis of apo C's, apo A-II, and serum amyloid (SAA) proteins. (A) Protein (300 μg) obtained from human chylomicrons isolated from plasma of nonfasting subject. (B) Protein (100 μg) obtained from human VLDL. (C) Protein (150 μg) obtained from thoracic duct lymph chylomicrons. The positions of apo CIII, apo CII, apo A-II, and SAA are indicated. Note the different forms of apo CIII-0 and apo CIII-1.

gene is located approximately 2.6 kb downstream of the 3′ end of the apo A-I gene. It appears that the coding-like DNA sequences of the two genes are on opposite DNA strands, which would require convergent transcription of these two genes (Fig. 4C).[309] As previously noted, both genes are located on human chromosome 11.[309a]

Apo D

Apo D, originally designated apo A-III,[347] is a glycoprotein found in HDL and the $d > 1.21$ g/ml fraction[348] and contains 18% carbohydrate by weight.[349] Earlier reports indicated a molecular weight of 22,000[347,350]; however, recent estimates indicate that the protein has a molecular weight of 32,500–35,000[49,152] and is composed of three isoproteins.[49] There are conflicting reports on the role of apo D in the activation of

LCAT[140,351,352] as well as on its function in the transfer of cholesteryl esters.[49,152,155] Thus, the physiological significance of this apoprotein remains uncertain.

Apo E

Apolipoprotein E (apo E) was first identified in 1973 in human VLDL[353] and has subsequently been found in various lipoprotein classes of all mammalian species studied.[354,355] It is a single polypeptide chain composed of 299 amino acid residues of known sequence.[356] Apo E synthesis has been demonstrated in liver, kidney, adrenal gland, and reticuloendothelial cells.[10,11,18,19,25,28,31-33,42] High-resolution 2D-PAGE of human plasma apo E has shown it to consist of several isoproteins that differ in size and/or charge. This complexity of human apo E is the result of both genetic variation of apo E in the human population and post-translational modification of apo E with carbohydrate chains containing sialic acid.[357,358] The genetic polymorphism of apo E is further discussed in section II, (p. 166). Present evidence indicates that human apo E is synthesized as a 317-amino acid-long preprotein and undergoes intracellular proteolysis and glycosylation[42] and extracellular desialation[25,28,42,355,358] to attain the major asialo apo E isoprotein form observed in plasma (Figs. 1E to 1I). Apo E desialation may play an important as yet undefined role in lipoprotein metabolism.[25,28,42,359] Recent studies have shown that apo E mediates lipoprotein catabolism by both extrahepatic[208,245,246] and hepatic tissues.[237,256,258] Extrahepatic tissues catabolize apo E-containing lipoproteins by the LDL (apo B/E) receptor.[208,245,246] Hepatic tissues catabolize apo E-containing lipoproteins by the LDL (apo B/E) receptor as well as by the chylomicron remnant (apo E) receptor.[237,256,258] Binding studies using phospholipid vesicles containing fragments of apo E (359a) as well as the inhibition of apo E binding by monoclonal antibodies [359b] have localized the receptor binding domain of apo E. This domain is in the region between residues 139 to 169. Structural mutations in apo E dramatically affect its recognition and catabolism by lipoprotein receptors.[360-364] Nutritional experiments involving cholesterol feeding in animals result in the accumulation in plasma of lipoprotein particles designated HDL with apo E, βVLDL, and IDL, which are enriched in cholesteryl ester and apo E[355,365-369] and have a high affinity for the LDL receptor and chylomicron remnant receptors.[208,237,245,246,256,258] Type II hyperlipoproteinemia patients on normal diets show alterations in plasma lipoproteins similar to those seen after cholesterol feeding, including increased plasma apo E content and β VLDL.[275-279,298,299,355,370,371] The accumulation of apo E-rich lipoproteins in plasma observed following cholesterol feeding of experimental animals or in type III hyperlipoproteinemia patients on normal diets may reflect either increased apo E synthesis,[372] saturation of the clearance mechanism for apo E-containing lipoproteins,[354] or a combination of both processes.[253] The gene for human apo E has been isolated and characterized, and is approximately 3.6 kb long and contains at least three intervening sequences.[373] Similar to apo A-I, human apo E contains six tandemly repeated, 66-bp regions corresponding to amino acids 62–239. These regions are highly homologous to each other and may have originated by an internal gene duplication.[373] Human apo E has been mapped to chromosome 19.[374]

Other Apoproteins

Apo F and apo G are minor proteins present in HDL. The former has a molecular weight of 26,000–32,000 and isoelectric point of 3.7,[375] and the latter has a molecular weight of 72,000.[376] Apo H or β2-glycoprotein-I[377-379] is a glycoprotein of molecular weight 40,000–43,000 present in HDL and the $d > 1.21$ g/ml fraction.[377] It is composed of 18% carbohydrate by weight and contains sialic acid.[380] Apo H binds with high affinity to chylomicrons and artificial triglyceride emulsions[381] and acts synergistically with apo CII in the activation of lipoprotein lipase.[378] Proline-rich protein (PRP) has been isolated from chylomicrons and has a molecular weight of 74,000.[382] A group of two major and four minor proteins designated as serum amyloid A proteins (SAA) have been found as components of HDL and intestinal chylomicrons (Fig. 5B; V. I. Zannis et al., unpublished data).[383-387] The proteins are synthesized by the liver[386] and intestine (V. I Zannis et al., unpublished data). They have approximately the same molecular weight (11,000) but different isoelectric points. The two major human amyloid proteins, apo SAA_1 and apo SAA_2, have very similar amino acid compositions and N-terminal amino acid sequences. However, apo SAA_2 lacks the N-terminal arginine residue that is found in SAA_1.[387] Human apo SAA_1 is a polypeptide composed of 104 amino acids of known sequence.[388] Cleavage of the COOH-terminal hexapeptide 99–104 of SAA_1 generates the amyloid protein that accumulates in tissues in certain inflammatory conditions.[388] In contrast to the human proteins, a recent report indicates that the two SAA proteins of the mouse may be products of different genes.[389] The physiological significance of all these proteins for lipoprotein metabolism and their firm classification as apoproteins require further investigation.

MUTATIONS IN THE PATHWAY OF LIPOPROTEIN METABOLISM

Mutations in LDL Receptor Pathway

Familial hypercholesterolemia (FH) is an autosomal dominant disorder characterized by elevated plasma LDL levels, xanthomas, and premature atherosclerosis.[206,390,391] The estimated frequency of heterozygotes with this disease is 1/500 and of homozygotes 1/1,000,000.[206,392] Cells from patients with FH have a defect in the LDL receptor pathway.[204,206,393–396] Based on LDL binding to cultured fibroblasts, Brown, Goldstein, and colleagues originally described three different types of LDL receptor defects.[204] Evidence indicates that these are the result of mutations at a single genetic locus that specifies the LDL receptor.[206,219,220,222] The most common type, designated receptor negative R^{b0}, specifies a receptor that has no detectable binding activity.[202,206,229,230] The second most frequent type, designated receptor defective R^{b-}, specifies a receptor that has markedly reduced (2–30% of normal) binding activity.[206,393] The third type, designated internalization defective $R^{b+,i0}$, is rare and specifies a receptor that has normal binding activity but cannot transport the LDL–receptor complex into the cell.[206,394,395] Fibroblast cultures from homozygotes for the R^{b0} allele fail to bind LDL and also fail to suppress HMG-CoA reductase activity and stimulate ACAT activity when LDL is added to the cell culture medium.[202,229,230] Ultrastructural studies confirm the fact that LDL receptors, which are normally located in fuzzy coated regions of the fibroblast surface, are not present in such mutant cells.[211] Fibroblasts from patients homozygous for the R^{b-} allele or from phenotypic homozygotes who are genetic compounds for R^{b-} and R^{b0} alleles[206,393] display 2–30% of normal LDL binding activity.[204,206] The

LDL-induced suppression of HMG-CoA reductase activity and stimulation of ACAT activity in mutant fibroblast cultures correlates with their residual LDL binding activity.[393,397] Diminished LDL binding activity in mutant fibrobalst is due either to decreased number or reduced affinity of LDL receptors.[397] Fibroblasts from subjects heterozygous for one normal and either the R^{b0} or R^{b-} alleles have approximately half normal LDL binding activity.[206,398,399] Their LDL binding activity correlates with their ability to suppress HMG-CoA reductase activity and stimulate ACAT activity when LDL is added to the culture medium. Analysis of fibroblasts from three probands with phenotypic homozygous FH and their families has revealed an internalization defective allele for the LDL receptor locus, designated $R^{b+,i0}$.[206,394–396] Fibroblasts from phenotypic homozygotes are either homozygous for the $R^{b+,i0}$ allele[396] or genetic compounds for the $R^{b+,i0}$ and R^{b0} alleles[206,394,395] and show normal LDL binding but fail to internalize LDL, suppress HMG-CoA reductase stimulate ACAT, or regulate LDL binding when LDL is added to the culture medium. Ultrastructural studies indicate that bound LDL does not cluster in the coated pit region but is randomly distributed along the cell membrane.[400,401] On the basis of these biochemical, ultrastructural, and genetic studies, Goldstein and Brown have proposed that the LDL receptor molecule has at least two active sites, one that mediates LDL binding on the external surface of the cell membrane and another that mediates LDL internalization on the cytoplasmic surface of the cell membrane.[206,221] Interaction of the internalization site with another membrane protein (possibly clathrin) may result in the clustering of receptors in the coated pit region of the membrane. According to this model, the product of the $R^{b+,i0}$ allele has a mutation that affects the internalization domain of the LDL receptor.

Further insight into the molecular basis of LDL receptor defects has been obtained by studies of the synthesis and intracellular post-translational modification of these receptors[219,220,222] by cultured fibroblasts from different individuals with phenotypic homozygous familial hypercholesterolemia. Three well-defined and possibly a fourth class of mutations have been identified in these studies:

1. Mutations in which no immunologically detectable receptor is synthesized.[219,222] These mutations result from a null allele designated RO. The relative frequency of this allele in the population of FH homozygotes was estimated to be $\geq 16\%$.

2. Mutations in which a receptor precursor (usually 120,000 molec-

ular weight) is synthesized but not processed to the mature form (usually 160,000 molecular weight).[219,222] Three different alleles have been found and designated $R100$, $R120$, and $R135$. They produce receptors of molecular weight 100,000, 120,000, and 135,000, respectively, which cannot be transported to the cell surface.[222] These defects may represent a structural mutation in the LDL receptor domain involved in post-translational modification or in the signal sequences that are necessary for the transport of the receptors from the endoplasmic reticulum to the cell surface.[222]

3. Mutations in which the receptor is synthesized, processed normally, but either cannot bind LDL normally or be internalized.[219,222] Three alleles have been defined in this category and have been designated $R100 \rightarrow 140$, $R120 \rightarrow 160$, and $R170 \rightarrow 210$. These alleles synthesize receptors of 100,000, 120,000, and 170,000 molecular weight, which are processed to 140,000, 160,000, and 210,000 molecular weight, respectively, and are transported to the cell surface.[220,222] In this category also belongs the product of the $R^{b+,i0}$ allele of one of the LDL internalization defective patients which is indistinguishable from normal by two-dimensional gel electrophoresis.[220,393,396] Finally, 31 patients representing 40% of the FH homozygotes studied[222] have both the precursor (120,000 molecular weight) and the mature (160,000 molecular weight) form of the LDL receptor. This may result from homozygosity for a new type of mutant allele that produces a form of 120,000-molecular weight receptor that is processed slowly to a 160,000 molecular weight form. Alternatively, the patients may be heterozygous, having an $R120$ and an $R120 \rightarrow 160$ mutant allele. It is obvious from these studies that considerable genetic heterogeneity exists in the structural LDL receptor locus.

The originally defined R^{b0}, R^{b-}, and $R^{b+,i0}$ alleles, detected on the basis of LDL binding and internalization assays, represent three families of alleles each with different mutations. The newly defined RO, $R100$, $R120$, $R135$, and the $R100 \rightarrow 140$ structural alleles correspond to the R^{b0} allele. The majority (76%) of the $R120 \rightarrow 160$ mutant alleles, the alleles that are processed slowly, as well as the $R170 \rightarrow 210$ alleles correspond to the R^{b-} allele. As already mentioned, one of the $R^{b+,i0}$ alleles corresponds to one of the $R120 \rightarrow 160$ mutant structural alleles.[220] The detailed relationship of the functional R^{b0}, R^{b0}, and $R^{b+,i0}$ alleles to the structural alleles is provided in Ref. 222. At present, there are no known mutations in the other types of lipoprotein receptors described.

Mutations in Apoproteins

Tangier Disease: A defect in the Apo A-I Isoprotein 2 to Apo A-I Isoprotein 4 Conversion?*

Tangier disease, first described by Fredrickson *et al.* in 1961,[402] is a rare autosomal recessive disorder of lipoprotein metabolism characterized by extremely low levels of plasma HDL cholesterol and extensive tissue cholesteryl ester storage.[5,402,403] Previous studies have shown that Tangier plasma contains very low levels of apo A-I, of which over 90% is found in the $d > 1.21$ g/ml fraction.[5,404,409] In contrast, Tangier intestinal epithelial cells contain normal amounts of apo A-I, as demonstrated by immunofluorescent antibody techniques.[17,410] These observations suggest that the defect in Tangier disease might not be in apo A-I synthesis but rather in apo A-I post-translational modification, resulting in enhanced apo A-I catabolism.[25,27,28] To further explore this possibility, plasma and intestinal apo A-I isoproteins of normal subjects and Tangier patients were studied.[80] As shown in Figs. 6A and 6B, this comparison, and similar ones involving three other cases of Tangier disease, indicate that 40–70% of Tangier apo A-I consists of isoprotein 2, whereas this isoprotein represents <2% of total plasma apo A-I in normal subjects (Fig. 6A). These experiments suggest that the defect in Tangier disease may involve apo A-I post-translational modification. In further experiments, Tangier intestine in organ culture[27,28] secreted normal amounts of apo A-I with an apo A-I isoprotein pattern indistinguishable from normal by 2D-PAGE (Figs. 6C and 6D).[80] This finding rules out the possibility of a type of apo A-I structural gene mutation in Tangier disease that produces an even more basic set of intestinal isoproteins, which upon subsequent normal post-translational modification might generate the predominately more basic than normal plasma apo A-I isoproteins seen in Tangier patients. The apparent accumulation of apo A-I$_2$ in the plasma of Tangier patients could be the result of a structural mutation in the apo A-I gene that results in a slower apo A-I$_2$ to apo A-I$_4$ conversion or an unstable conversion product. Alternatively, the Tangier defect could be the result of a defective apo A-I$_2$ to apo A-I$_4$ converting protease.[27,28,39,80] Apo A-I from the two obligate heterozygous children of one of the Tangier patients has a normal isoprotein composition but half-normal HDL and apo A-I levels.[80] This observation implies that the apo A-I$_2$ to apo A-I$_4$

conversion is rate-limiting in Tangier homozygotes as well as heterozygotes or that the product of the mutant apo A-I allele is unstable and hypercatabolized. Since Tangier patients are characterized by very low levels of plasma HDL, these observations would suggest that apo A-I$_2$ to apo A-I$_4$ conversion may be necessary for maintaining normal plasma apo A-I and HDL levels.

Other Human Genetic Variations in Apo A-I and HDL

The first structural mutation of apo A-I described was found in Italy and has been called apo A-I Milano.[411,412] Subsequently, other apo A-I variants were described and named apo A-I Giessen and apo A-I Marburg.[5,413] The patient with apo A-I Marburg had hypertriglyceridemia

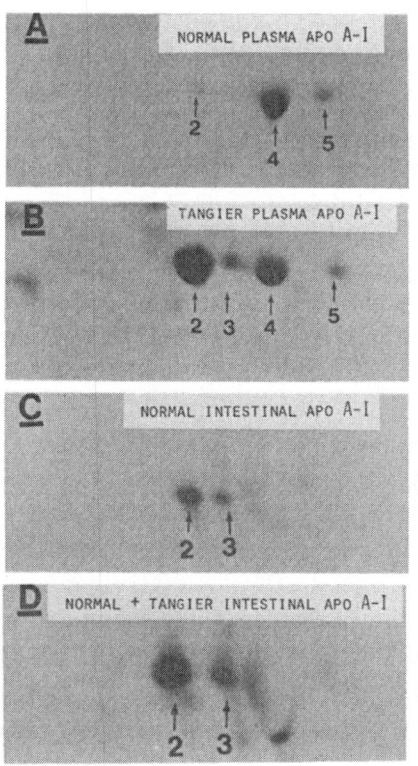

Fig. 6. Comparison of normal and Tangier plasma and intestinal apo A-I by 2D-PAGE and/or autoradiography. Aliquots of normal and Tangier lipoprotein-free ($d > 1.21$ g/ml) plasma were immunoprecipitated with anti-apo A-I antibodies as explained in Ref. 80. The resulting immunoprecipitates were analyzed by 2D-PAGE. (A,B) Normal (15 μg) and Tangier (35 μg) apo A-I immunoprecipitated from lipoprotein-free plasma. (C,D) Normal and Tangier intestinal apo A-I isoproteins by 2D-PAGE and autoradiography. Aliquots of medium obtained from intestinal organ cultures grown in media containing ^{35}S-methionine were mixed with carrier HDL, immunoprecipitated, and analyzed as explained in Refs. 27, 28, and 80. (C) An autoradiogram derived from 2D-PAGE analysis of an immunoprecipitate obtained from organ cultures of normal intestine. The same pattern was obtained by analyzing an immunoprecipitate obtained from organ culture of Tangier intestine.[80] (D) An autoradiogram derived from 2D-PAGE analysis of a mixture of the two immunoprecipitates derived from normal and Tangier intestinal organ cultures. Each immunoprecipitate contained 15,000 cpm. Note that the normal and Tangier apo A-I isoproteins overlap.

and reduced HDL cholesterol levels.[413] Subjects with apo A-I Milano have low HDL cholesterol and apo A-I levels, but do not appear to suffer from premature atherosclerotic disease.[411] Further analysis indicated that the mutant apo A-I Milano allele results from a structural mutation that causes a 173 arg → cys substitution.[414] The product of the variant apo A-I allele is more acidic by one charge unit than the product of the normal allele. Affected individuals appear to be heterozygotes and carry one normal and one variant apo A-I allele.[414] Four other heterozygote variants of apo A-I have been described recently. Three of these variants have resulted from a Asp103 → Asn, Pro3 → His, and Pro4 → Arg substitution, respectively, and the fifth has resulted from a deletion of Lys107.[414a] Patients with the other apo A-I variants, apo A-I Marburg and apo A-I Giessen, also represent heterozygosity for one normal and one variant allele. The variant alleles of apo A-I Marburg and apo A-I Giessen produce a gene product that differs from wild type by −1 and + 1 charges, respectively. The apo A-I Giessen results from a Pro143 → Arg substitution and is deficient in its ability to activate LCAT.[414a] Screening of approximately 400 human subjects in our laboratory revealed one heterozygote apo A-I phenotype with low HDL levels. This phenotype is similar to apo A-I Giessen, although it may represent a different mutation (Figs. 7A and 7B). Following the nomenclature system adopted for human apo E,[415] and assuming that the apo A-I phenotypes observed originate from α-14, and α-13, and α-12 alleles, apo A-I phenotypes can be designated A-13/3 (the common phenotype), apo A-14/3 (the Giessen phenotype), and apo A-13/2 (the Milano and Marburg phenotypes). The relationships of the isoelectric points of the major normal and variant apo A-I isoproteins are shown in Fig. 7C.

Several cases have been described in the literature, distinct from Tangier disease, with apo A-I and HDL deficiency. In one family Norum[416] described two sisters with severe premature atherosclerosis, HDL, apo A-I, and apo CIII deficiency. Analysis of the apo A-I gene structure of these individuals revealed that they have at least a 6.5-kb insertion in the coding region adjacent to the 3' end of the third intervening sequence in the apo A-I gene (Fig. 3B).[417,418] Other cases of familial HDL cholesterol deficiency have been described.[419,423] One of these conditions was associated with severe premature atherosclerosis,[423] and another, known as Fish Eye disease, was associated with atherosclerosis at old age.[421] Recent studies have also shown that low levels of HDL cholesterol and apo A-I can be inherited in an autosomal dominant

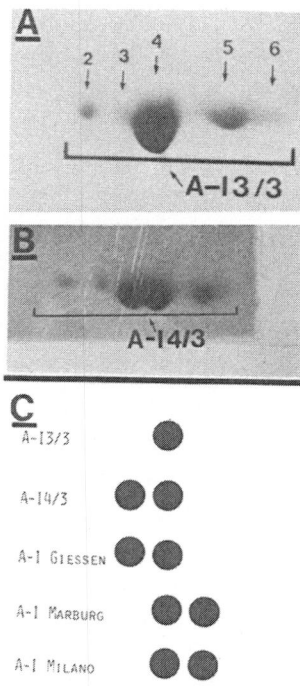

Fig. 7. Two-dimensional PAGE patterns of the different apo A-I phenotypes observed in humans. (A) Homozygous phenotype A-I3/3. (B) Heterozygous phenotype A-I4/3. (C) Schematic presentation of the relationship of apo A-I phenotypes shown in A and B and those described in Refs. 411–414. Only the major plasma apo A-I isoproteins produced by the different alleles are shown. Differences exist in the relative concentration of the major isoproteins of some of the heterozygous phenotypes.[411–414] For simplicity, the concentration of these isoproteins is arbitrarily presented as equal.

mode. This condition has been named hypoalphalipoproteinemia and is associated with premature atherosclerosis.[424] It is also interesting that human subjects have been identified who have high levels of plasma HDL cholesterol and apo A-I. This condition has been named hyperalphalipoproteinemia,[425–428] is inherited in an autosomal dominant mode,[427] and is thought to protect individuals from atherosclerosis.[426] It is possible that some of these hyper- or hypoalphalipoproteinemias may represent structural or regulatory apo A-I gene mutations.

Apolipoprotein E and Type III Hyperlipoproteinemia (Type III HLP)

Genetic Variation and Post-Translational Modification of Human Apo E. Recent studies have shown that human apo E consists of several isoproteins that differ in size and/or charge. In the early stages of these studies, two distinct electrophoretic patterns of apo E were observed and were designated apo E classes β and α (Figs. 8A and 8B).[357,358,429] Following a recently adopted uniform nomenclature,[415] the apo E classes (and subclasses) we had described are now referred to as apo E phenotypes. The α phenotype has two major asialo apo E isoproteins, of apparent molecular weight 38,000 (determined by SDS polyacrylamide gel electrophoresis in 12% gels), and at least six sialo apo E (apo E_s) isoproteins. In contrast, the β phenotype has only one major asialo apo E isoprotein, of apparent molecular weight 38,000 and at least three sialo apo E isoproteins. The sialo apo E isoproteins, which are more acidic and have slightly higher molecular weight than the asialo apo E isoproteins, are converted to the corresponding asialo isoprotein forms upon treatment of apo E with *Clostridium perfringens* neuraminidase (Figs. 8C and 8D).[25,28,358] We have found that newly secreted apo E has a higher sialo content than plasma apo E (81 $\pm$ 11% versus 24 $\pm$ 6%) (Figs. 1H and 1I).[25,28,42,359] Increased sialation is also observed in apo E secreted by perfused monkey and guinea pig livers and cultured human and mouse monocyte-macrophages.[32,369] Extracellular desialation must therefore occur as a normal step in apo E metabolism, and we have recently shown that apo E from the plasma of four Tangier patients contains excessive amounts of sialo apo E.[359] This observation suggests that the metabolic defect in Tangier disease, which is believed to be an inability to convert apo A-I from its secreted form to the mature plasma form,[80] disrupts the normal phys-

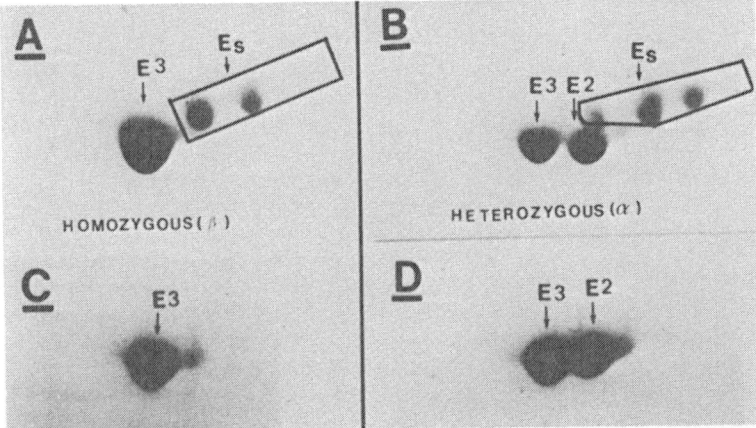

Fig. 8. Two-dimensional PAGE patterns of two easily distinguishable β and α apo E phenotypes. (A) The homozygous (β) and (B) heterozygous (α) apo E phenotypes. Note the multiplicity of apo E isoproteins that comprise the β and α apo E phenotypes. Also shown are (C) homozygous (β) and (D) heterozygous (α) phenotypes following treatment with *C. perfringens* neuraminidase.

iological events leading to apo E desialation in plasma. This finding is also consistent with the hypothesis that apo E is secreted as sialo apo E *in vivo* and that the increased sialation of newly secreted apo E observed in the organ and cell culture experiments is not an artifact of the culture conditions. The physiological significance of apo E sialation is not known. One possibility is that sialation is required for apo E secretion; another is that sialation may prevent liver cells from recognizing, internalizing, and catabolizing apo E just after it has been secreted.

Genetic Polymorphism of Human Apo E Is Explained by Three Common Alleles at a Single Genetic Locus. Comparison of apo E patterns between human subjects revealed additional genetic heterogeneity within the α and β apo E phenotypes. A total of six different apo E phenotypes were established by mixing equal quantities of VLDL obtained from different subjects with either α or β apo E patterns and analyzing the mixture by 2D-PAGE. These experiments allows us to distinguish three homozygous (β) and three heterozygous (α) phenotypes of apo E. The homozygous phenotypes have been designated E4/4 (βII), E3/3 (βIII), E2/2 (βIV), and the heterozygous phenotypes E4/3 (αII), E3/2 (αIII), and E4/2 (αIV) (Fig. 9).[357,358,429] Typical mixing experiments of dif-

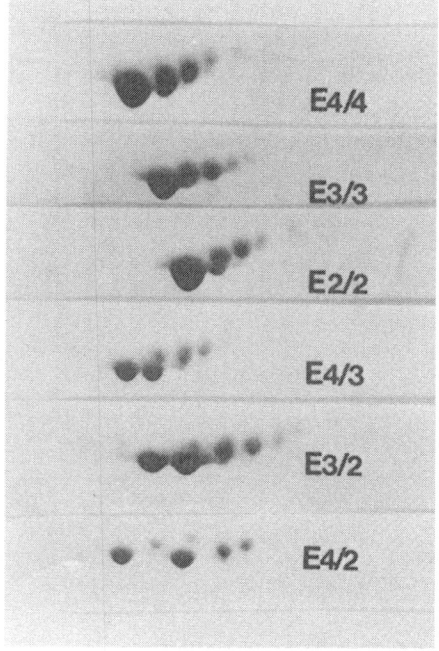

Fig. 9. Two-dimensional PAGE patterns of the six pattern apo E phenotypes observed in humans. The designations are indicated.

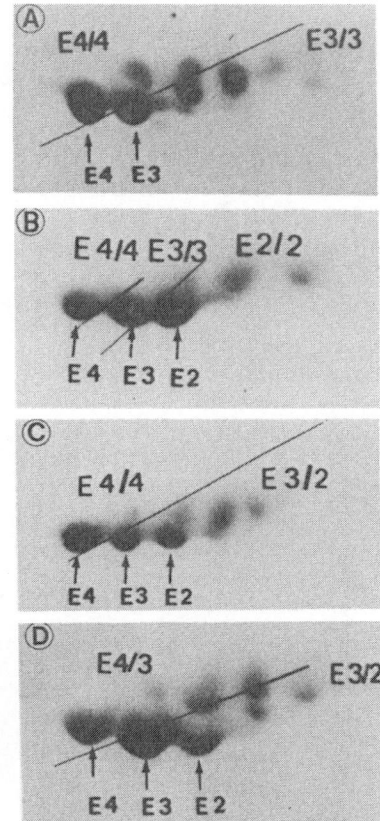

Fig. 10. Two-dimensional PAGE of mixtures of VLDL fractions obtained from individuals with different apo E phenotypes: (A) 25 μg of E4/4 and 15 μg of E3/3; (B) 20 μg of E4/4, 20; μg of E3/3, and 30 μg of E2/2; (C) 20 μg of E4/4 and 20 μg of E3/2; (D) 20 μg of E4/3 and 20 μg of E3/2. The phenotypes that were mixed and the major isoproteins of each phenotype are indicated.

ferent apo E phenotypes are shown in Figs. 10A–10D. These experiments showed that a defined homology of isoelectric points and molecular weights existed between isoproteins belonging to different apo E phenotypes.

The observation that the α phenotypes could be mimicked by mixing two different β phenotypes suggested that the apo E phenotypes were genetically determined and that the α and β phenotypes represented heterozygosity and homozygosity, respectively, for various apo E alleles. To substantiate this hypothesis, we have studied the inheritance of apo E phenotypes in 34 families where both parents and total of 84 children were phenotyped. These studies, summarized in Table IV, are compatible with the following genetic model (Fig. 11A). Apo E phenotypes are specified at a single structural gene locus with three alleles: ε4 (εII), ε3, (εIII), and ε2 (εIV). Individuals homozygous for alleles ε4, ε3, and ε2 have the

Table IV. Expected Versus Observed Apo E Phenotypes of Offspring in Families Where Both Parents Were Sampled

Family	Parents	Number of children	Children (observed)	Children (expected)
1	E4/3, E3/2	2	1 E4/2, 1 E4/3	0.5 E4/3, 0.5 E3/2, 0.5 E4/2, 0.5 E3/3
2	E3/3, E4/2	2	1 E4/3, 1E3/2	1 E4/3, 1 E3/2
3	E4/3, E4/3	2	1 E4/3, 1 E3/3	1 E4/3, 0.5 E4/4, 0.5 E3/3
4	E4/4, E4/3	2	1 E4/3, 1E4/4	1 E4/3, 1 E4/4
5	E3/3, E3/2	6	4 E3/2, 2 E3/3	3 E3/2, 3 E3/3
6	E3/2, E3/3	4	3 E3/2, 1 E3/3	2 E3/2, 2 E3/3
7	E3/3, E3/3	3	3 E3/3	3 E3/3
8	E3/2, E3/2	2	1 E3/2, 1 E2/2	0.5 E3/3, 1 E3/2, 0.5 E2/2
9	E4/2, E4/3	3	2 E4/4, 1 E4/2	0.75 E4/4, 0.75 E4/3, 0.75 E3/2, 0.75 E4/2
10	E2/2, E3/3	5	5 E3/2	5 E3/2
11	E4/2, E3/3	2	2 E3/2	1 E4/3, 1 E3/2
12	E2/2, E4/2	3	1 E4/2, 2 E2/2	1.5 E4/2, 1.5 E2/2
13	E2/2, E4/2	5	3 E4/2, 2 E2/2	2.5 E4/2, 2.5 E2/2
14	E2/2, E3/2	2	2 E3/2	1 E3/2, 1 E2/2
15	E2/2, E3/2	2	2 E3/2	1 E3/2, 1 E2/2
16	E3/2, E3/2	3	2 E3/2, 1 E2/2	0.75 E3/3, 1.5 E3/2, 0.75 E2/2
17	E3/2, E3/3	2	2 E3/3	1 E3/3, 1 E3/2
18	E2/2, E3/3	2	2 E3/2	2 E3/2
19	E3/2, E4/2	2	1 E4/2, 1 E2/2	0.5 E4/3, 0.5 E3/2, 0.5 E4/2, 0.5 E2/2
20	E2/2, E4/3	2	2 E4/2	1 E4/2, 1 E3/2
21	E2/2, E4/3	2	2 E3/2	1 E4/2, 1 E3/2
22	E3/3, E2/2	2	2 E3/2	2 E3/2
23	E3/3, E2/2	2	2 E3/2	2 E3/2
24	E2/2, E4/3	1	1 E3/2	0.5 E4/2 0.5 E3/2
25	E2/2, E3/3	2	2 E3/2	2 E3/2
26	E4/2, E3/2	3	1 E4/3, 1 E3/2, 1 E2/2	0.75 E4/3, 0.75 E4/2, 0.75 E3/2, 0.75 E2/2
27	E3/3, E2/2	1	1 E3/2	1 E3/2
28	E3/3, E3/2	3	2 E3/2, 1 E3/3	1.5 E3/2, 1.5 E3/3
29	E3/2, E3/3	4	2 E3/2, 2 E3/3	2 E3/2, 2 E3/3
30	E3/2, E3/2	1	1 E2/2	0.25 E3/3, 0.5 E3/2, 0.25 E2/2
31	E2/2, E3/3	3	3 E3/2	3 E3/2
32	E2/2, E3/2	2	2 E3/2	1 E3/2, 1 E2/2
33	E3/3, E2/2	1	1 E3/2	1 E3/2
34	E3/3, E2/2	1	1 E3/2	1 E3/2

	E4/4	E3/3	E2/2	E4/3	E3/2	E4/2	Total
Expected[a]	2.25	15.00	9.75	6.50	41.50	9.00	84
Observed	3.00	12.00	9.00	5.00	46.00	9.00	84

[a] χ^2 analysis with five degrees of freedom indicated that the expected and observed apo E phenotypes were compatible with a χ^2 of 1.74 ($0.8 < p < 0.9$).

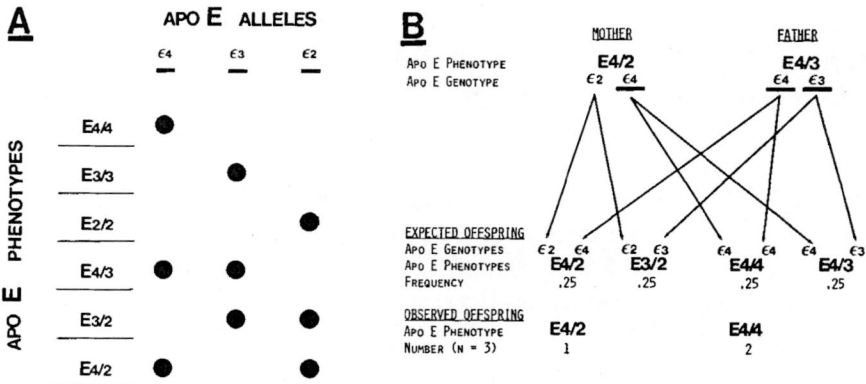

Fig. 11. (A) Schematic representation of the single-structural gene-locus, three-allele model of apo E inheritance. Closed circles represent the major asialo apo E isoproteins. (B) Schematic representation of the inheritance of apo E phenotypes based on the single-structural gene-locus, three-allele model of apo E inheritance.

apo E phenotypes E4/4, E3/3, and E2/2, respectively. Individuals heterozygous for apo E alleles have the apo E phenotypes E4/3, E3/2, and E4/2, which correspond to genotypes $\epsilon4;\epsilon3$, $\epsilon3;\epsilon2$, and $\epsilon4,\epsilon2$, respectively. Examples of inheritance of apo E phenotypes are shown in Fig. 11B and Table IV. Figure 11B also shows that parents with phenotypes E4/3 and E4/2 (heterozygous for the $\epsilon4$ allele) can produce offspring with the apo E phenotype E4/4. This observation provides direct evidence that the apo E allele $\epsilon4$ is at the same locus as the apo E allele, $\epsilon3$ and $\epsilon2$. In the 34 families studied, the frequencies of the apo E phenotypes in the children are compatible with the model proposed. In addition, there were no families that produced offspring that had apo E phenotypes incompatible with the proposed model.

In further studies, we have analyzed the apo E phenotypes of 152 normal volunteers (individuals without hyperlipidemia or atherosclerosis). The phenotype frequencies were E4/4 = 0.03, E3/3 = 0.58, E2/2 = 0.013, E4/3 = 0.14, E3/2 = 0.22, and E4/2 = 0.02. Therefore, in this population, the apo E alleles occurred with frequencies of $\epsilon4$ = 0.12, $\epsilon3$ = 0.75, and $\epsilon2$ = 0.13. If we assume a Hardy–Weinberg distribution of the apo E alleles, the apo E phenotype frequencies should be E4/4 = 0.014, E3/3 = 0.56, E2/2 = 0.017, E4/3 = 0.18, E3/2 = 0.195, and E4/2 = 0.031. The genetic model we proposed has been verified in independent studies by three other groups.[430–432] The apo E allele frequencies have also been assessed by others. In Germany apo E phenotypes were assessed in 1031 blood bank donors and the apo E allele frequencies were

$\epsilon4 = 0.15$, $\epsilon3 = 0.77$, and $\epsilon2 = 0.08$.[430] An analysis of 426 blood bank donors in New Zealand gave apo E allele frequencies of $\epsilon4 = 0.16$, $\epsilon3 = 0.72$, and $\epsilon2 = 0.12$.[431] The minor differences in apo E allele frequencies among these studies may be due to selection bias or reflect true genetic differences between the populations studied.

Apo E Phenotypes Demonstrated to Be the Result of Structural Mutations in the Apo E Gene.* The first evidence of genetic polymorphism of human apo E was obtained by Utermann and colleagues.[433-435] On the basis of the family studies and the 2D-PAGE experiments presented above, we had proposed that the apo E phenotypes were the result of structural mutations in the apo E gene. This hypothesis has been verified recently by amino acid sequence analysis of apo E obtained from individuals with homozygous apo E phenotypes.[356,364,436] The protein sequence studies have identified four polymorphic amino acid sites at positions 112, 145, 146, and 158. In the most common apo E polypeptide E3, specified by the $\epsilon3$ allele, these sites have the following amino acids: 112 Cys, 145 Arg, 146 Lys, and 158 Arg.[356,436] The polypeptide one charge unit more basic than E3, specified by the $\epsilon4$ allele, differs from E3 by a 112 Cys to Arg substitution.[356,436] The polypeptides one charge unit more acidic than E3 differ from E3 by either a 158 Arg to Cys, a 145 Arg to Cys, or a 146 Lys to Gln substitution.[364,437] These alleles have been designated $\epsilon2$, $\epsilon2^*$, and $\epsilon2^{**}$, respectively.[364,437] Individuals may possess the E2/2 phenotype with any combination of the $\epsilon2$, $\epsilon2^*$, and $\epsilon2^{**}$ alleles. An electrophoretic variant of apo E designated apo E1 has been found in heterozygote E3/1[437a,b] and E2/1 phenotypes.[437b, and Zannis et al., unpublished data] One of the apo E1 proteins results from a Gly127 → Asp and an Arg158 → Cys substitution. These data show that within a given apo E phenotype there can be genetic heterogeneity. This concept is further supported by data to be discussed in section II,2C5 that show the association of apo E phenotypes other than E2/2 with type III HLP.[438] In addition to structural mutations, other significant variations may exist in the apo E gene, as suggested by the recent report of an individual with undetectable amounts of plasma apo E who presented with a type III HLP phenotype.[439]

In recent studies, DNA inserts carrying the apo E gene were obtained from cDNA and genomic clones. DNA sequence analysis of the human apo E gene also supports the concept that the apo E alleles are due to mutations in the apo E structural gene. These studies show that at the polymorphic amino acid sites, the codons specifying the most common apo E allele $\epsilon3$ were residue 112 TGC, 145 CGT, 146 AAG, and 158

Allele	Codon at the Polymorphic Site				Base Substitution Relative To ε3 Allele		Amino Acid Substitution Relative To E3/3 Phenotype	Diagram of Apo E Sequence Variations
	112	145	146	158				
ε3	TGC	CGT	AAG	CGC	None		None	Cys-112 Arg-145 Lys-146 Arg-158
ε4	CGC	Same	Same	Same	T	C	112Cys Arg	Arg-112 Arg-145 Lys-146 Arg-158
ε2	Same	Same	Same	TGC	C	T	158Arg Cys	Cys-112 Arg-145 Lys-146 Cys-158
ε2*	Same	TGT	Same	Same	C	T	145Arg Cys	Arg-112 Cys-145 Lys-146 Arg-158
ε2**	Same	Same	CAG	Same	A	C	146Lys Gln	Cys-112 Arg-145 Gln-146 Arg-158

Fig. 12. Schematic representation of the human apo E alleles. The polymorphic sites, nucleotides, and corresponding amino acid substitutions are indicated.[354,437,441]

CGC.[440] A single base substitution in the first nucleotide of each of these codons could account for the amino acid substitutions observed by protein sequence analysis of the variant apo E gene products. A TGC (Cys) to CGC (Arg) substitution has been recently observed in the sequence corresponding to amino acid 112 of the plasma apo E (J. L. Breslow *et al.*, unpublished data). The specific nucleotide and amino acid changes that lead to the different apo E phenotypes and genotypes are shown in Fig. 12.

Apo E Phenotype E2/2 Is Associated with Type III HLP. Familial type III HLP, also called familial dysbetalipoproteinemia, broad β, or floating β disease, is characterized by premature atherosclerosis, xanthomas, elevated cholesterol and triglyceride levels, cholesterol enriched βVLDL and IDL particles, and increased plasma apo E levels.[441−444] The most reliable criterion used in the past for diagnosis of this disease was an increase in the ratio of VLDL cholesterol to total triglyceride ($r >$ 0.30) and a triglyceride concentration between 150 and 1000 mg/ dl.[443,445,446] The frequency of the disease was estimated to be 0.1–0.01% in the population.[444,447]

In 1975, Utermann and colleagues described an apparent apo E4 and apo E3 isoprotein deficiency in patients with type III hyperlipoproteinemia.[433,434] Subsequent work established that the apo E phenotype observed in type III HLP patients (E2/2) is not deficient in any isoprotein, but rather is shifted to a more acidic isoelectric point as a result of a structural mutation that changes the net charge of apo E.[337,358,429] In a recent study, we determined the clinical symptoms and lipoprotein patterns in 17 individuals with type III HLP and their relatives and spouses, and used the apo E phenotype E2/2 as a molecular marker to study the transmission as well as the phenotypic expression of the disease.[438] We found that the apo E phenotype E2/2 occurred in 15 type III HLP probands and the apo E phenotype E4/2 in two probands. In another study still in progress of the families of 17 additional probands, we found that the E2/2 phenotype occurred in 16 and the E3/2 phenotype in one proband. Thus, in these studies, the apo E phenotype E2/2 was found in 91% of probands with type III HLP, where it would be expected to occur in only 1–2% of the normal population.[438] These studies and others show a very strong association of the E2/2 phenotype with type III HLP. However, there are individuals who apparently have this condition but do not have this apo E phenotype. It is possible that other mutations in a functional domain of apo E may occur that do not change the net charge of this apoprotein but affect its biological function(s). It is also possible that individuals may have an altered apo E receptor[237] or mutations in other, still undefined steps of apo E metabolism (Figs. 1E–1I and 2B)[42] that could result in the type III HLP phenotype. For example, an important step prior to apo E secretion where mutations may occur is the post-translational glycosylation of apo E. As mentioned above, a patient with an apparent deficiency in plasma apo E has been described who also displays the clinical symptoms of type III HLP.[439] The exact nature of this apo E mutation remains unknown.

Mode of Inheritance of Type III HLP. Type III HLP was believed to be a single-gene disorder on the basis of the occurrence of this disease in siblings in certain families and in a parent and one or more children in other families.[390,441,444,448,449] Since the former suggests recessive inheritance and the latter dominant, confusion has existed as to the true mechanism of inheritance of this disease. The recognition that the apo E phenotype E2/2 is a marker for most patients with type III HLP, along with an understanding of the inheritance of the apo E phenotypes, now allows a better understanding of the genetic transmission of this disease. Individuals with the apo E phenotype E2/2 are homozygotes for the apo E allele ε2, and the genetic tendency for type III HLP would in most cases be recessive. This is indicated by non-type III HLP parents, who carry the apo E allele ε2 and produce offspring with type III HLP and the apo E phenotype E2/2. In addition, type III HLP parents with the apo E phenotype E2/2 who marry individuals who do not carry the apo E allele $\epsilon2$ produce no children with type III HLP and the apo E phenotype E2/2. In some families, an individual with type III HLP and the apo E phenotype E2/2 marries a phenotypically normal individual who carries the apo E allele $\epsilon2$. These individuals can have the apo E phenotypes E3/2 or E4/2 and, based on the apo E allele frequencies, comprise 20% and 3% of the population, respectively. Half of the offspring of these marriages would be homozygous for the apo E allele $\epsilon2$ and possess the apo E phenotype E2/2 and the genetic tendency to type III HLP. The vertical transmission of type III HLP in such families suggests dominant inheritance, but this is a pseudodominant pattern due to the common frequency of the $\epsilon2$ allele in the population (13%). Finally, as mentioned above, we have found some individuals with type III HLP and the apo E phenotypes E4/2 and E3/2 who have only one copy of the $\epsilon2$ gene and may inherit the tendency to type III HLP in a truly dominant fashion.

Reduced Binding to Lipoprotein Receptors of Apo E Derived from Individuals with the E2/2 Phenotype May Underlie Type III HLP. As discussed earlier, apo E is one of the apoproteins that, as a component of lipoprotein particles and liposomes, binds to cell surface receptors and mediates the catabolism of lipoproteins by hepatic and extrahepatic tissues.[208,237,245,246,256,258] Turnover studies showed that the catabolism of ^{125}I-labeled apo E derived from an individual with type III HLP and the E2/2 phenotype was slower than when apo E from normal individuals was used.[360,361] In addition to these *in vivo* studies, extensive experiments involving fibroblast cultures and membrane preparations have shown that apo E of different phenotypes in phospholipid complexes displays variable degrees of competition for the LDL receptor.[362–364] Apo E from individuals with the E3/3 and E4/4 phenotypes displays the same competition for the LDL receptor as described previously.[363] However, apo E derived from individuals with the E2/2 phenotype does not compete as well for the LDL receptor.[362,364] Mahley and colleagues have noted functional heterogeneity in this regard within the E2/2 phenotype.[364] These studies have shown that apo E that has arisen from a 158 Arg → Cys substitution competes very inefficiently, whereas apo E that has arisen from a 145 Arg → Cys substitution competes almost normally for the LDL receptor (Fig. 13).[364] Apo E from individuals with the apo E phenotype E2/2, who are genetic compounds for these two alleles, shows an intermediate binding defect. In other studies, apo E of the E2/2 phenotype with a severe receptor binding defect was functionally restored by

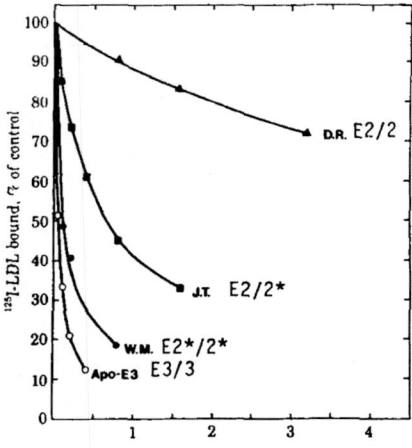

Fig. 13. Displacement of ^{125}I-LDL from monolayers of cultured fibroblasts by apo E phospholipid vesicles. The phenotype of the apo E used is indicated. (From Rall et al.[364] Reproduced by permission of the authors.)

treatment with cysteamine.[363] This treatment restores the positive charge at amino acid 158.[363] These findings indicate that a positively charged amino acid at residue 158 is crucial to apo E-receptor binding.[363] These binding experiments are consistent with earlier observations showing accumulation of remnant lipoproteins in the plasma of patients with type III HLP which are enriched in cholesteryl esters and apo E.[276–279,298,299,355,370,371] These apo E-rich lipoprotein remnants are apparently the result of slow clearance *in vivo* of the apo E-containing lipoproteins due to the described structural defect in apo E.

Factors Affecting the Phenotypic Expression of Type III HLP. Numerous studies suggest that the E2/2 phenotype alone is not sufficient to cause type III HLP and that other genetic factors may be required for the phenotypic expression of the disease.[390,441,444,448–451] In order to assess the influence of other factors that might contribute to the phenotypic expression of type III HLP, we analyzed the plasma lipids and lipoproteins in 69 relatives of 15 type III HLP probands according to their apo E phenotypes.[438] These studies showed that relatives of type III HLP probands had normal cholesterol and HDL cholesterol levels but triglyceride levels that were almost twice normal. The cause of this could be either environmental or genetic and the latter could be either monogenic or polygenic. As shown in Fig. 14, the frequency distribution of triglyceride levels in all first-degree relatives or in those 25 years or older did not yield a bimodal distribution. This suggests that the cause of the hypertriglyceridemia in these families was in most cases not due to a single dominant gene. These findings do not rule out the contribution of a single dominant hyperlipidemia gene to the expression of type III HLP in some of the families studied. However, proof that this has actually occurred will probably await the recognition of a suitable molecular marker for these familial hyperlipidemias.

These as well as previous studies indicate that in most cases type III HLP is expressed in families with a tendency to hypertriglyceridemia based on environmental or other genetic factors or some combination of the two. The concept that other genetic and/or environmental factors may be required for the expression of type III HLP has received direct biochemical support by recent studies of Rall *et al.*[455] These investigators have shown that apo E from subjects with the apo E2/2 phenotype who are normolipidemic and even hypolipidemic behave the same in competition experiments and presumably have the same molecular defect as apo E from patients with the E2/2 phenotype (158 Cys) who express type III HLP. In conclusion, the genetic and biochemical data involving human apo E cannot completely account for the lipid and lipoprotein abnormalities observed in patients with type III HLP. Future studies should be directed toward other genetic and environmental factors that trigger the onset of this disease. Such studies will require a long-term followup of asymptomatic subjects with the E2/2 phenotype in order to assess what environmental factors may trigger the onset of the disease. In

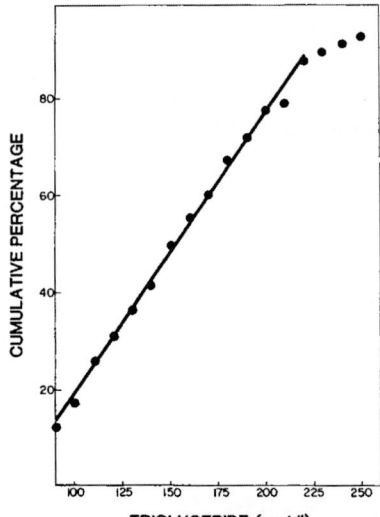

Fig. 14. Frequency distribution of the adjusted triglyceride levels in all first-degree relatives of type III HLP probands.

addition, it will require suitable genetic markers to assess the contribution of other monogenic hyperlipidemias to the expression of type III HLP.

The $\epsilon2$ Apo E Allele Affects Plasma Lipoprotein Levels in the General Population. In addition to the contribution of the apo E phenotype to the expression of type III HLP, it has been suggested by Uterman *et al.*[452] that the apo E phenotype is involved in determining plasma lipoprotein levels in the general population. There are now five studies in the literature whose data can be used to reflect on this problem.[299,431,432,438,452] Although all of the studies do not agree on every point, the following trends appear:

The $\epsilon2$ allele exerts a stepwise gene dosage effect on lowering the LDL cholesterol levels. The $\epsilon2$ allele also appears to affect the VLDL fraction and result in an increase in cholesterol and triglyceride, which presumably is the result of increased remnants of triglyceride-rich lipoproteins in the circulation (βVLDL). The data are less clear for a stepwise gene dosage effect for the number of $\epsilon2$ apo E alleles on this phenomenon. Thus, carriage of the apo E allele $\epsilon2$, which occurs in approximately 23% of people, may play a significant role in the regulation of plasma lipoprotein levels in the general population. The lipoprotein alterations appear to be a decrease in LDL cholesterol, which may protect against atherosclerosis, and an increase in VLDL cholesterol and triglycerides, which, in the form of βVLDL, are thought to be atherogenic.[456] The net effect of these two alterations on an individual's susceptibility to atherosclerosis remains to be determined.

Variants in Other Apoproteins

Apo A-IV. Heterozygous variants in apo A-IV have been described by two laboratories.[413,457] Screening of 212 subjects in our laboratory revealed three common phenotypes (Figs. 15A–15C). Following the nomenclature system adopted for human apo E,[415] and based on the data of Fig. 15 and Ref. 424, we assume that the A-IV phenotypes result from two alleles, apo α-IV3 and apo α-IV4. These alleles give rise to two homozygous (A-IV4/4 and A-IV3/3) phenotypes and one heterozygous (A-IV4/3) phenotype (Figs. 15A–15C). The observed phenotype frequencies are A-IV4/4 = 0.01, A-IV3/3 = 0.90, and A-IV4/3 = 0.094. Therefore, in this population, the apo A-IV allele frequency is α-IV4 = 0.057 and α-

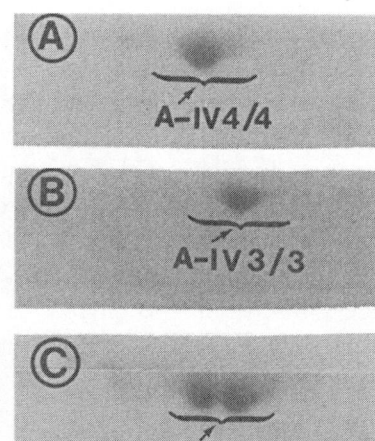

Fig. 15. Two-dimensional PAGE patterns of the different apo A-IV phenotypes. (A) homozygous A-IV4/4 phenotype. (B) Homozygous A-IV3/3 phenotype. (C) Heterozygous A-IV4/3 phenotype.

IV3 = 0.943. If we assume a Hardy–Weinberg distribution of the apo E alleles, the apo E phenotype frequencies should be A-IV4/4 = 0.003, A-IV3/3 = 0.89, and A-IV4/3 = 0.107.

Apo B. *Abetalipoproteinemia.* Abetalipoproteinemia is a rare autosomal recessive disorder characterized by fat malabsorption, failure to thrive, ataxic neuropathy, retinitis pigmentosa, and acanthocytosis.[5] Approximately 50 cases with abetalipoproteinemia have been reported to date.[5] These patients are characterized by low plasma cholesterol and triglycerides[458] and complete absence of plasma apo B, VLDL, and LDL, and chylomicrons.[459] Severe deficiency of apo CIII-1 has also been observed in this condition.[460,461] In abetalipoproteinemia, all the other apoproteins are found in the HDL fraction.[355] Immunofluorescence techniques have shown absence of apo B in intestinal biopsies obtained from patients with abetalipoproteinemia.[462] It is possible that these cases of abetalipoproteinemia result from apo B gene mutations that prevent synthesis of apo B or produce an unstable aberrant apo B particle.[462]

Genetically Altered Betalipoprotein Levels. Individuals with half normal LDL and betalipoprotein levels have been described. These people are said to have hypobetalipoproteinemia and are usually phenotypically normal. Patients homozygous for hypobetalipoproteinemia have been described who lack plasma apo B, VLDL, LDL, and chylomicrons and are phenotypically indistinguishable from patients with abetalipoproteinemia. The only difference appears to be that parents of these patients have half normal LDL levels,[463-467] whereas parents of abetali-poproteinemia patients have normal LDL levels.[468-470] Recently, a patient has been described who lacks plasma VLDL and LDL but has chylomicrons. This individual has a selective deficiency of the B-100 form of apo B,[327] which suggests that the B-100 and B-48 forms of apo B may be under the control of different genes. Another distinct case of hypobetalipoproteinemia has been reported which was characterized by very low, but not absent, LDL cholesterol levels (4–8 mg/dl) and complete absence of apo CIII-1. The apo B of this patient has not been characterized.[471] The latter two cases responded differently to a high-carbohydrate diet. After carbohydrate feeding, the B-100-deficient patient increased plasma triglycerides twofold, whereas the other patient decreased triglyceride levels.[327,471] The molecular basis of these diseases is not known. They may result from either mutation in the apo B gene and/or defective intracellular modification of this apoprotein. Whatever the nature of the defect, these diseases demonstrate the requirement of apo B synthesis in the cellular secretion of chylomicrons and VLDL. Similar conclusions can be drawn from recent tissue culture experiments in which blockage of apo B synthesis by cycloheximide prevents the secretion of VLDL.[22,74,75] Further studies of apo B synthesis and secretion by intestinal or hepatic biopsies obtained from patients with these conditions may provide meaningful new information.[462]

Numerous population studies indicate that elevated LDL cholesterol levels are associated with increased risk of coronary heart disease.[472,473] In contrast, it has been suggested that moderately decreased LDL cholesterol levels are associated with longevity.[426] Finally, subjects have been described having a condition characterized as hyperapobetalipoproteinemia.[474] These people have elevated LDL apo B but normal LDL cholesterol levels and are at increased risk for developing coronary atherosclerosis.[474] Some of the variations in LDL cholesterol and apo B levels observed in these subjects may be the result of as yet unidentified structural apo B abnormalities.

Apo CII.* As discussed earlier, apo CII is a cofactor for LDL that catalyzes the hydrolysis of triglycerides in chylomicrons and VLDL.[85-91] Nineteen patients originating from four different kindred[108,109,475-477] have been reported who have an inherited apo CII deficiency. This causes a functional LDL deficiency and results in the accumulation of chylomicrons and VLDL in the plasma of these patients. The addition of apo CII to LPL from these patients results in normal lipolytic activity.[109] The disease is transmitted as an autosomal recessive, and obligate heterozygotes usually have normal lipid and lipoprotein concentrations.[475–478] Three patients with lipemia and xanthomas have been described who have a normal as well as a variant form of apo CII.[334,479] The variant apo CII form, which differs by -1 charge from the normal form, appears to result from a structural apo CII gene mutation. This mutation causes a lysine to glutamine substitution.[479] The variant apo CII activates LPL normally, which leaves uncertain the nature of the relationship of this variant with hyperlipidemia. It remains to be established whether the variant apo CII form results from a structural apo CII mutation or a post-translational modification.

Apo CIII. As mentioned above, a kindred has been recently described with two sisters who have severe atherosclerosis and HDL, apo A-I, and apo CIII deficiency.[416] These patients appear to be homozygous for a DNA insertion in the coding region of their apo A-I gene (Fig. 4). Genomic blotting analysis of the patients' DNA digested with various restriction enzymes shows that the apo CIII gene is not grossly altered.[417,418] This suggests that the apo CIII deficiency may not be caused by a structural mutation of the apo CIII gene, but by an impairment in the expression of the apo CIII gene that results from a gross alteration in the neighboring apo A-I gene.[418] Finally, a nucleotide polymorphism in the 3' untranslated region of the apo CIII gene has been observed in humans,[309] which occurs at greater frequency in hypertriglyceridemic patients.[480] This polymorphism results from a C to G substitution and generates a sequence in the DNA that is cleaved by the *Sac*I enzyme (Fig. 4). Patients with type III, type IV, and type V hyperlipoproteinemia have elevated plasma apo CIII levels.[442] Variations in the relative concentration of apo CIII isoproteins have been observed that deviate from normal values.[5,342,460,461,481] Thus, patients with type V hyperlipoproteinemia are reported to have statistically lower relative apo CIII-0 concentrations.[481] Patients with abetalipoproteinemia and one type of hypobetalipoproteinemia have been found to lack the apo CIII-1 isoprotein form.[5,460,461] Finally, normal subjects have been found with familial preponderance of apo CIII-0.[482] These abnormal apo CIII isoprotein patterns may result from selective synthesis and/or secretion of one isoprotein form, preferential catabolism of one isoprotein form, or defective apo CIII isoprotein conversion.

Proposed Nomenclature of Variant Apoprotein Phenotypes and Genotypes. It is obvious from the above that extensive genetic heterogeneity exists in the different human apoproteins. The fast progress in the discovery of new apoprotein variants necessitates that a uniform nomenclature system be used for their description. In this section, we would like to expand the recently proposed nomenclature system for human apo E[415] to one that more precisely describes the genetic variation of this apoprotein. In addition, we would like to use this system as a model in order to describe the genetic variation that exists in other apoproteins. The existing apo E nomenclature is as follows. The common apo E alleles are called $\epsilon 4$, $\epsilon 3$, and $\epsilon 2$. The major asialo apo E isoproteins seen in plasma by two-dimensional gel electrophoresis are designated apo E4, apo E3, and apo E2, respectively. Apo E4 is the most basic and apo E2 is the most acidic isoprotein. The minor plasma apo E isoproteins, which are eliminated by treatment with neuraminidase, have been collectively designated apo E_s. Thus, the sialo apo E isoproteins of apo E4, apo E3, and apo E2 are designated apo $E4_s$, apo $E3_s$, and apo $E2_s$, respectively.[415] The model of apo E inheritance of three alleles at a single genetic locus provides for six genotypes and phenotypes that have been recognized and designated: $\epsilon 4;\epsilon 4$ = E4/4, $\epsilon 3;\epsilon 3$ = E3/3, $\epsilon 2;\epsilon 2$ = E2/2, $\epsilon 4;\epsilon 3$ = E4/3, $\epsilon 3;\epsilon 2$ = E3/2, and $\epsilon 4;\epsilon 2$ = E4/2 (Figs. 9 and 11A). Recent studies have shown additional genetic heterogeneity in the apo E gene locus and that different genotypes may give the same apparent apo E phenotype. To differentiate among the various genotypes that have the same phenotype, we propose the following modifications in the original nomenclature. We define arbitrarily the most common allele $\epsilon 3$ as the reference allele. We assume that this allele corresponds to the published apo E sequence.[356] All other alleles will be designated on the basis of the phenotype they produce and the amino acid substitution(s) they introduce. For example, the alleles that generate the E4/4 phenotype will be designated $\epsilon 4_{arg-112}$, the alleles generate the E2/2 phenotype, previously designated $\epsilon 2$, $\epsilon 2^*$, and $\epsilon 2^{**}$, will be referred to as $\epsilon 2_{cys-158}$, $\epsilon 2_{cys-145}$, and $\epsilon 2_{gln-146}$, respectively (Fig. 12). A conceptually similar adaptation of the apo E nomenclature system has been introduced recently by Rall *et al.*[437,437a] In this nomenclature system, the phenotype that is produced by the $\epsilon 2$ and $\epsilon 2^{**}$ alleles will be designated E2(Arg158 → Cys) and E2(Lys146 → Gln), respectively.

The genetic variation in apo A-I can be described in a similar fashion. The apo A-I isoproteins seen by two-dimensional gel electrophoresis will be designated A-I$_2$, A-I$_3$, A-I$_4$, A-I$_5$, A-I$_6$, from basic to acidic (Fig. 7A). The A-I$_2$ is the major nascent and A-I$_4$ is the major plasma apo A-I isoprotein.[27,28,80] The apo A-I alleles are called α-I4, α-I3, and α-I2. Homozygosity for the α-I3 allele generates the common apo A-I phenotype designated A-I3/3 (Fig. 7A). Homozygosity for the α-I4 and α-I2 alleles would generate the putative phenotypes designated A-I4/4 and A-I2/2, respectively, which have not yet been observed. Heterozygosity for the apo A-I alleles will produce A-I4/3 (Fig. 7B and apo A-I Giessen[413]) and A-I3/2 (apo A-I Milano and apo A-I Marburg[411−414]). When the mutant apo A-I protein or gene sequence is elucidated, the mutant alleles can be specified more precisely according to the specific amino acid substitution that produces the variant phenotype. For instance, the variant allele of the apo A-I Milano will be designated as α-I2$_{cys-173}$.[414] The alleles specifying the common apo CI, apo CII, apo CIII, apo A-II, and apo A-IV phenotypes will be designated γ-I3, γ-II3, γ-III3, α-II3, and α-IV3, respectively. Homozygosity for γ-I3, γ-II3, γ-III3, α-II3, and α-IV3 will give rise to the phenotypes CI3/3, CII3/3, CIII3/3, A-II3/3, and A-IV3/3, respectively. Alleles that generate phenotypes differing by $+1$ or -1 charges relative to the common phenotype (for example, CI) will be designated γ-I4 and γ-I2, respectively, and the corresponding homozygous phenotypes will be designated CI4/4 and CI2/2, respectively. Heterozygous phenotypes will be named in accordance with the examples provided for apo E and apo A-I. As explained in section II, 2D and in Figs. 15A–15C, variant homozygous A-IV4/4 and heterozygous A-IV4/3 phenotypes for apo A-IV occur with relatively high frequency in the population. Figures 16A and 16B show a schematic presentation of normal and variant apoprotein phenotypes as seen by 2D-PAGE. Figure 16C shows the analysis of all the common apoproteins on a single two-dimensional gel.

Mutations in Enzymes Participating in Lipoprotein Catabolism

Mutations in LPL and HTL

Familial lipoprotein lipase deficiency is a rare autosomal recessive disorder characterized by greatly increased plasma triglyceride and chy-

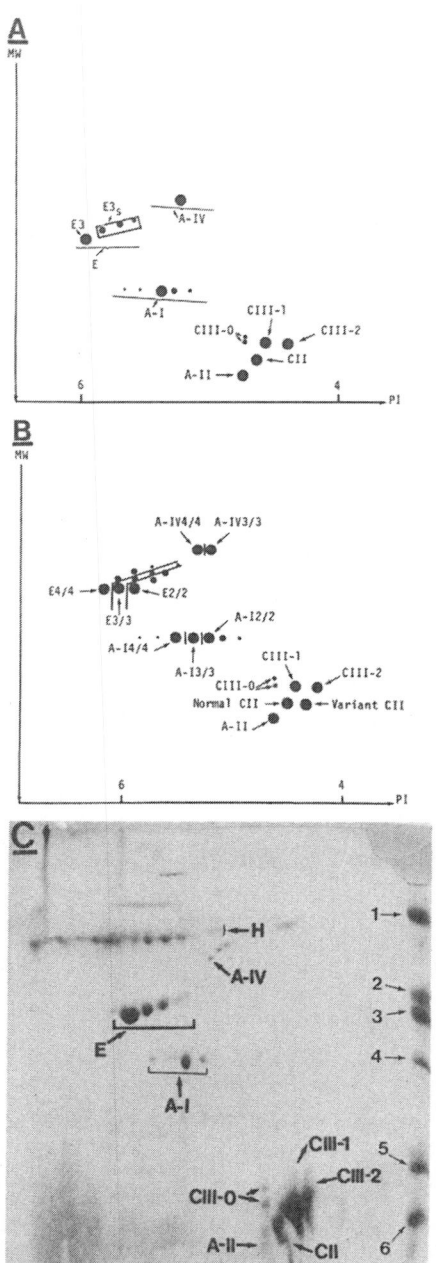

Fig. 16. (A) Schematic representation of the 2D-PAGE patterns of normal human apoproteins. The apoproteins and their corresponding isoproteins are designated by dots. (B) Schematic representation of 2D-PAGE patterns of a mixture of normal and variant human apoproteins. The variant apoproteins focus in a different position than those of normal apoproteins and can be recognized by comparison of the patterns in A and B. (C) Two-dimensional gel electrophoresis of a mixture of VLDL and apo A-I and apo A-II immunoprecipitated with specific antibodies. The various apoproteins are indicated. H indicates heavy IgG chains. The numbers 1–6 at the right side of panel C indicate protein molecular weight markers as follows: (1) bovine serum albumin (68,000), (2) ovalbumin (43,000), (3) aldolase (40,000), (4) human apo A-I (28,000), (5) trypsin inhibitor (19,000), (6) egg white lysozyme (14,300). The cathode is on the left and the anode is on the right.

lomicrons, decreased plasma HDL and LDL, xanthomatosis, hepatosplenomegaly, and recurrent attacks of pancreatitis.[108,390,483−485] Sixty patients with primary LPL deficiency have been reported and there is evidence of genetic heterogeneity in the disease.[486] The molecular nature of primary LPL deficiencies is not known, but may result from either mutations in the LPL gene or possibly defective post-translational modifications of LPL.[486] Recently, a patient with severe deficiency of HTL (5% normal) has been described,[117] who had xanthomatosis and elevated levels of plasma cholesterol and triglycerides. In contrast with LPL-deficient patients, this individual has elevated plasma HDL, βVLDL, and increased concentration of triglycerides and phospholipids in his LDL and HDL.[117] The unusual lipoprotein particles that accumulate in the plasma of these patients may constitute the natural substrates of normal HTL.

Mutations in LCAT

Familial LCAT deficiency is a rare autosomal recessive disorder characterized by lipoproteins of abnormal shape and composition, with numerous tissue and organ abnormalities, which probably result from excessive amounts of unesterified cholesterol and lecithin in plasma.[78,181,487,488] The most serious complications of the disease are renal failure and atherosclerosis.[78,489−491] Quantitation of plasma LCAT mass in deficient patients by radioimmunoassay revealed 0–20% of normal amounts of LCAT. This observation is consistent with structural mutations in the LCAT gene that inactivate the enzyme and affect to various degrees the synthesis and/or the stability of the mutant LCAT protein.[492,493] The lipoprotein abnormalities that result from LCAT deficiency include βVLDL, large- and intermediate-size LDL_2, and the discoidal HDL particles[77,78] with abnormal lipid and apoprotein composition. The patients' VLDL has increased apo E and apo CI and decreased apo CII and apo CIII concentrations.[78,494] The large- and intermediate-size LDL_2 have an increased concentration of cholesterol and lecithin and decreased concentration of cholesteryl esters.[78] Finally, the discoidal HDL particles have a high apo E to apo A-I ratio and increased concentration of unesterified cholesterol and phospholipid compared to normal HDL.[78] These particles resemble the nascent HDL particles secreted by the intestine and liver.[10,15,18] These abnormal lipoprotein particles found in the plasma of LCAT-deficient patients may be intermediates of lipoprotein metabolism that do not reach significant concentrations in normal plasma.

Mutations in Intracellular Cholesteryl Ester Hydrolysis (Wolman Disease and Cholesteryl Ester Storage Disease)

Wolman Disease[495] and cholesteryl ester storage disease[496] are two autosomal recessive disorders characterized by accumulation of cholesteryl esters and neutral lipids in several tissues.[495,497,498] It is believed that both conditions result from different mutations in the locus controlling the enzyme acid cholesteryl ester hydrolase (commonly known as acid lipase or acid esterase).[499,500] Wolman disease is associated with adrenal calcification[498,501,502] and is fatal in the first year of life.[495,497] Cholesteryl ester storage disease is more benign and two of the reported patients survived beyond the age of 40.[498] Cholesteryl ester acid hydrolase is a lysosomal enzyme that hydrolyzes the cholesteryl esters and triglycerides of LDL and other lipoproteins that enter the cell through receptor-mediated pathways. The enzyme acts upon its substrate following fusion of endosomes, which carry the lipoprotein receptor complex, with the lysosomes.[221,503] Cultured fibroblasts of patients with cholesteryl ester storage disease bind and internalize LDL but fail to hydrolyze its cholesteryl ester moiety and thus accumulate cholesteryl esters in their lysosomes.[227] The human enzyme has been recently purified to near homogeneity.[504] The purified enzyme appears to be a tetramer with a subunit molecular weight of approximately 30,000. The purified enzyme maintains hydrolytic activity for both cholesteryl esters and triglycerides.[504]

Mutations in Other Steps of Lipoprotein Metabolism

As explained in section II,2A, Tangier disease may result from a defective conversion of nascent apo A-I$_2$ to plasma apo A-I$_4$.[80] This conversion could be the result of a structural mutation in apo A-I$_2$ that precludes its conversion to apo A-I$_4$. Alternatively, Tangier patients may have normal apo A-I$_2$ but a defective A-I$_2$ to apo A-I$_4$ converting protease.

In the latter case, Tangier disease should be classified with the group of mutations listed in this section. Other mutations in the various steps of lipoprotein metabolism described in section I,2A–C have not been described at the present time.

FUTURE DIRECTIONS

Despite the impressive amount of knowledge that has been acquired during the last 30 years, the pathways of lipoprotein metabolism are not completely elucidated. Much remains to be learned about processes such as intracellular and extracellular modification of apoproteins, assembly and secretion of lipoproteins, exchange and transfer of lipid and protein moieties of lipoproteins, spectrum and physiological role of other receptors beside the LDL receptor, function of several apoproteins, structure of apo B, and finally, other still unidentified steps of lipoprotein metabolism. As has been the case in the past, this knowledge has to be acquired by systematic application of advanced techniques of biochemistry and molecular biology in the study of these problems. In addition, a systematic screening of diseases of lipoprotein metabolism and/or creation of experimental animal models may provide knowledge about mutations in known or as yet unrecognized steps of lipoprotein metabolism that will be useful for further biochemical and physiological studies. These studies will hopefully provide knowledge of the structure and function of all the enzymes and proteins that participate in lipoprotein metabolism. The use of existing recombinant DNA technology will permit the determination of the gene structure of normal and variant genes of these proteins. Such studies are currently underway in several laboratories and are expected to proceed at a faster pace in the near future.[41,43,306,307,505,506] It may not be unrealistic to predict that when these studies are completed, we will be able to describe most of the human disorders of lipoprotein metabolism at the molecular level, as has been the case with the human hemoglobinopathies.[507,508]

ACKNOWLEDGMENTS. This work was supported by grants from the National Institutes of Health (HL33952), March of Dimes Birth Defects

Foundation (1-817), and the American Heart Association (83-963). Dr. Jan L. Breslow and Dr. Vassilis I. Zannis are Established Investigators of the American Heart Association. We would like to thank Dr. Thomas Innerarity, Dr. Julian Marsh, and Dr. Sandra Erickson for reviewing this manuscript, and Ms. Lorraine M. Duda for her expert assistance.

REFERENCES*

1. Morrisett, J. D., Jackson, R. L., and Gotto, A. M., Jr., Lipoproteins: Structure and function, *Annu. Rev. Biochem.* **44**:183 (1975).
2. Atkinson, D., Davis, M. A. F., and Leslie, R. B., The structure of a high density lipoprotein (HDL₃) from porcine plasma, *Proc. R. Soc. Lond. B* **186**:165 (1974).
3. Laggner, P., Kostner, G. M., Rakusch, U., and Worcester, D., Neutron small angle scattering on selectively deuterated human plasma low density lipoproteins, *J. Biol. Chem.* **255**:11832 (1981).
4. Smith, L. C., Pownall, H. J., and Gotto, A. M., The plasma lipoproteins: Structure and metabolism, *Annu. Rev. Biochem.* **47**:751 (1978).
5. Herbert, P. N., Assmann, G., Gotto, A. M., Jr., and Fredrickson, D. S., Familial lipoprotein deficiency: Abetalipoproteinemia, hypobetalipoproteinemia, and Tangier disease, in: *The Metabolic Basis of Inherited Disease*, 5th ed. (J. B. Stanbury, J. B. Wyngaarden, D. S. Fredrickson, J. L. Goldstein, and M. D. Brown, eds.), pp. 589–651, McGraw-Hill, New York (1982).
6. Scanu, A. M., Byrne, R. E., and Mihovilovic, M., Functional roles of plasma high density lipoproteins, *CRC Crit. Rev. Biochem.* **13**:109 (1982).
7. Alaupovic, P., Conceptual development of the classification systems of plasma lipoproteins, in: *Protides of the Biological Fluids* (H. Peeters, ed.), pp. 9–20, Pergamon, Oxford (1971).
8. Windmueller, H. G., Herbert, P. N., and Levy, R. I., Biosynthesis of lymph and plasma lipoprotein apoproteins by isolated perfused rat liver and intestine, *J. Lipid Res.* **14**:215 (1973).
9. Marsh, J. B., Apoproteins of the lipoproteins in a nonrecirculating perfusate of rat liver, *J. Lipid Res.* **17**:85 (1976).
10. Hamilton, R. L., Williams, M. C., Fielding, C. J., and Havel, R. J., Discoidal bilayer structure of nascent high density lipoproteins from perfused rat liver, *J. Clin. Invest.* **58**:667 (1976).
11. Felker, T. E., Fainaru, M., Hamilton, R. L., and Havel, R. J., Secretion of the arginine rich and A-I apolipoproteins by the isolated perfused rat liver, *J. Lipid Res.* **18**:465 (1977).

* This chapter attempts to provide a comprehensive review of genetic mutations that affect human lipoprotein metabolism, with special emphasis on mutations in apoproteins. It covers a wide range of topics, and is intended to introduce the reader to the subject matter, rather than to provide an in-depth review of these topics. For this reason recent reviews covering specific topics are cited in the place of individual references.

12. Glickman, R. M., and Green, P. H. R., The intestine as a source of apolipoprotein A-I, *Proc. Natl. Acad. Sci. USA* **74**:2569 (1977).
13. Wu, A. L., and Windmueller, H. G., Identification of circulating apolipoproteins synthesized by rat small intestine *in vivo, J. Biol. Chem.* **253**:2525 (1978).
14. Imaizumi, K., Havel, R. J., Fainaru, M., and Vigne, J. L., Origin and transport of the A-I and arginine-rich apolipoproteins in mesenteric lymph of rats, *J. Lipid Res.* **19**:1038 (1978).
15. Green, P. H. R., Tall, A. R., and Glickman, R. M., Rat intestine secretes discoid high density lipoproteins, *J. Clin. Invest.* **61**:528 (1978).
16. Schonfeld, G., Bell, E., and Alpers, D. H., Intestinal apoproteins during fat absorption, *J. Clin. Invest.* **61**:1539 (1978).
17. Glickman, R. M., Green, P. H. R., Lees, R. S., and Tall, A., Apoprotein A-I synthesis in normal intestinal mucosa and in Tangier disease, *N. Engl. J. Med.* **2399**:1424 (1978).
18. Hamilton, R. L., Hepatic secretion and metabolism of high density lipoproteins, in: *Disturbances in Lipid and Lipoprotein Metabolism* (J. Dietschy, A. M. Gotto, Jr., and J. A. Ontko, eds.), pp. 155–171, Clinical Physiology Series, American Physiology Society, Baltimore (1978).
19. Wu, A. L., and Windmueller, H. G., Relative contribution by liver and intestine to individual plasma apolipoproteins in the rat, *J. Biol. Chem.* **254**:7316 (1979).
20. Windmueller, H. G., and Wu, A. L., Biosynthesis of plasma apolipoproteins by rat small intestine without dietary biliary fat, *J. Biol. Chem.* **256**:3012 (1981).
21. Tarlow, D. M., Watkins, P. A., Reed, R. E., Miller, R. S., Zwergel, E. E., and Lane, D., Lipogenesis and the synthesis and secretion of very low density lipoprotein by avian liver cells in nonproliferating monolayer culture, *J. Cell Biol.* **73**:332 (1977).
22. Davis, R. A., Engelhorn, S. C., Pangburn, S. H., Weinstein, D. B., and Steinberg, D., Very low density lipoprotein synthesis and secretion by cultured rat hepatocytes, *J. Biol. Chem.* **254**:2010 (1979).
23. Dashti, N., McConathy, W. J., and Ontka, J. A., Production of apolipoprotein E and apolipoprotein A-I by rat hepatocytes in primary culture, *Biochim. Biophys. Acta* **618**:347 (1980).
24. Kempen, H. J. M., Lipoprotein secretion by isolated rat hepatocytes: Characterization of the lipid-carrying particles and modification of their release, *J. Lipid Res.* **21**:671 (1980).
25. Zannis, V. I., Breslow, J. L., SanGiacomo, T. R., Aden, D. P., and Knowles, B. B., Characterization of the major apolipoproteins secreted by two human hepatoma cell lines, *Biochemistry* **20**:7089 (1981).
26. Rachmilewitz, D., Albers, J. J., Saunders, D. R., and Fainaru, M., Apoprotein synthesis by human duodenojejunal mucosa, *Gastroenterology* **75**:677 (1978).
27. Zannis, V. I., Breslow, J. L., and Katz, A. J., Isoproteins of human apolipoprotein A-I demonstrated in plasma and intestinal organ culture, *J. Biol. Chem.* **255**:8612 (1980).
28. Zannis, V. I., Kurnit, D., and Breslow, J. L., Hepatic apo A-I and apo E and intestinal apo A-I are synthesized in precursor isoprotein forms by organ cultures of human fetal tissues, *J. Biol. Chem.* **257**:536 (1982).
29. Blue, M. L., Protter, A. A., and Williams, D. L., Biosynthesis of apolipoprotein B in rooster kidney, intestine, and liver, *J. Biol. Chem.* **255**:10048 (1980).
30. Blue, M. L., Ostapchuk, P., Gordon, J. S., and Williams, D. L., Synthesis of apolipoprotein A-I by peripehral tissues of the rooster, *J. Biol. Chem.* **257**:11151 (1982).
31. Basu, S. K., Brown, M. S., Ho, Y. K., Havel, R. J., and Goldstein, J. L., Mouse mac-

rophages synthesize and secrete a protein resembling apolipoprotein E, *Proc. Natl. Acad. Sci. USA* **78**:7545 (1981).

32. Basu, S. K., Ho. Y. K., Brown, M. S., Bilheimer, D. W., Anderson, R. G. W., and Goldstein, J. L., Biochemical and genetic studies of the apoprotein E secreted by mouse macrophages and human monocytes, *J. Biol. Chem.* **257**:9788 (1982).

33. Blue, M. L., Williams, D. L., Zucker, S., Khan, S. A., and Blum, C. B., Apolipoprotein E synthesis in human kidney, adrenal gland, and liver, *Proc. Natl. Acad. Sci. USA* **80**:283 (1983).

34. Blobel, G., Walter, P., Chang, C. N., Goldman, B., Erickson, A. H., and Lingappa, V. R., Translocation of proteins across membranes: The signal hypothesis and beyond, in: *Symposium of the Society of Experimental Biology (Great Britain)*, Vol. 33 (C. R. Hopkins and C. J. Duncan, eds.), pp. 9–36, Cambridge University Press, London (1979).

35. Inouye, M., and Halegoua, S., Secretion and membrane localization of proteins in *Escherichia coli, CRC Crit. Rev. Biochem.* **7**:339 (1980).

36. Blobel, G., and Dobberstein, B., Transfer of proteins across membranes. II. Reconstitution of functional rough microsomes from heterologous components, *J. Cell Biol.* **67**:852 (1975).

37. Lingappa, V. R., Lingappa, J. R., and Blobel, G., Chicken ovalbumin contains an internal signal sequence, *Nature* **281**:117 (1979).

38. Gordon, J. I., Smith, D. P., Andy, R., Alpers, D. H., Schonfeld, G., and Strauss, A. W., The primary translation product of rat intestinal apolipoprotein A-I mRNA is an unusual preproprotein, *J. Biol. Chem.* **257**:971 (1982).

39. Zannis, V. I., Karathanasis, S. K., Keutmann, H. T., Goldberger, G., and Breslow, J. L., Intracellular and extracellular processing of human apolipoprotein A-I: Secreted apolipoprotein A-I isoprotein 2 is a propeptide, *Proc. Natl. Acad. Sci. USA* **80**:2574 (1983).

40. Gordon, J. I., Sims, H. F., Lentz, S. R., Edelstein, C., Scanu, A. M., and Strauss, A. W., Proteolytic processing of human preproapolipoprotein A-I. A proposed defect in the conversion of pro A-I to A-I in Tangier's disease, *J. Biol. Chem.* **258**:4037 (1983).

41. McLean, J. W., Fukazawa, C., and Taylor, J. M., Rat apolipoprotein E mRNA. Cloning and sequencing of double-stranded cDNA, *J. Biol. Chem.* **258**:8993 (1983).

42. Zannis, V. I., McPherson, J., Goldberger, G., Karathanasis, S. K., and Breslow, J. L., Synthesis, intracellular processing and signal peptide of human apo E, *J. Biol. Chem.*, **259**:5495 (1984).

42a. Gordon, J. I., Budelier, K. A., Sims, H. F., Edelstein, C., Scanu, A. M., and Strauss, A. W., Biosynthesis of human preproapolipoprotein A-II, *J. Biol. Chem.* **258**:14054 (1983).

43. Gordon, J. I., Smith, D. P., Alpers, D. H., and Strauss, A. W. Proteolytic processing of the primary translation product of rat intestinal apolipoprotein A-IV mRNA. Comparison with preproapolipoprotein A-I processing, *J. Biol. Chem.* **257**:8418 (1982).

43a. Karathanasis, S. K., Zannis, V. I., and Breslow, J. L., Isolation and sequence of human apo CIII cDNA clones specifying two different alleles, *J. Lipid Res.*, in press (1984).

44. Jackson, C., and Breslow, J. L., Isolation of a human apo CII cDNA clone, *Arteriosclerosis* **3**:514a (1983).

45. Brewer, H. B., Shulman, R., Herbert, P., and Ronan, R., The complete amino acid sequence of alanine apolipoprotein (apo C-III), an apolipoprotein from human plasma very low denstiy lipoproteins, *J. Biol. Chem.* **249**:4975 (1974).

46. Lee, P., and Breckenridge, W. C., Isolation and carbohydrate composition of glyco-peptides of human apo low-density lipoprotein from normal and type II hyperlipo-proteinemic subjects, *Can. J. Biochem.* **54**:829 (1976).
47. Swaminathan, N., and Aladjem, F., The monosaccharide composition and sequence of the carbohydrate moiety of human serum low density lipoproteins, *Biochemistry* **15**:1516 (1976).
48. Jain, R. S., and Quarfordt, S. H., The carbohydrate content of apolipoprotein E from human very low density lipoproteins, *Life Sci.* **25**:1315 (1979).
49. Albers, J. J., Cheung, M. C., Ewens, S. L., and Tollefson, J. H., Characterization and immunoassay of apolipoprotein D, *Atherosclerosis* **39**:395 (1981).
50. Zannis, V. I., Fraser, P., Rooney, V., and Breslow, J. L., Use of electrophoretic tech-niques for detection of molecular defects of lipoprotein metabolism, in: *CRC Hand-book of Electrophoresis 1983* (L. A. Lewis, ed.), Vol. III, pp. 319–348, CRC Publishing Co. (1983).
51. Lo, C. H., and Marsh, J. B., The synthesis of plasma lipoproteins: Incorporation of ^{14}C-glucosamine by cells and subcellular fractions of rat liver, *J. Biol. Chem.* **245**:5001 (1970).
52. Bizzi, A., and Marsh, J. B., Further observations on the attachment of carbohydrate to lipoproteins by rat liver Golgi membranes, *Proc. Soc. Exp. Biol. Med.* **144**:762 (1973).
53. Wetmore, S., Mahley, R. W., Brown, W. V., and Schachter, H., Incorporation of sialic acid into sialidase-treated apolipoprotein of human very low density lipoprotein by a pork liver sialytransferase, *Can. J. Biochem.* **52**:655 (1974).
54. Siuta-Mangano, P., Howard, S. C., Lennarz, W. J., and Lane, M. D., Synthesis, pro-cessing, and secretion of apolipoprotein B by the chick liver cell, *J. Biol. Chem.* **257**:4292 (1982).
55. Struck, D. K., Siuta, P. B., Lane, M. D., and Lennarz, W. J., Effect of tunicamycin on the secretion of serum proteins by primary cultures of rat and chick hepatocytes, *J. Biol. Chem.* **253**:5332 (1978).
56. Green, P. H. R., Lefkowitch, J. H., Glickman, R. M., Riley, J. W., Quinet, E., and Blum, C. B., Apolipoprotein localization and quantitation in the human intestine, *Gastroenterology* **83**:1223 (1982).
57. Wu, A. L., and Windmueller, H. G., Variant forms of plasma polipoprotein B. Hepatic and intestinal biosynthesis and heterogeneous metabolism in the rat, *J. Biol. Chem.* **256**:3615 (1981).
58. Ockner, R. K., and Manning, J. A., Fatty acid binding proteins. Role in esterification of absorbed long chain fat in rat intestine, *J. Clin. Invest.* **58**:632 (1976).
59. Cardell, R. R., Jr., Badenhausen, S., and Porter, K. R., Intestinal triglyceride absorp-tion in the rat: An electron microscopical study, *J. Cell Biol.* **34**:123 (1967).
60. Kessler, T. E., Narcessian, P., and Maudlin, D. P., Biosynthesis of lipoprotein by intestinal epithelium. Site of synthesis and sequence of association of lipid sugar and protein moiety, *Gastroenterology* **68**:1058 (1975).
61. Alexander, C. A., Hamilton, R. L., and Havel, R. J., Subcellular localization of B apoprotein of plasma lipoproteins in rat liver, *J. Cell Biol.* **69**:241 (1976).
62. Rubin, E. C., Perkins, W. D., Surawicz, C. M., McDonald, G. B., and Albers, J. J., Ultrastructural apoprotein B localization within human jejunal absorption cells dur-ing fat absorption, *Gastroenterology* **78**:1248 (1980).
63. Glickman, R. M., Kirsch, K., and Isselbacher, K. J., Fat absorption during inhibition of protein synthesis: Studies in lymph chylomicrons, *J. Clin. Invest.* **51**:356 (1972).
64. Soutar, A. K., Myant, N. B., and Thompson, G. R., Simultaneous measurement of

apolipoprotein B turnover in very low and low density lipoproteins in familial hyper-cholesterolemia, *Atherosclerosis* **28**:247 (1977).

65. Fainaru, M., Felker, T. E., Hamilton, R. L., and Havel, R. J., Evidence that a separate particle containing B-apoprotein is present in high density lipoproteins from perfused rat liver, *Metabolism,* **26**:999 (1977).

66. Nakaya, N., Chung, B. H., Patsch, J. R., and Taunton, O. D., Synthesis and release of low density lipoproteins by the isolated perfused pig liver, *J. Biol. Chem.* **252**:7530 (1977).

67. Berman, M., Hall, M., III, Levy, R. I., Eisenberg, S., Bilheimer, D. W., Phair, R. D., and Goebel, R. H., Metabolism of apo B and apo C lipoproteins in man: Kinetic studies in normal and hyperlipoproteinemic subjects, *J. Lipid Res.* **19**:38 (1978).

68. Soutar, A. K., Myant, N. B., and Thompson, G. R., Metabolism of apolipoprotein B-containing lipoproteins in familial hypercholesterolaemia, *Atherosclerosis* **32**:315 (1979).

69. Stein, O., and Stein, Y., Synthesis and intracellular degradation of serum lipopro-teins, in: *Fettstoffwechsel* (G. Schettler, H. Greten, G. Schlierf, and D. Seidel, eds.), p. 197, Springer-Verlag, New York (1976).

70. Mahley, R. W., Hamilton, R. L., and Lequire, V. S., Characterization of lipoprotein particles isolated from the Golgi apparatus of rat liver, *J. Lipid Res.* **10**:433 (1969).

71. Mahley, R. W., Bersot, T. P., Lequire, V. S., Levy, R. I., Windmueller, H. G., and Brown, W. V., Identity of very low density lipoprotein apoproteins of plasma and liver Golgi apparatus, *Science* **168**:380 (1970).

72. Chapman, M. J., Mills, G. L., and Taylaur, C. E., The effect of a lipid-rich diet on the properties and composition of lipoprotein particles from the Golgi apparatus of guinea pig liver, *Biochem. J.* **131**:177 (1973).

73. Swift, L. L., Manowitz, N. R., Dunn, G. D., and Lequire, V. S., Isolation and char-acterization of hepatic Golgi lipoproteins from hypercholesterolemic rats, *J. Clin. Invest.* **66**:415 (1980).

74. Davis. R. A., and Boogaerts, J. R., Intrahepatic assembly of very low density lipo-proteins. Effect of fatty acids on triacylglycerol and apolipoprotein synthesis, *J. Biol. Chem.* **257**:10908 (1982).

75. Suita-Mangano, P., Janero, D. R., and Lane, M. D., Association and assembly of triglyceride and phospholipid with glycosylated and unglycosylated apoproteins of very low density lipoprotein in the intact liver cell, *J. Biol. Chem.* **257**:11463 (1982).

76. LeMarchand, Y., Singh, A., Assimacopoulos-Jeannet, F., Orci, L., Rouiller, C., and Jeanrenaud, B., A role for the microtubular system in the release of very low density lipoprotein by perfused mouse livers, *J. Biol. Chem.* **248**:6862 (1973).

77. Mitchell, C. D., King, W. C., Applegate, K. R., Forte, T., Glomset, J. A., Norum, K. R., and Gjone, E., Characterization of apolipoprotein E-rich high density lipoproteins in familial lecithin:cholesterol acyltransferase deficiency, *J. Lipid Res.* **21**:625 (1980).

78. Glomset, J. A., Norum, K. R., and Gjone, E., Familial lecithin:cholesterol acyltrans-ferase deficiency, in: *The Metabolic Basis of Inherited Disease,* 5th ed. (J. B. Stanbury, J. B. Wyngaarden, D. S. Fredrickson, J. L. Goldstein, and M. S. Brown, eds.), pp. 643–654, McGraw-Hill, New York (1982).

79. Sigurdsson, G., Nicoll, A., and Lewis, B., Conversion of very low density lipoprotein to low density lipoprotein. A metabolic study of apolipoprotein B kinetics in human subjects, *J. Clin. Invest.* **56**:1481 (1975).

80. Zannis, V. I., Lees, A. M., Lees, R. S., and Breslow, J. L., Abnormal apo A-I iso-protein composition in patients with Tangier disease, *J. Biol. Chem.* **257**:4978 (1982).

80a. Stoffel, W., Kurger, E., and Deutzmann, R., Cell free translation of human liver apo-lipoprotein A-I and A-II mRNA. Processing of primary translation product, *Hoppe-Seyler's Z. Physiol. Chem.* **364**:227 (1983).

81. Breslow, J. L., Zannis, V. I., Nicolosi, R. J., and Hayes, K. C., Apolipoprotein E (apo E) isoproteins in nonhuman primates, *Fed Proc.* **40**:1635 (1981).

82. Attie, A. D., Weinstein, D. B., Freeze, H. H., Pittman, R. C., and Steinberg, D., Unal-tered catabolism of desialylated low-density lipoprotein in the pig and in cultured rat hepatocytes, *Biochem. J.* **180**:647 (1979).

83. Filipovic, I., Schwarzmann, G., Mraz, W., Weigandt, H., and Buddecke, E., Sialic-acid content of low-density lipoproteins controls their binding and uptake by cultured cells, *Eur. J. Biochem.* **93**:51 (1979).

84. Fielding, C. J., and Havel, R. J., Lipoprotein lipase, *Arch. Pathol. Lab. Med.* **101**:225 (1977).

85. Nilsson-Ehle, P., Lypolytic enzymes and plasma lipoprotein metabolism, *Annu. Rev. Biochem.* **49**:667 (1980).

86. Scow, R. O., and Egelrud, T., Hydrolysis of chylomicron phosphatidylcholine *in vitro* by lipoprotein lipase, phospholipase A_2, and phospholipase C, *Biochim. Biophys. Acta* **431**:538 (1976).

87. Eisenberg, S., and Olivectrona, I., Very low density lipoprotein. Fate of phospho-lipids, cholesterol, and apoliprotein C during lipolysis *in vitro*, *J. Lipid Res.* **20**:614 (1979).

88. Havel, R. J., Shore, V. G., Shore, B., and Bier, D. M., Role of specific glycopeptides of human serum lipoproteins in the activation of lipoprotein lipase, *Circ. Res.* **27**:595 (1970).

89. LaRosa, J. C., Levy, R. I., Herbert, P., Lux, S. E., and Fredrickson, D. S., A specific apoprotein activator for lipoprotein lipase, *Biochem. Biophys. Res. Commun.* **41**:57 (1970).

90. Miller, A. L., and Smith, L. C., Activation of lipoprotein lipase by apolipoprotein glutamic acid, *J. Biol. Chem.* **248**:3359 (1973).

91. Chung, J., and Scanu, A. M., Isolation, molecular properties, and kinetic character-ization of lipoprotein lipase from rat heart, *J. Biol. Chem.* **252**:4202 (1977).

92. Augustin, J., Freeze, H., Tejada, P., and Brown, W. V., A comparison of molecular properties of hepatic triglyceride lipase and lipoprotein lipase from human post-hep-arin plasma, *J. Biol. Chem.* **253**:2912 (1978).

93. Shimada, K., Gill, P. J., Silbert, J. E., Douglas, W. H. J., and Fanburg, B. L., Involve-ment of cell surface heparin sulfate in the binding of lipoprotein lipase to cultured bovine endothelial cells, *J. Clin. Invest.* **68**:995 (1981).

94. Cunningham, V. J., and Robinson, D. S., Clearing factor lipase in adipose tissue. Distinction of different states of the enzyme and the possible role of the fat cell in the maintenance of tissue activity, *Biochem. J.* **112**:203 (1969).

95. Hernell, O., Egelrud, T., and Olivecrona, T., Serum-stimulated lipases (lipoprotein lipases). Immunological crossreaction between the bovine and the human enzymes, *Biochim. Biophys. Acta* **381**:233 (1975).

96. Kompiang, I. P., Bensadoun, A., and Yan, M. W. W., Effect of an antilipoprotein lipase serum on plasma triglyceride removal, *J. Lipid Res.* **17**:498 (1976).

97. Schotz, M. C., Twu, J. S., Pedersen, M. E., Chen, C. H., Garfinkel, A. S., and Bor-ensztajn, J., Antibodies to lipoprotein lipase. Application of perfused heart, *Biochem. Biophys. Acta* **489**:214 (1977).

98. Chajek, T., Stein, O., and Stein, Y., Rat heart in culture as a tool to elucidate the cellular origin of lipoprotein lipase, *Biochim. Biophys. Acta* **488**:140 (1977).

99. Khoo, J. C., Mahoney, E. M., and Witztum, J. L., Secretion of lipoprotein lipase by macrophages in culture, *J. Biol. Chem.* **256:**7105 (1981).

100. Fielding, C. J., Lipoprotein lipase: Evidence for high- and low-affinity enzyme sites, *Biochemistry* **15:**879 (1976).

101. Fielding, P. E., Shore, V. G., and Fielding, C. J., Lipoprotein lipase, isolation and characterization of a second enzyme species from postheparin plasma, *Biochemistry* **16:**1896 (1977).

102. Nilsson-Ehle, P., Carlstrom, S., and Belfrage, P., Rapid effects on lipoprotein lipase activity in adipose tissue of humans after carbohydrate and lipid intake. Time course and relation to plasma glycerol, triglyceride and insulin levels, *Scand. J. Clin. Lab. Invest.* **35:**373 (1975).

103. Pykalisto, O. J., Smith, P. H., and Brunzell, J. D., Determinations of human adipose tissue lipoprotein lipase. Effect of diabetes and obesity on basal- and diet-induced activity, *J. Clin. Invest.* **56:**1108 (1975).

104. Lithell, H., Boberg, J., Hellsing, K., Lundqvist, G., and Vessby, B., Lipoprotein-lipase activity in human skeletal muscle and adipose tissue in the fasting and the fed states, *Atherosclerosis* **30:**89 (1978).

105. Zinder, O., Hamosh, M., Fleck, T. R. C., and Scow, R. O., Effect of prolactin on lipoprotein lipase in mammary gland and adipose tissue of rats, *Am. J. Physiol.* **226:**744 (1974).

106. Eckel, R. H., Fujimoto, W. Y., and Brunzell, J. D., Gastric inhibitory polypeptide enhanced lipoprotein lipase activity in cultured preadipocytes, *Diabetes* **28:**1141 (1979).

107. Wasada, T., McCorkle, K., Harris, V., Kawai, K., Howard, B., and Unger, R. H., Effect of gastric inhibitory polypeptide on plasma levels of chylomicron triglycerides in dogs, *J. Clin. Invest.* **68:**1106 (1981).

108. Nikkila, E. A., Familial lipoprotein lipase deficiency and related disorders of chylomicron metabolism, in: *The Metabolic Basis of Inherited Disease,* 5th ed. (J. B. Stanbury, J. B. Wyngaarden, D. S. Fredrickson, J. L. Goldstein, and M. S. Brown, eds.), pp. 622–642, McGraw-Hill, New York (1982).

109. Breckenridge, W. C., Little, J. A., and Steiner, G., Hypertriglyceridemia associated with deficiency of apolipoprotein C-II, *N. Engl. J. Med.* **298:**1265 (1978).

110. Stalenhoef, A. F., Casparie, A. F., Demacker, P. N., Stouten, T., Ltterman, J. A., and Van't Laar, A., Combined deficiency of apolipoprotein C-II and lipoprotein lipase in familial hyperchylomicronemia, *Metabolism* **30:**919 (1981).

111. Kuusi, T., Nikkila, E. A., Virtanen, I., and Kinnunen, P. K. J., Localization of the heparin-releasable lipase *in situ* in the rat liver, *Biochem. J.* **181:**245 (1979).

112. LaRosa, J. C., Levy, R. I., Windmueller, H. G., and Fredrickson, D. S., Comparison of the triglyceride lipase of liver, adipose tissue, and post heparin plasma, *J. Lipid Res.* **13:**356 (1972).

113. Jansen, H., VanZuylen-VanWiggen, A., and Hulsmann, W. C., Lipoprotein lipase from heart and liver: An immunological study, *Biochem. Biophys. Res. Commun.* **55:**30 (1973).

114. Jansen, H., VanBerkel, T. J. C., Hulsmann, W. C., Binding of liver lipase to parenchymal and non-parenchymal rat liver cells, *Biochem. Biophys. Res. Commun.* **85:**148 (1978).

115. Krauss, R. M., Levy, R. I., and Fredrickson, D. S., Selective measurement of two lipase activities in postheparin plasma from normal subjects and patients with hyperlipoproteinemia, *J. Clin. Invest.* **54:**1107 (1974).

116. Greten, H., DeGrella, R., Klose, G., Rascher, W., DeGennes, J. L., and Gjone, E., Measurement of two plasma triglyceride lipases by an immunochemical method: Studies in patients with hypertriglyceridemia, *J. Lipid Res.* **17**:203 (1976).

117. Breckenridge, W. C., Little, J. A., Alaupovic, P., Wang, C. S., Kuksis, A., Kakis, G., Lindgren, F., and Gardiner, G., Lipoprotein abnormalities associated with a familial deficiency of hepatic lipase, *Atherosclerosis* **45**:161 (1982).

118. Baginsky, M. L., and Brown, W. V., A new method for the measurement of lipoprotein lipase in postheparin plasma using sodiumdodecyl sulfate for the inactivation of hepatic triglyceride lipase, *J. Lipid Res.* **20**:548 (1979).

119. Ostlund-Lindqvist, A. M., Properties of salt-resistant lipase and lipoprotein lipase purified from human post-heparin plasma, *Biochem. J.* **179**:555 (1979).

120. Kuusi, T., Kinnunen, P. K. J., and Nikkila, E. A., Hepatic endothelial lipase antiserum influences rat plasma low and high density lipoproteins *in vivo*, *FEBS Lett.* **104**:314 (1979).

121. Paterniti, J. R., Jr., Brown, W. V., Ginsberg, H. N., and Artzt, K., Combined lipase deficiency (cld): A lethal mutation on chromosome 17 of the mouse, *Science* **221**:167 (1983).

122. VanTol, A., VanGent, I., and Jansen, H., Degradation of high density lipoprotein by heparin releaseable liver lipase, *Biochem. Biophys. Res. Commun.* **94**:101 (1980).

123. Nikkila, E. A., Huttunen, J. K., and Ehnholm, G., Low postheparin plasma hepatic lipase activity in familial type IIa hyperlipoproteinemia, *Ann. Clin. Res.* **8**:63 (1976).

124. Mordasini, R., Frey, F., Flury, W., Klosc, G., and Greten, H., Selective deficiency of hepatic triglyceride lipase in uremic patients, *N. Engl. J. Med.* **297**:1362 (1977).

125. Freeman, M., Kuiken, I., Ragland, J. B., and Sabesin, S. M., Hepatic triglyceride lipase deficiency of liver disease, *Lipids* **12**:443 (1977).

126. Murase, T., and Itakura, H., Accumulation of intermediate density lipoprotein in plasma after intravenous administration of hepatic triglyceride lipase antibody in rats, *Atherosclerosis* **39**:293 (1981).

127. Jansen, H., VanTol, A., and Hulsmann, W. C., On the metabolic function of heparin releaseable liver lipase, *Biochem. Biophys. Res. Commun.* **92**:53 (1980).

127a. Landin, B., Nilsson, A., Twu, J. S., and Schotz, M. C., A role for hepatic lipase in chylomicron and HDL phospholipid metabolism, *Circulation* **68III**:231 (1983).

128. Glomset, J. A., The plasma lecithin:cholesterol acyltransferase reaction, *J. Lipid Res.* **9**:155 (1968).

129. Fielding, P. E., and Fielding, C. J., A cholesteryl ester transfer complex in human plasma, *Proc. Natl. Acad. Sci. USA* **77**:3327 (1980).

130. Sgoutas, D. S., Fatty acid specificity of plasma phosphatidylcholine:cholesterol acyltransferase, *Biochemistry* **11**:293 (1972).

131. Assmann, G., Schmitz, G., Donath, N., and Lekim, D., Phosphatidylcholine substrate specificity of lecithin:cholesterol acyltransferase, *Scand. J. Clin. Lab. Invest.* **38**(150):16 (1978).

132. Fielding, C. J., and Fielding, P. E., Purification and substrate specificity of lecithin-cholesterol acyl transferase from human plasma, *FEBS Lett.* **15**:355 (1971).

133. Fielding, C. J., Shore, V. G., and Fielding, P. D., A protein cofactor of lecithin:cholesterol acyltransferase, *Biochem. Biophys. Res. Commun.* **46**:1943 (1972).

134. Soutar, A. K., Garner, C. W., Baker, H. N., Sparrow, J. T., Jackson, R. L., Gotto, A. M., and Smith, L. C., Effect of the human plasma apolipoproteins and phosphatidylcholine acyl donor on the activity of lecithin:cholesterol acyltransferase, *Biochemistry* **14**:3057 (1975).

135. Fukushima, D., Yokoyama, S., Kroon, D. J., Kezdy, F. J., and Kaiser, T., Chain length–function correlation of amphiphilic peptides, *J. Biol. Chem.* **255**:10651 (1980).

136. Subbaiah, P. V., Albers, J. J., Chen, C. H., and Bagdade, J. D., Low density lipoprotein-activated lysolecithin acylation by human plasma lecithin-cholesterol acyltransferase. Identity of lysolecithin acyltransferase and lecithin-cholesterol acyltransferase, *J. Biol. Chem.* **255**:9275 (1980).

137. Aron, L., Jones, S., and Fielding, C. J., Human plasma lecithin:cholesterol phospholipase activity, *J. Biol. Chem.* **253**:7220 (1978).

138. Simon, J. B., and Boyer, J. L., Production of lecithin:cholesterol acyltransferase by the isolated perfused rat liver, *Biochim. Biophys. Acta* **218**:549 (1971).

139. Nordby, G., Berg, T., Nilsson, M., and Norum, K. R., Secretion of lecithin:cholesterol acyltransferase from isolated rat hepatocytes, *Biochim. Biophys. Acta* **450**:69 (1976).

140. Albers, J. J., Lin, J. T., and Roberts, G. T., Effect of human plasma apolipoproteins on the activity of purified lecithin:cholesterol acyltransferase, *Artery* **5**:61 (1979).

141. Chung, J., Abano, D. A., Fless, G. M., and Scanu, A. M., Isolation, properties, and mechanism of *in vitro* action of lecithin:cholesterol acyltransferase from human plasma, *J. Biol. Chem.* **254**:7459 (1979).

142. Fielding, C. J., and Fielding, P. E., Regulation of human plasma lecithin:cholesterol acyltransferase activity by lipoprotein acceptor cholesteryl ester content, *J. Biol. Chem.* **256**:2102 (1981).

143. Barter, P. J., Hopkins, G. J., and Calvert, G. D., Transfers and exchanges of esterified cholesterol between plasma lipoproteins, *Biochem. J.* **208**:1 (1982).

144. Zilversmit, D. B., Hughes, L. B., and Balmer, J., Stimulation of cholesterol ester exchange by lipoprotein-free rabbit plasma, *Biochim. Biophys. Acta* **409**:393 (1975).

145. Pattnaik, N. M., Montes, A., Hughes, L. B., and Zilversmit, D. B., Cholesteryl ester exchange protein in human plasma: Isolation and characterization, *Biochim. Biophys. Acta* **530**:428 (1978).

146. Barter, P. J., and Lally, J. I., The activity of an esterified cholesterol transferring factor in human and rat serum, *Biochim. Biophys. Acta* **531**:233 (1978).

147. Barter, P. J., and Jones, M. E., Rate of exchange of esterified cholesterol between human plasma low and high density lipoproteins, *Atherosclerosis* **34**:67 (1979).

148. Barter, P. J., and Jones, M. E., Kinetic studies of the transfer of esterified cholesterol between human plasma low and high density lipoproteins, *J. Lipid Res.* **21**:238 (1980).

149. Barter, P. J., Ha, Y. C., and Calvert, G. D., Studies of esterified cholesterol in subfractions of plasma high density lipoproteins, *Atherosclerosis* **38**:165 (1981).

150. Ha, Y. C., Calvert, G. D., McIntosh, G. H., and Barter, P. J., A physiologic role for the esterified cholesterol transfer protein: *In vivo* studies in rabbits and pigs, *Metabolism* **30**:380 (1981).

151. Ha, Y. C., and Barter, P. J., Differences in plasma cholesteryl ester transfer activity in sixteen vertebrate species, *Comp. Biochem. Physiol. Ser. B* **71**:265 (1982).

152. Chajek, T., and Fielding, C. J., Isolation and characterization of a human serum cholesteryl ester transfer protein, *Proc. Natl. Acad. Sci. USA* **75**:3445 (1978).

153. Nestel, P. J., Reardon, M., and Billington, T., *In vivo* transfer of cholesteryl esters from high density lipoproteins to very low density lipoproteins in man, *Biochim, Biophys. Acta* **573**:403 (1979).

154. Hopkins, G. J., and Barter, P. J., Transfers of esterified cholesterol and triglyceride

between high density and very low density lipoproteins: *In vitro* studies of rabbits and humans, *Metabolism* **29**:546 (1980).

155. Morton, R. E., and Zilversmit, D. B., The separation of apolipoprotein D from cholesteryl ester transfer protein, *Biochim. Biophys. Acta* **663**:350 (1981).

156. Barter, P. J., Gorjatschko, L., and Calvert, G. D., Net mass transfer of esterified cholesterol from human low density lipoproteins to very low density lipoproteins incubated *in vitro, Biochim. Biophys. Acta* **619**:436 (1980).

157. Hopkins, G. J., and Barter, P. J., Dissociation of the *in vitro* transfers on esterified cholesterol and triglyceride between human lipoproteins, *Metabolism* **31**:78 (1982).

158. Barter, P. J., Gooden, J. M., and Rajaram, O. V., Species differences in the activity of a serum triglyceride transferring factor, *Atherosclerosis* **33**:165 (1979).

159. Morton, R. E., and Zilversmit, D. B., Purification and characterization of lipid transfer protein(s) from human lipoprotein-deficient plasma, *J. Lipid Res.* **23**:1058 (1982).

160. Barter, P. J., Lally, J. I., and Wattchow, D., Metabolism of triglyceride in rabbit plasma low and high density lipoproteins: Studies *in vivo* and *in vitro, Metabolism* **28**:614 (1979).

161. Rajaram, O. V., White, G. H., and Barter, P. J., Partial purification and characterization of a triacylglycerol-transfer protein from rabbit serum, *Biochim. Biophys. Acta* **617**:383 (1980).

162. Ellsworth, J. L., and McVittie, L., Dissociation of human plasma lipid transfer activities by a sulfhydryl reagent, *Fed. Proc.* **40**:1695 (1981).

163. Pattnaik, N. M., and Zilversmit, D. B., Interaction of chol-ester exchange protein with human plasma lipoproteins and phospholipid vessicles, *J. Biol. Chem.* **254**:2782 (1979).

164. Brewster, M. E., Ihm, J., Brainard, J. R., and Harmony, J. A. K., Transfer of phosphatidylcholine facilitated by a component of human plasma, *Biochim. Biophys. Acta* **529**:147 (1978).

165. Ihm, J., Harmoney, J. A. K., Ellsworth, J., and Jackson, R. L., Simultaneous transfer of cholesteryl ester and phospholipid by protein(s) isolated from human lipoprotein-free plasma, *Biochem. Biophys. Res. Commun.* **93**:1114 (1980).

166. Morton, R. E., and Zilversmit, D. B., A plasma inhibitor of triglyceride and cholesteryl ester transfer activities, *J. Biol. Chem.* **256**:11992 (1981).

167. Havel, R. J., Kane, J. P., and Kashyap, M. L., Interchange of apolipoproteins between chylomicrons and high density lipoproteins during alimentary lipemia in man, *J. Clin. Invest.* **52**:32 (1973).

168. Green, P. H. R., Glickman, R. M., Sauder, C. D., Blum, C. B., and Tall, A. R., Human intestinal lipoproteins. Studies in chyluric subjects, *J. Clin, Invest.* **64**:233 (1979).

169. Green, P. H. R., Glickman, R. M., Riley, J. W., and Quinet, E., Human apolipoprotein A-IV. Intestinal origin and distribution in plasma, *J. Clin. Invest.* **65**:911 (1980).

170. Fidge, N. H., The redistribution and metabolism of iodinated apolipoprotein A-IV in rats, *Biochim. Biophys. Acta* **169**:129 (1980).

171. Sheperd, J., Patsch, J. R., Packard, C. J., Gotto, A. M., Jr., and Taunton, O. D., Dynamic properties of human high density lipoprotein apoproteins, *J. Lipid Res.* **19**:383 (1978).

172. Grow, T. E., and Fried, M., Interchange of apoprotein components between the human plasma high density lipoprotein subclases HDL$_2$ and HDL$_3$ *in vitro, J. Biol. Chem.* **253**:8034 (1978).

173. Glomset, J. A., Mitchell, C. D., King, W. C., Applegate, K. R., Forte, T., Norum, K.

R., and Gjone, E., *In vitro* effects of lecithin:cholesterol acyltransferase on apolipoprotein distribution in familial lecithin:cholesterol acyltransferase deficiency, *Ann. N.Y. Acad. Sci.* **348:**224 (1980).

174. Kushwaha, R. S., and Hazzard, W. R., Catabolism of very low density lipoproteins in the rabbit. Effect of changing composition and pool size, *Biochim. Biophys. Acta* **528:**176 (1978).

175. Eisenberg, S., Effect of temperature and plasma on the exchange of apolipoproteins and phospholipids between rat plasma very low and high density lipoproteins, *J. Lipid Res.* **19:**229 (1978).

176. Patsch, J. R., Gotto, A. M., Jr., Olivecrona, T., and Eisenberg, S., Formation of high density lipoprotein$_2$-like particles during lipolysis of very low density lipoproteins *in vitro, Proc. Natl. Acad. Sci. USA* **75:**4519 (1978).

177. Redgrave, T. G., and Small, D. M., Quantitation of the transfer of surface phospholipid of chylomicrons to the high density lipoprotein fraction during the catabolism of chylomicrons in the rat, *J. Clin, Invest.* **64:**162 (1979).

178. Blum, C., Dynamics of apolipoprotein E metabolism in humans, *J. Lipid Res.* **23:**1308 (1982).

179. Cooper, A. D., and Yu, P. Y. S., Rates of removal and degradation of chylomicron remnants by isolated perfused rat liver, *J. Lipid Res.* **19:**635 (1978).

180. Sherrill, B. C., and Dietschy, J. M., Characterization of the sinusoidal transport process responsible for uptake of chylomicrons by the liver, *J. Biol. Chem.* **253:**1859 (1978).

180a. Dory, L., Boquet, L. M., Hamilton, R. L., Sloop, C. H., and Roheim, P. S., Presence of an HDL$_c$ precursor in the peripheral lymph of cholesterol-fed dogs, *Circulation* **68III:**117 (1983).

181. Glomset, J. A., and Norum, K. R., The metabolic role of lecithin:cholesterol acyltransferase: Perspectives from pathology, *Adv. Lipid Res.* **2:**1 (1973).

182. Lux, S. E., Kirz, R., Shrager, R. L., and Gotto, A. M., The influence of lipid on the conformation of human plasma high density apolipoproteins, *J. Biol. Chem.* **247:**2598 (1972).

183. Norum, K. R., Glomset, J. A., Nichols, A. V., Forte, T., Albers, J. J., King, W. C., Mitchell, C. D., Applegate, K. R., Gong, E. L., Cabana, V., and Gjone, E., Plasma lipoproteins in familial lecithin:cholesterol acyltransferase deficiency. Effects of incubation with lecithin:cholesterol acyltransferase deficiency *in vitro, Scand. J. Clin. Lab. Invest.* **35**(Suppl. 142):31 (1975).

184. Roheim, P. S., Rachmilewitz, D., Stein, O., and Stein, Y., Metabolism of iodinated high density lipoproteins in the rat: Half life in the circulation and uptake by organs, *Biochim. Biophys. Acta* **248:**315 (1971).

185. Nakai, T., Otto, P. S., Kennedy, D. L., and Whayne, T. F., Jr., Rat high density lipoprotein subfraction (HDL$_3$) uptake and catabolism by isolated rat liver parenchymal cells, *J. Biol. Chem.* **251:**4914 (1976).

186. Kovanen, P. T., Brown, M. S., and Goldstein, J. L., Increased binding of low density lipoprotein to liver membranes from rats treated with I-a-ethinyl estradiol, *J. Biol. Chem.* **254:**11367 (1979).

187. Chen, Y. D., Kroemer, F. B., and Reaven, G. M., Identification of specific high density lipoprotein-binding sites in rat testis and regulation of binding by human chorionic gonadotropin, *J. Biol. Chem.* **255:**9162 (1980).

188. Gwynne, J. T., and Hess, B., The role of high density lipoproteins in rat adrenal cholesterol metabolism and steroidogenesis, *J. Biol. Chem.* **255:***10875 (1980).*

189. Kovanen, P. T., Schneider, W. J., Hillman, G. M., Goldstein, J. L., and Brown, M.

S., Separate mechanism for the uptake of high and low density lipoprotein by mouse adrenal gland *in vivo, J. Biol. Chem.* **254**:5498 (1979).

190. Turley, S. D., and Dietschy, J. M., Cholesterol metabolism and excretion, in: *The Liver: Biology and Pathobiology* (I. Arias, H. Popper, D. Schachter, and D. A. Shafritz, eds.), pp. 468–487, Raven Press, New York (1982).

191. Stein, O., and Stein, Y., The removal of cholesterol from landschultz ascites cells by high-density apolipoprotein, *Biochim. Biohys. Acta* **326**:232 (1973).

192. Oram, J. F., Albers, J. J., and Bierman, E. L., Rapid regulation of the activity of the low density lipoprotein receptor of cultured human fibroblasts, *J. Biol. Chem.* **255**:475 (1980).

193. Oram, J. F., Albers, J. J., Cheung, M. C., and Bierman, E. L., The effects of subfractions of high density lipoprotein on cholesterol efflux from cultured fibroblasts. Regulation of low density lipoprotein receptor activity, *J. Biol. Chem.* **256**:8348 (1981).

194. Biesbroeck, R., Oram, J. F., Albers, J. J., and Bierman, E. L., Specific high-affinity binding of high density lipoproteins to cultured human skin fibroblasts and arterial smooth muscle cells, *J. Clin. Invest.* **71**:525 (1983).

195. Goldstein, J. L., Ho, Y. K., Basu, S. K., and Brown, M. S., Binding site on macrophages that mediates uptake and degradation of acetylated low density lipoprotein, producing massive cholesterol deposition, *Proc. Natl. Acad. Sci. USA* **76**:333 (1979).

196. Brown, M. S., Goldstein, J. L., Krieger, M., Ho, Y. K., and Anderson, R. G. W., Reversible accumulation of cholesteryl esters in macrophages incubated with acetylated lipoproteins, *J. Cell Biol.* **82**:597 (1979).

197. Ho, Y. K., Brown, M. S., and Goldstein, J. L., Hydrolysis and excretion of cytoplasmic cholesteryl esters by macrophages, stimulation of high density lipoprotein and other agents, *J. Lipid Res.* **21**:391 (1980).

198. Brown, M. S., Ho, Y. K., and Goldstein, J. L., The cholesteryl ester cycle in macrophage foam cells, *J. Biol. Chem.* **255**:9344 (1980).

199. Basu, S. K., Goldstein, J. L., and Brown, M. S., Independent pathways for secretion of cholesterol and apolipoprotein E by macrophages, *Science* **219**:871 (1982).

199a. Gordon, V., Innerarity, T. L., and Mahley, R. W., Formation of cholesterol- and apoprotein E-enriched high density lipoproteins in vitro, *J. Biol. Chem.* **258**:6202 (1983).

200. Miller, G. J., High density lipoproteins and atherosclerosis, *Annu. Rev. Med.* **31**:97 (1980).

201. Castelli, W. P., Doyle, J. T., Gordon, T., Hames, C. G., Hjortland, M. C., Hulley, S. B., Kagan, A., and Zukel, W. J., HDL cholesterol and other lipids in coronary heart disease. The Cooperative Lipoprotein Phenotyping Study, *Circulation* **55**:767 (1977).

202. Goldstein, J. L., and Brown, M. S., Binding and degradation of low density lipoproteins by cultured human fibroblasts: Comparison of cells from a normal subject and from a patient with homozygous familial hypercholesterolemia, *J. Biol. Chem.* **249**:5153 (1974).

203. Brown, M. S., and Goldstein, J. L., Regulation of the activity of the low density lipoprotein receptor in human fibroblasts, *Cell* **6**:307 (1975).

204. Goldstein, J. L., and Brown, M. S., The low density lipoprotein pathway and its relation to atherosclerosis, *Annu. Rev. Biochem.* **46**:897 (1977).

205. Brown, M. S., Kovanen, P. T., and Goldstein, J. L., Regulation of plasma cholesterol by lipoprotein receptors, *Science,* **212**:628 (1981).

206. Goldstein, J. L., and Brown, M. S., Familial hypercholesterolemia, in: *The Metabolic Basis of Inherited Disease,* 5th ed. (J. B. Stanbury, J. B. Wyngaarden, D. S. Fredrickson, J. L. Goldstein, and M. S. Brown, eds.), pp. 672–712, McGraw-Hill, New York (1982).

207. Goldstein, J. L., Basu, S. K., Brunschede, G. Y., and Brown, M. S., Release of low density lipoprotein from its cell surface receptor by sulfated glycosamino glycans, *Cell* **7**:85 (1976).

208. Pitas, E., Innerarity, T. L., Arnold, K. S., and Mahley, R. W., Rate equilibrium constants for binding of apo-E HDL$_c$ (a cholesterol-induced lipoprotein) and low density lipoproteins to human fibroblasts. Evidence for multiple receptor binding of apo-E HCL$_c$, *Proc. Natl. Acad. Sci. USA* **76**:2311 (1981).

209. Anderson, R. G. W., Goldstein, J. L., and Brown, M. S., Localization of low density lipoprotein receptors on plasma membrane of normal human fibroblasts and their absence in cells from a familial hypercholesterolemia homozygote, *Proc. Natl. Acad. Sci. USA* **73**:2434 (1976).

210. Anderson, R. G. W., Brown, M. S., and Goldstein, J. L., Role of the coated endocytic vesicle in the uptake of receptor-bound low density lipoprotein in human fibroblasts, *Cell* **10**:351 (1977).

211. Orci, L., Carpenter, J. L., Perrelet, A., Anderson, R. G. W., Goldstein, J. L., and Brown M. S., Occurrence of low density lipoprotein receptors within large pits on the surface of human fibroblasts as demonstrated by freeze-etching, *Exp. Cell. Res.* **113**:1 (1978).

212. Anderson, R. G. W., Brown, M. S., Beisiegel, U., and Goldstein, J. L., Surface distribution and recycling of the low density lipoprotein receptor as visualized with antireceptor antibodies, *J. Cell Biol.* **93**:523 (1982).

213. Basu, S. K., Goldstein, J. L., Anderson, R. G. W., and Brown, M. S., Degradation of cationized low density lipoprotein and regulation of cholesterol metabolism in homozygous familial hypercholesterolemia fibroblasts, *Proc. Natl. Acad. Sci. USA* **73**:3178 (1976).

214. Mahley, R. W., Innerarity, T. L., Pitas, R. E., Weisgraber, K. H., Brown, J. H., and Gross, E., Inhibition of lipoprotein binding to cell surface receptors of fibroblasts following selective modification of arginyl residues in arginine rich and B-apoproteins, *J. Biol. Chem.* **252**:7279 (1977).

215. Weisgraber, K. H., Innerarity, T. L., and Mahley, R. W., Role of the lysine residues of plasma lipoproteins in high affinity binding to cell surface receptors, *J. Biol. Chem.* **253**:9053 (1978).

216. Basu, S. K., Goldstein, J. L., and Brown, M. S., Characterization of the low density lipoprotein receptor in membranes prepared from human fibroblasts, *J. Biol. Chem.* **253**:3852 (1978).

217. Schneider, W. J., Goldstein, J. L., and Brown, M. S., Partial purification and characterization of the low density lipoprotein receptor from bovine adrenal cortex, *J. Biol. Chem.* **255**:11442 (1980).

218. Schneider, W. J., Beisiegel, U., Goldstein, J. L., and Brown, M. S., Purification of the low density lipoprotein receptor, an acidic glycoprotein of 164,000 molecular weight, *J. Biol. Chem.* **257**:2664 (1982).

219. Tolleshaug, H., Goldstein, J. L., Schneider, W. J., and Brown, M. S., Posttranslational processing of the LDL receptor and its genetic disruption in familial hypercholesterolemia, *Cell* **30**:715 (1982).

220. Beisiegel, U., Schneider, W. J., Brown, M. S., and Goldstein, J. L., Immunoblot analysis of low density lipoprotein receptors in fibroblasts from subjects with familial hypercholesterolemia, *J. Biol. Chem.* **257**:13150 (1982).

221. Brown, M. S., Anderson, R. G. W., and Goldstein, J. L., Recycling receptors: The round-trip itinerary and migrant membrane proteins, *Cell* **32**:663 (1983).

222. Tolleshaug, H., Hobgood, K. K., Brown, M. S., and Goldstein, J. L., The LDL receptor locus in familial hypercholesterolemia: Multiple mutations disrupt transport and processing of a membrane receptor, *Cell* **32**:941 (1983).

223. Beisiegel, U., Kita, T., Anderson, R. G. W., Schneider, W. J., Brown, M. S., and Goldstein, J. L., Immunologic cross-reactivity of the low density lipoprotein receptor from bovine adrenal cortex, human fibroblasts, canine liver and adrenal gland, and rat liver, *J. Biol. Chem.* **256**:4071 (1981).

224. Beisiegel, U., Schneider, W. J., Goldstein, J. L., Anderson, R. G. W., and Brown, M. S., Monoclonal antibodies to the low density lipoprotein receptor as probes for study of receptor-mediated endocytosis and the genetics of familial hypercholesterolemia, *J. Biol. Chem.* **256**:11923 (1981).

225. Goldstein, J. L., Anderson, R. G. W., and Brown, M. S., Coated pits, coated vesicles, and receptor-mediated endocytosis, *Nature* **279**:679 (1979).

226. Basu, S. K., Goldstein, J. L., Anderson, R. G. W., and Brown, M. S., Monensin interrupts the recycling of low density lipoprotein receptors in human fibroblasts, *Cell* **24**:493 (1981).

227. Goldstein, J. L., Dana, S. E., Faust, J. R., Beaudet, A. L., and Brown, M. S., Role of lysosomal acid lipase in the metabolism of plasma low density lipoprotein: Observations in cultured fibroblasts from a patient with cholesteryl ester storage disease, *J. Biol. Chem.* **250**:8487 (1975).

228. Brown, M. S., Faust, J. R., and Goldstein, J. L., Role of the low density lipoprotein receptor in regulating the content of free and esterified cholesterol in human fibroblasts, *J. Clin. Invest.* **55**:783 (1975).

229. Brown, M. S., Dana, S. E., and Goldstein, J. L., Regulation of 3-hydroxy-3-methylglutaryl coenzyme A reductase activity in cultured human fibroblasts: Comparison of cells from a normal subject and from a patient with homozygous familial hypercholesterolemia, *J. Biol. Chem.* **249**:789 (1974).

230. Goldstein, J. L., Dana, S. E., and Brown, M. S., Esterification of low density lipoprotein in human fibroblasts and its absence in homozygous familial hypercholesterolemia, *Proc. Natl. Acad. Sci. USA* **71**:4288 (1974).

231. Ho, Y. K., Brown, M. S., Kayden H. J., and Goldstein, J. L., Binding, internalization, and hydrolysis of low density lipoproteins in long term lymphoid cell lines from a normal subject and a patient with homozygous familial hypercholesterolemia, *J. Exp. Med.* **144**:444 (1976).

232. Ho. Y. K., Brown, M. S., Bilheimer, D. W., and Goldstein, J. L., Regulation of low density lipoprotein receptor activity in freshly isolated human lymphocytes, *J. Clin. Invest.* **58**:1465 (1976).

233. Goldstein, J. L., and Brown, M. S., Lipoprotein receptors, cholesterol metabolism, and atherosclerosis, *Arch. Pathol.* **99**:181 (1975).

234. Albers, J. J., and Bierman, E. L., The effect of hypoxia on uptake and degradation of low density lipoproteins by cultured human arterial smooth muscle cells, *Biochim. Biophys. Acta* **424**:422 (1976).

235. Stein, O., and Stein, Y., High density lipoproteins reduce the uptake of low density lipoproteins by human endothelial cells in culture, *Biochim. Biophys. Acta* **431**:363 (1976).

236. Chao, Y., Windler, E. E., Chen, C. G., and Havel, R. J., Hepatic catabolism of rat and human lipoproteins in rats treated with 17a-ethinyl estradiol, *J. Biol. Chem.* **254**:11360 (1979).

237. Hui, D. Y., Innerarity, T. L., and Mahley, R. W., Lipoprotein binding to canine hepatic membranes, *J. Biol. Chem.* **256**:5646 (1981).

238. Goldstein, J. L., The estradiol-stimulated lipoprotein receptor of rat liver, *J. Biol. Chem.* **255**:10464 (1980).
239. Shepherd, J., Packard, C. J., Bicker, S., Lawrie, T. D. V., and Morgan, H. G., Cholestrylamine promotes receptor-mediated low-density lipoprotein catabolism, *N. Engl. J. Med.* **302**:1219 (1980).
240. Slater, H. R., Packard, C. J., Bicker, S., and Shepherd, J., Effects of cholestyramine on receptor-mediated plasma clearance and tissue uptake of human low density lipoproteins in the rabbit, *J. Biol. Chem.* **255**:10210 (1980).
241. Tanzawa, K., Shinada, Y., Kuroda, M., Tsujiota, Y., Arai, M., and Watanabe, Y., WHHL-rabbit: A low density lipoprotein receptor-deficient animal model for familial hypercholesterolemia, *FEBS Lett.* **118**:81 (1980).
242. Attie, A. D., Pittman, R. C., Watanabe, Y., and Steinberg, D., Low density lipoprotein receptor deficiency in cultured hepatocytes of the WHHL rabbit. Further evidence of two pathways for catabolism of exogenous proteins, *J. Biol. Chem.* **256**:9789 (1981).
243. Kita, T., Brown, M. S., Watanabe, Y., and Goldstein, J. L., Deficiency of low density lipoprotein receptors in liver and adrenal gland of the WHHL rabbit, an animal model of familial hypercholesterolemia, *Proc. Natl. Acad. Sci. USA* **78**:2268 (1981).
244. Mahley, R. W., Innerarity, T. L., Weisgraber, K. H., and Fry, D. L., Accumulation of lipid by aorticmedial cells *in vivo* and *in vitro, Am. J. Pathol.* **87**:205 (1977).
245. Bersot, T. P., Mahley, R. W., Brown, M. S., and Goldstein, J. L., Interaction of swine lipoproteins with the low density lipoprotein receptor in human fibroblasts, *J. Biol. Chem.* **251**:2395 (1976).
246. Innerarity, T. L., and Mahley, R. W., Enhanced binding by cultured human fibroblasts of apo-E-containing lipoproteins as compared with low density lipoproteins, *Biochemistry* **17**:1440 (1978).
247. Mahley, R. W., Weisgraber, K. H., and Innerarity, T. L., Interaction of plasma lipoprotein containing apolipoproteins B and E with heparin and cell surface receptors, *Biochim. Biophys. Acta* **575**:81 (1979).
248. Innerarity, T. L., Pitas, R. E., and Mahley, R. W., Binding of arginine-rich (E) apoprotein after recombination with phospholipid vesicles to the low density lipoprotein receptors of fibroblasts, *J. Biol. Chem.* **254**:4186 (1979).
249. Pitas, R. E., Innerarity, T. L., and Mahley, R. W., Cell surface receptor binding of phospholipid–protein complexes containing different ratios of receptor-active and -inactive E apoprotein, *J. Biol. Chem.* **255**:5454 (1980).
250. Gianturco, S. H., Gotto, A. M., Jr., Jackson, R. L., Patsch, J. R., Sybers, H. D., Taunton, O. D., Yeshurin, D. L., and Smith, L. C., Control of 3-hydroxy-3-methyl glutaryl-CoA reductase activity in cultured human fibroblasts by very low density lipoproteins of subjects with hypertriglyceridemia, *J. Clin. Invest.* **61**:320 (1978).
251. Innerarity, T. L., Pitas, R. E., and Mahley, R. W., Disparities in the interaction of rat and human lipoproteins with cultured rat fibroblasts and smooth muscle cells, *J. Biol. Chem.* **255**:11163 (1980).
252. Floren, C. H., Albers, J. J., Kudchodkar, B., and Bierman, E. L., Receptor-dependent uptake of human chylomicron remnants by cultured skin fibroblasts, *J. Biol. Chem.* **256**:425 (1981).
253. Kovanen, P. T., Brown, M. S., Basu, S. K., Bilheimer, D. W., and Goldstein, J. L., Saturation and suppression of hepatic lipoprotein receptors: A mechanism for the hypercholesterolemia of cholesterol-fed rabbits, *Proc. Natl. Acad. Sci. USA* **78**:1396 (1981).
254. Van'tHooft, F., and Havel, R. J., Metabolism of chromatographically separated rat

serum lipoproteins specifically labeled with ^{125}I-apolipoprotein E, *J. Biol. Chem.* **256**:3963 (1981).

255. Steinmetz, A., Kushwaha, R., Foster, D., Unune, A., and Hazzard, W., The differential catabolism of apolipoprotein E in very low and high density lipoproteins, *Circulation* **66**(II):12 (1982).

256. Carrela, M., and Cooper, A. D., High affinity binding of chylomicron remnants to rat liver plasma membranes, *Proc. Natl. Acad. Sci. USA* **76**:338 (1979).

257. Windler, E., Chao, Y., and Havel, R. J., Determinants of hepatic uptake of triglyceride-rich lipoproteins and their remnants in the rat, *J. Biol. Chem.255:*5475 (1980).

258. Sherrill, B. C., Innerarity, T. L., and Mahley, R. W., Rapid hepatic clearance of the canine lipoproteins containing only the E apoprotein by a high affinity receptor, *J. Biol. Chem.* **255**:1804 (1980).

259. Mahley, R. W., Weisgraber, K. H., Innerarity, T. L., and Windmueller, H. G., Accelerated clearance of low density and high density lipoproteins and retarded clearance of E apoprotein-containing lipoproteins from the plasma of rats after modification of lysine residues, *Proc. Natl. Acad. Sci. USA* **76**:1746 (1979).

260. Mahley, R. W., Weisgraber, K. H., Melchio, G. W., Innerarity, T. L., and Holcome, K. S., Inhibition of receptor-mediated clearance of lysine and arginine modified lipoproteins from the plasma of rats and monkeys, *Proc. Natl. Acad. Sci. USA* **77**:225 (1980).

261. Shelburne, F., Hanks, J., Meyers, W., and Quarfordt, S., Effect of apoproteins on hepatic uptake of drug emulsions in the rat, *J. Clin. Invest.* **65**:652 (1980).

262. Windler, E., Chao, Y., and Havel, R. J., Regulation of the hepatic uptake of triglyceride-rich lipoproteins in the rat, *J. Biol. Chem.* **255**:8303 (1980).

263. Quarfordt, S. H., Michalopoulos, G., and Schirmer, B., The effect of human C apolipoproteins on the *in vitro* hepatic metabolism of triglyceride emulsions in the rat, *J. Biol. Chem.* **257**:14642 (1982).

264. Sparks, C. E., and Marsh, J. B., Metabolic heterogeneity in apolipoprotein B in the rat, *J. Lipid Res.* **22**:519 (1981).

265. Sparks, C. E., Huatink, O., and Marsh, J. B., Hepatic and intestinal contribution of two forms of apolipoprotein B to plasma lipoprotein fractions in the rat, *Can. J. Biochem.* **59**:693 (1981).

266. Elovson, J., Huang, Y. O., Baker, N., and Kannan, R., Apolipoprotein B is structurally and metabolically heterogeneous in the rat, *Proc. Natl. Acad. Sci. USA* **78**:157 (1981).

267. Van't Hooft, F. M., and Hardman, D. A., Kane, J. P., and Havel, R. J., Apolipoprotein B (B-48) of rat chylomicrons is not a precursor of the apolipoprotein of low density lipoproteins, *Proc. Natl. Acad. Sci. USA* **79**:179 (1982).

268. Carey, M. C., Small, D. M., and Bliss, C. M., Lipid digestion and absorption, *Annu. Rev. Physiol.* **45**:637 (1983).

269. Kane, J. P., Hardman, D. A., and Paulus, H. E., Heterogeneity of apolipoprotein B: Isolation of a new species from human chylomicrons, *Proc. Natl. Acad. Sci. USA* **77**:2465 (1980).

269a. Hui, D. Y., Innerarity, T. L., Ehnholm, C., and Mahley, R. W., Protein determinants for B-very low density lipoprotein and chylomicron remnant binding to hepatic and extrahepatic receptors, *Circulation* **68III**:118 (1983).

270. Havel, R. J., Goldstein, J. L., and Brown, M. S., Lipoproteins and lipid transport, in: *Metabolic Control and Disease* (P. K. Bondy and L. L. Rosenberg, eds.), pp. 393–494, Saunders, Philadelphia (1980).

271. Kita, T., Brown, M. S., Bilheimer, D. W., and Goldstein, J. L., Delayed clearance of

very low density and intermediate density lipoproteins with enhanced conversion to low density lipoprotein in WHHL rabbits, *Proc. Natl. Acad. Sci. USA* **79**:5693 (1982).

272. Kita, T., Goldstein, J. L., Brown, M. S., Watanabe, Y., Hornick, C. A., and Havel, R. J., Hepatic uptake of chylomicron remnants in WHHL rabbits: A mechanism genetically distinct from the low density lipoprotein receptor, *Proc. Natl. Acad. Sci. USA* **79**:3623 (1982).

273. Goldstein, J. L., Kita, T., and Brown, M. S., Defective lipoprotein receptors and atherosclerosis, *N. Engl. J. Med.* **308**:288 (1983).

274. Goldstein, J. L., Ho, Y. K., Brown, M. S., Innerarity, T. L., and Mahley, R. W., Cholesteryl ester accumulation in macrophages resulting from receptor-mediated uptake and degradation of hypercholesterolemic canine B-very low density lipoproteins, *J. Biol. Chem.* **2155**:1839 (1980).

275. Mahley, R. W., Innerarity, T. L., Brown, M. S., Ho, Y. K., and Goldstein, J. L., Cholesteryl ester synthesis in macrophages: Stimulation by B-very low density lipoproteins from cholesterol-fed animals of several species, *J. Lipid Res.* **21**:970 (1980).

276. Fainaru, M., Mahley, R. W., Hamilton, R. L., and Innerarity, T. L., Structural and metabolic heterogeneity of B-very low density lipoprotein from cholesterol-fed dogs and from humans with type III hyperlipoproteinemia, *J. Lipid Res.* **23**:7092 (1982).

277. Havel, R. J., and Kane, J. L., Primary dysbetalipoproteinemia: Predominance of a specific apoprotein species in triglyceride rich lipoproteins, *Proc. Natl. Acad. Sci. USA* **70**:2015 (1973).

278. Hazzard, W. R., and Bierman, E. L., Delayed clearance of chylomicron remnants following vitamin A containing oral fat loads in broad-B disease (type III hyperlipoproteinemia), *Metabolism* **25**:777 (1976).

279. Chait, A., Hazzard, W. R., Albers, J. J., Kushwaha, R. P., and Brunzell, J. D., Impaired very low density lipoprotein and triglyceride removal in broad beta disease: Comparison with endogenous hypertriglyceridemia, *Metabolism* **27**:1055 (1978).

280. Mahley, R. W., Dietary fat, cholesterol, and accelerated atherosclerosis, *Atheroscler. Rev.* **5**:1 (1979).

281. Faggiotto, A., Ross, R., and Harker, L., Early arterial changes in the hypercholesterolemic non-human primate, *Circulation* **66**(II):225 (1982).

282. Mahley, R. W., Atherogenic hyperlipoproteinmia. The cellular and molecular biology of plasma lipoproteins altered by dietary fat and cholesterol, in: *Medical Clinics of North America: Lipid Disorders,* Vol. 66 (R. J. Havel, ed.), pp. 375–402, W. B. Saunders, Philadelphia (1982).

283. Pitas, R. E., Innerarity, T. L., and Mahley, R. W., Foam cells in explants of atherosclerotic rabbit aortas have receptors for B-very low density lipoproteins and modified low density lipoproteins, *Arteriosclerosis* **3**:2 (1983).

284. Mahley, R. W., and Innerarity, T. L., Lipoprotein receptors and cholesterol homeostasis, *Biochim. Biophys. Acta* **737**:197 (1983).

285. VanLenten, B. J., Fogelman, A. M., Hokom, M. M., Benson, L., Haberland, M. E., and Edwards, P. A., Regulation of the uptake and degradation of B-VLDL in human monocyte-macrophages, *J. Biol. Chem.* **258**:5151 (1983).

285a. Baker, D., Van Lenten, B. J., Fogelman, A. M., Edwards, P. A., and Berliner, J. A., Identification and characterization of a B-VLDL receptor on adult aortic endothelial cells, *Circulation* **68**III:49 (1983).

286. Goldstein, J. L., and Brown, M. S., Atherosclerosis: The low-density lipoprotein receptor hypothesis, *Metabolism* **26**:1257 (1977).

287. Fogelman, A. M., Schechter, I., Seager, J., Hokom, M., Child, J. S., and Edwards, P. A., Malondialdehyde alteration of low density lipoproteins leads to cholesteryl ester

accumulation in human monocyte-macrophages, *Proc. Natl. Acad. Sci. USA* **77**:2214 (1980).

288. Brown, M. S., and Goldstein, J. L., Lipoprotein metabolism in the macrophage: Implications for cholesterol deposition in atherosclerosis, *Annu. Rev. Biochem.* **52**:223 (1983).

289. Via, D. P., Dresel, H. A., and Gotto, A. M., Jr., Isolation and characterization of the murine macrophage acetyl LDL receptor, *Circulation* **66**(II):37 (1982).

289a. Wong, H., Fogelman, A. M., Haberland, M. E., and Edwards, P. A., Identification of the scavenger receptor from rabbit aveolar macrophages, *Circulation* **68III**:50 (1983).

289b. Via, D. P., Vignale, S., and Gotto, A. M., Jr., Recycling of the acetyl-LDL receptor in murine macrophage cell line P388D$_1$, *Circulation* **68III**:74 (1983).

290. Henriksen, T., Mahoney, E. M., and Steinberg, D., Enhanced macrophage degradation of low density lipoprotein previously incubated with cultured endothelial cells: Recognition by receptors for acetylated low density lipoproteins, *Proc. Natl. Acad. Sci. USA* **78**:6499 (1981).

291. Drevon, C. A., Berg, T., and Norum, K. R., Uptake and degradation of cholesterol ester-labelled rat plasma lipoproteins in purified rat hepatocytes and non-parenchymal liver cells, *Biochim. Biophys. Acta* **487**:122 (1977).

292. Ose, L., Roken, I., Norum, K. R., Drevon, C. A., and Berg, T., The binding of high density lipoproteins to isolated rat hepatocytes, *Scand. J. Clin. Invest.* **41**:63 (1981).

293. Wandel, M., Norum, K. R., Berg, T., and Ose, L., Binding, uptake, and degradation of ^{125}I-labeled high-density lipoproteins in isolated non-parenchymal rat liver cells, *Scand. J. Gastroenterol.* **16**:71 (1981).

293a. Brinton, E. A., Oram, J. F., Chen, C. H., Albers, J. J., and Bierman, E. L., Ligand characterization of the HDL receptor in cultured fibroblasts, *Circulation* **68III**:215 (1983).

294. Miller, N. E., Weinstein, D. B., and Steinberg, D., Binding, internalization, and degradation of high density lipoprotein by cultured normal human fibroblasts, *J. Lipid Res. 18:438 (1977).*

295. Wu, J. D., Butler, J., and Bailey, J. M., Lipid metabolism in cultured cells. XVIII. Comparative uptake of low density and high density lipoprotein by normal, hypercholesterolemic, and tumor-transformed human fibroblasts, *J. Lipid Res.* **20**:472 (1979).

296. Brinton, E. A., Oram, J. F., and Bierman, E. L., Regulation of high-density-lipoprotein receptor activity of cultured human fibroblasts, *Circulation* **66**(II):101 (1982).

297. Sparrow, J. T., Morrisett, J. D., Pownall, H. J., Jackson, R. L., and Gotto, A. M., Jr., The mechanism of lipid binding by the plasma lipoproteins: Synthesis of model peptides, in: *Peptides: Chemistry, Structure and Biology* (R. Walter and J. Meinenhofer, eds.), p. 597–602, Ann Arbor Science, Ann Arbor, Michigan (1975).

298. Blum, C. B., Aron, L., and Sciacca, R., Radioimmunoassay studies of human apolipoprotein E, *J. Clin. Invest.* **66**:1240 (1980).

299. Havel, R., Kotite, J. L., Vigne, J. L., Kane, J. P., Tun, P., Phillips, N., and Chen, G. C., Radioimmunoassay of human arginine rich apolipoprotein, apoprotein E, *J. Clin. Invest.* **6**:1351 (1980).

300. Schonfeld, G., Patsch, W., Rudel, L. L., Nelson, C., Epstein, M., and Olson, R. E., Effects of dietary cholesterol and fatty acids on plasma lipoproteins, *J. Clin. Invest.* **69**:1072 (1982).

301. Carlson, L. A., and Holmquist, L., Concentrations of apolipoproteins B, C-I, C-II, C-III and E in sera from normal men and their relation to serum lipoprotein levels, *Clin. Chim. Acta* **124**:163 (1982).

301a. Bisgaier, C., Sachdev, O., Megna, L., and Glickman, R., Plasma distribution of human apo A-IV, *Circulation* **68III**:215 (1983).

302. Brewer, H. B., Jr., Fairwell, T., Larue, A., Ronan, R., Houser, A., and Bronzert, T., The amino acid sequence of human apo A-I, an apoprotein isolated from high density lipoproteins, *Biochem. Biophys. Res. Commun.* **80**:623 (1978).

303. Albers, J. J., Albers, L. V., and Aladjem, F., Isoelectric heterogeneity of the major polypeptide human serum high density lipoproteins, *Biochem. Med.* **5**:48 (1971).

304. Lux, S. E., and John, K. M., Further characterization of the polymorphic forms of a human high density apolipoprotein, apoLP-Gln-I (apo A-I), *Biochim. Biophys. Acta* **278**:266 (1972).

305. Ghiselli, G., Brewer, H. B., Jr., and Windmueller, H. G., Apolipoprotein A-I isoprotein synthesis by the perfused rat liver, *Biochem. Biophys. Res. Commun.* **107**:144 (1982).

306. Karathanasis, S. K., Zannis, V. I., and Breslow, J. L., Isolation and characterization of the human apolipoprotein A-I gene, *Proc. Natl. Acad. Sci USA,* **80**:6147–6151 (1983).

307. Shoulders, C. C., and Baralle, F. E., Isolation of the human HDL apoprotein AI gene, *Nucl. Acids Res.* **10**:4873 (1982).

308. Lin-Su, M. H., Lin-Lee, Y. C., Bradley, W. A., and Chan, L., Characterization, cell-free synthesis, and processing of apolipoprotein A-I of rat high-density lipoproteins, *Biochemistry* **20**:2470 (1981).

309. Karathanasis, S. K., and Breslow, J. L., Linkage of human apolipoproteins A-I and C-III genes, *Nature* **304**:371 (1983).

309a. Bruns, G. A. P., Karathanasis, S. K., and Breslow, J. L., The human apolipoprotein AI-CIII gene complex is located on chromosome 11, *Arteriosclerosis,* **4**:97 (1984).

310. McLachlin, A. D., Repeated helical pattern in apolipoprotein A-I, *Nature* **267**:465 (1977).

311. Barker, W. C., and Dayhoff, M. O., Evolution of lipoproteins deduced from protein sequence data, *Comp. Biochem. Physiol.* **57B**:309 (1977).

312. Brewer, H. B., Jr., Lux, S. E., Ronan, R., and John, K. M., Amino acid sequence of human apoLp-Gln-II (apo A-II), an apolipoprotein isolated from the high density lipoprotein complex, *Proc. Natl. Acad. Sci. USA* **69**:1304 (1972).

313. Weisgraber, K. H., and Mahley, R. W., Apoprotein (E-A-II) complex of human plasma lipoproteins. I. Characterization of this mixed disulfide and its identification in a high density lipoprotein subfraction, *J. Biol. Chem.* **253**:6281 (1978).

314. Jackson, R. L., Mao, S. J. T., and Gotto, A. M., Jr., Effects of maleylation on the lipid-binding and immunochemical properties of human plasma high density apolipoprotein A-II, *Biochem. Biophys. Res. Commun.* **61**:1317 (1974).

315. Mao, S. J. T., Sparrow, J. T., Gilliam, E. B., Gotto, A. M., Jr., and Jackson, R. L., Mechanism of lipid–protein interaction in the plasma lipoproteins: Lipid-binding properties of synthetic fragments of apolipoprotein A-II, *Biochemistry* **16**:4150 (1977).

316. Mao, S. J. T., Jackson, R. L., Gotto, A. M., Jr., and Sparrow, J. T., Mechanism of lipid–protein interaction in the plasma lipoproteins: Identification of a lipid-binding site in apolipoprotein A-II, *Biochemistry* **20**:1676 (1981).

317. Shinomiya, M., Sasaki, N., Barnhart, R. L., Shirai, K., and Jackson, R. L., Effect of apolipoproteins on the hepatic lipase-catalyzed hydrolysis of human plasma high density lipoprotein$_2$-triacylglycerols, *Biochim. Biophys. Acta* **713**:292 (1982).

318. Jahn, C. E., Osborne, J. C., Jr., Schaefer, E. J., and Brewer, H. B., Jr., Activation of enzymatic activity of hepatic lipase by apolipoprotein A-II, *Eur. J. Biochem. 131:25 (1983).*

319. Lagocki, P. A., and Scanu, A. M., *In vitro* modulation of the apolipoprotein composition of high density lipoprotein, *J. Biol. Chem.* **255**:3701 (1980).
320. Swaney, J. B., Reese, H., and Eder, H. A., Polypeptide composition of rat high density lipoprotein: Characterization by SDS-gel electrophoresis, *Biochem. Biophys. Res. Commun.* **59:513 (1974).**
321. Weisgraber, K. H., Bersot, T. P., Mahley, R. W., Isolation and characterization of an apoprotein from the $d < 1.006$ lipoproteins of human and canine lymph homologous with the rat A-IV apoprotein, *Biochem. Biophys. Res. Commun.* **85**:287 (1978).
322. Beisiegel, U., and Utermann, G., An apolipoprotein homolog of rat apolipoprotein A-IV in human plasma: Isolation and partial characterization, *Eur. J. Biochem.* **93**:601 (1979).
323. Zannis, V. I., Fraser, P., Rooney, V., and Breslow, J. L., Human lymph chylomicron apolipoproteins examined at the isoprotein level, *Arteriosclerosis* **2**:426a (1982).
323a. Weinberg, R. B., and Spector, M. S., Human apolipoprotein A-IV: Displacement from the surface of triglyceride-rich particles by HDL_2 associated C-apoproteins, *Circulation* **68III**:116 (1983).
324. Lee, D. M., Valente, A. J., Keuo, W. H., and Maeda, H., Properties of apolipoprotein B in urea and in aqueous buffers, the use of glutathione and nitrogen in its solubilization, *Biochim. Biophys. Acta* **666**:133 (1981).
325. Kane, J. P., Richards, E. G., and Havel, R. J., Subunit heterogeneity in human serum beta lipoprotein, *Proc. Natl. Acad. Sci. USA* **66**:1075 (1970).
326. Chen, C. H., and Aladjem, F., Subunit structure of the apoprotein of human serum low density lipoproteins, *Biochem. Biophys. Res. Commun.* **60**:549 (1974).
327. Malloy, M. J., Kane, J. P., Hardman, D. A., and Hamilton, R. L., Absence of the B-100 apolipoprotein. Normotriglyceridemic, abetalipoproteinemia, *J. Clin. Invest.* **67**:1441 (1981).
328. Krishnaiah, K. V., Walker, L. F., Borensztajn, J., Schonfeld, G., and Getz, G. S., Apolipoprotein B variant derived from rat intestine, *Proc. Natl. Acad. Sci. USA* **77**:3806 (1980).
329. Jackson, R. L., Sparrow, J. T., Baker, H. N., Morriset, J. D., Taunton, O. D., and Gotto, A. M., Jr., The primary structure of apolipoprotein-serine, *J. Biol. Chem.* **249**:5308 (1974).
330. Shulman, R. S., Herbert, P. N., Wehrly, K., and Fredrickson, D. S., The complete amino acid sequence of CI (apo Lp-Ser), an apolipoprotein from human very low density lipoprotein, *J. Biol. Chem.* **250**:182 (1975).
331. Jackson, R. L., Morrisett, J. D., Sparrow, J. T., Segrest, J. P., Pownall, H. J., Smith, L. C., Hoff, H. F., and Gotto, A. M., Jr., The interaction of apolipoprotein-serine with phosphatidylcholine, *J. Biol. Chem.* **249**:5314 (1974).
332. Ganesan, D., Bradford, R. H., Alaupovic, P., and McConathy, W. J., Differential activation of lipoprotein lipase from human post-heparin plasma, milk and adipose tissue by polypeptides of human serum apolipoprotein C, *FEBS Lett.* **15**:205 (1971).
333. Jackson, R. I., Baker, H. N., Gilliam, E. B., and Gotto, A. M., Primary structure of very low density apolipoprotein C-II of human plasma, *Proc. Natl. Acad. Sci. USA* **74**:1942 (1977).
334. Havel, R. J., Kotite, L., and Kane, J. P., Isoelectric heterogeneity of the cofactor protein of lipoprotein lipase in human blood plasma, *Biochem. Med.* **21**:121 (1979).
335. Morrisett, J. D., Jackson, R. L., and Gotto, A. M., Jr., Lipid–protein interactions in the plasma lipoproteins, *Biochim. Biophys. Acta* **472**:93 (1977).
336. Mantulin, W. W., Rohde, M. F., Gotto, A. M., Jr., and Pownall, H., The conformational properties of human plasma apolipoprotein C-II, *J. Biol. Chem.* **255**:8185 (1980).

337. Musliner, T. A., Church, E. C., Herbert, P. N., Kingston, M. J., and Shulman, R. S., Lipoprotein lipase cofactor activity of a carbosyl-terminal peptide of apolipoprotein C-II, *Proc. Natl. Acad. Sci. USA* **74:**5358 (1977).
338. Kinnunen, P. K. J., Jackson, R. L., Smith, L. C., Gotto, A. M., Jr., and Sparrow, J. T., Activation of lipoprotein lipase by native and synthetic fragments of human plasma apolipoprotein C-II, *Proc. Natl. Acad. Sci. USA* **74:**4848 (1977).
339. Musliner, T. A., Herbert, P. N., and Church, E. C., Activation of lipoprotein lipase by native and acylated peptides of apolipoprotein C-II, *Biochim. Biophys. Acta* **573:**501 (1979).
340. Shulman, R. S., Herbert, P. N., Fredrickson, D. S., Wehrly, K., and Brewer, H. B., Jr., Isolation and alignment of the tryptic peptides of alanine apolipoprotein, an apolipoprotein from human plasma very low density lipoproteins, *J. Biol. Chem.* **249:**4969 (1974).
341. Zannis, V. I., and Breslow, J. L., Two dimensional maps of human apolipoproteins in normal and diseased states, in: *Electrophoresis 1979* (Radola, B. J., ed.), pp. 437–473, Walter de Gruyter, Berlin (1980).
342. Kashyap, M. L., Srivastava, L. S., Hynd, B. A., Gartside, P. S., and Perisutti, G., Quantitation of human apolipoprotein C-III and its subspecies by radioimmunoassay and analytical isoelectric focusing: Abnormal plasma triglyceride-rich lipoprotein apolipoprotein C-III subspecies concentrations in hypertriglyceridemia, *J. Lipid Res.* **22:**800 (1981).
343. Morrisett, J. D., David, J. S. K., Pownall, H. J., and Gotto, A. M., Jr., Interaction of an apolipoprotein (apolp-alanine) with phosphatidylcholine, *Biochemistry* **12:**1290 (1973).
344. Sparrow, J. T., Pownall, H. J., Hsu, F. J., Blumenthal, L. E., Culwell, A. R., and Gotto, A. M., Lipid binding by fragments of apolipoprotein C-III-1 obtained by thrombin cleavage, *Biochemistry* **16:**5427 (1977).
345. Brown, W. V., and Baginsky, M. L., Inhibition of lipoprotein lipase by an apoprotein of human very low density lipoprotein, *Biochem. Biophys. Res. Commun.* **46:**375 (1972).
346. Krauss, R. M., Herbert, P. N., Levy, R. I., and Fredrickson, D. S., Further observations on the activation and inhibition of lipoprotein lipase by apolipoproteins, *Circ. Res.* **33:**403 (1973).
347. Kostner, G. M., Studies of the composition and structure of human serum lipoproteins: Isolation and partial characterization of apolipoprotein A-III, *Biochim. Biophys. Acta* **336:**383 (1974).
348. Curry, M. D., McConathy, W. J., and Alaupovic, P., Quantitative determination of human apolipoprotein D by electroimmunoassay and radial immunodiffusion, *Biochim. Biophys. Acta* **491:**232 (1977).
349. McConathy, W. J., and Alaupovic, P., Studies on the isolation and partial characterization of apolipoprotein D and lipoprotein D of human plasma, *Biochemistry* **15:**515 (1976).
350. McConathy, W. J., and Alaupovic, P., Isolation and partial characterization of apolipoprotein D: A new protein moiety of the human plasma lipoprotein system, *FEBS Lett.* **37:**178 (1973).
351. Kostner, G., Studies on the cofactor requirement for lecithin:cholesterol acyltransferase, *Scand. J. Clin. Lab. Invest.* **33**(137):19 (1974).
352. Olofsson, S. O., and Gustafson, A., Degradation of high density lipoproteins (HDL) *in vitro, Scand. J. Clin. Lab. Invest.* **33**(137):57 (1974).
353. Shore, V. G., and Shore, B., Heterogeneity of human plasma very low density lipo-

proteins. Separation of species differing in protein components, *Biochemistry* **12**:502 (1973).

354. Mahley, R. W., Alterations in plasma lipoproteins induced by cholesterol feeding in animals including man, in: *Disturbances in Lipid and Lipoprotein Metabolism* (J. Dietschy, A. M., Gotto, Jr., and J. A. Ontko, eds.), pp. 181–197, Clinical Physiology Series, American Physiology Society (1978).

355. Zannis, V. I., and Breslow, J. L., Apolipoprotein E, *Mol. Cell. Biochem.* **42**:3 (1982).

356. Rall, S. C., Weisgraber, K. H., and Mahley, R. W., Human apolipoprotein E. The complete amino acid sequence, *J. Biol. Chem.* **257**:4171 (1981).

357. Zannis, V. I., Just, P. W., and Breslow, J. L., Human apolipoprotein E isoprotein subclasses are genetically determined, *Am. J. Hum. Genet.* **33**:11 (1981).

358. Zannis, V. I., and Breslow, J. L., Human VLDL apo E isoprotein polymorphism is explained by genetic variation and post-translational modification, *Biochemistry* **20**:1033 (1981).

359. Zannis, V. I., Blum, C., Lees, R., and Breslow, J. L., Plasma apo E in Tangier patients is mainly sialo-apo E, *Circulation* **66**(2):170 (1982).

359a. Innerarity, T. L., Friedlander, E. J., Rall, S. C., Jr., Weisgraber, K. H., and Mahley, R. W., The receptor-binding domain of human apolipoprotein E. Binding of apolipoprotein E fragments, *J. Biol. Chem.* **258**:12341 (1983).

359b. Weisgraber, K. H., Innerarity, T. L., Harder, K. J., Mahley, R. W., Milne, R. W., Marcel, Y. L., and Sparrow, J. T., The receptor-binding domain of human apolipoprotein E. Monoclonal antibody inhibition of binding, *J. Biol. Chem.* **258**:12348 (1983).

360. Havel, R. J., Chao, Y. S., Windler, E. E., Kotite, L., and Guo, L. S. S., Isoprotein specificity in the hepatic uptake of apolipoprotein E and the pathogenesis of familial dysbetalipoproteinemia, *Proc. Natl. Acad. Sci. USA* **77**:4349 (1980).

361. Gregg, M. E., Zech, L. A., Schaefer, E. J., and Brewer, M. B., Jr., Type III hyperlipoproteinemia: Defective metabolism of an abnormal apolipoprotein E, *Science* **211**:584 (1981).

362. Schneider, W. J., Kovanen, P. T., Brown, M. S., Goldstein, J. L., Utermann, G., Weber, W., Havel, R. J., Kotite, L., Kane, J. P., Innerarity, T. L., and Mahley, R. W., Familial dysbetalipoproteinemia. Abnormal binding of mutant apoprotein E to low density lipoprotein receptors of human fibroblasts and membranes from liver and adrenals of rats, rabbits, and cows, *J. Clin. Invest.* **68**:1075 (1981).

363. Weisgraber, K. H., Innerarity, T. L., and Mahley, R. W., Abnormal lipoprotein receptor-binding activity of the human apoprotein due to cysteine-arginine interchange at a single site, *J. Biol. Chem.* **257**:2518 (1982).

364. Rall, S. C., Jr., Weisgraber, K. H., Innerarity, T. L., and Mahley, R. W., Structural basis for receptor binding heterogeneity of apolipoprotein E from type III hyperlipoproteinemic subjects, *Proc. Natl. Acad. Sci. USA* **79**:4696 (1982).

365. Mahley, R. W., Weisgraber, K. H., Innerarity, T., Brewer, H. B., Jr., and Assmann, G., Swine lipoproteins and atherosclerosis. Changes in the plasma lipoproteins and apoproteins induced by cholesterol feeding, *Biochemistry* **14**:2817 (1975).

366. Mahley, R. W., Weisgraber, K. H., and Innerarity, T., Atherogenic hyperlipoproteinemia induced by cholesterol feeding in the patas monkey, *Biochemistry* **15**:2979 (1976).

367. Rodriguez, J. L., Ghiselli, G. C., Torreggiani, D., and Sirtoni, C. R., Very low density lipoproteins in normal and cholesterol fed rabbits: Lipid and protein composition and metabolism. Part I. Chemical compositions of very low density lipoproteins in rabbits, *Atherosclerosis* **23**:73 (1976).

368. Rudel, L. L., Shah, R., and Greene, D. G., Study of the atherogenic dyslipoprotei-
     nemia induced by dietary cholesterol in rhesus monkeys, *J. Lipid Res.* **20:**55 (1979).
369. Guo, L. S. S., Hamilton, R. L., Kane, J. P., Fielding, C. J., and Chen, G. C., Char-
     acterization and quantitation of apolipoproteins A-I and E of normal and cholesterol-
     fed guinea pigs, *J. Lipid Res.* **23:**531 (1982).
370. Curry, M. D., McConathy, W. J., Alaupovic, P., Ledford, J. H., and Popovic, M.,
     Determination of human apolipoprotein E by electro-immunoassay, *Biochim. Bio-
     phys. Acta* **439:**413 (1976).
371. Kushwaha, R. S., Hazzard, W. R., Wahl, R. W., and Hoover, J. J., Type 3 hyperlipo-
     proteinemia—Diagnosis of whole plasma by apolipoprotein E immunoassay, *Ann.
     Intern. Med.* **87:**509 (1977).
372. Wong, L., and Rubinstein, D., Turnover of apo E in normal and hypercholestero-
     lemic rats, *Atherosclerosis* **34:**249 (1979).
373. Breslow, J. L., McPherson, J., and Karathanasis, S. K., Apo E gene contains tandemly
     repeated 66bp DNA sequences highly homologous to similar repeated sequences in
     the apo A-I gene, *Arteriosclerosis,* **V3:**513 (1983).
374. Olaisen, B., Teisberg, P., and Gedde-Dahl, T., Jr., The locus for apolipoprotein E
     (apoE) is linked to the complement component C3 (C3) locus on chromosome 19 in
     man, *Hum. Genet.* **62:**233 (1982).
375. Olofsson, S. O., McConathy, W. J., and Alaupovic, P., Isolation and partial charac-
     terization of a new acidic apolipoprotein (apolipoprotein F) from high density lipo-
     proteins of human plasma, *Biochemistry* **17:**1032 (1978).
376. Ayrault-Jarrier, M., Alix, J. F., and Polonovsky, J., Une nouvelle proteine des lipo-
     proteines du serum humain: Isolement et caracterisation partielle d'une apolipopro-
     teine G, *Biochimie* **60:**65 (1978).
377. Polz, E., and Kostner, G. M., The binding of B2-glycoprotein-I to human serum lipo-
     proteins, *FEBS Lett.* **102:**183 (1979).
378. Nakaya, Y., Schaefer, E. J., and Brewer, H. B., Jr., Activation of human post heparin
     lipoprotein lipase by apolipoprotein H (B2-glycoprotein I), *Biochem. Biophys. Res.
     Commun.* **95:**1168 (1980).
379. Lee, N. S., Brewer, H. B., Jr., and Osborne, J. C., Jr., B2-Glycoprotein I. Molecular
     properties of an unusual apolipoprotein, apolipoprotein H, *J. Biol. Chem.* **258:**4765
     (1983).
380. Schultze, H. E., Heide, K., and Haupt, H., Uber ein bisher unbekanntes niedermo-
     lekulares B2-Globulin des Humanserums, *Naturwissenschaften* **48:**719 (1961).
381. Polz, E., and Kostner, G. M., Binding of B2-glycoprotein 1 to intralipid: Determi-
     nation of the dissociation constant, *Biochem. Biophys. Res. Commun.* **90:**1305
     (1979).
382. Sata, T., Havel, R. J., Kotite, L., and Kane, J. L., New protein in human blood
     plasma, rich in proline, with lipid-binding properties, *Proc. Natl. Acad. Sci. USA*
     73:1063 (1976).
383. Rosenthal, C. J., and Franklin, E. C., Variation with age and disease of an amyloid
     A protein-related serum component, *J. Clin. Invest.* **55:**746 (1975).
384. Benditt, E. P., and Eriksen, N., Amyloid protein SAA is associated with high density
     lipoprotein from human serum, *Proc. Natl. Acad. Sci. USA* **74:**4025 (1977).
385. Bausserman, L. L., Herbert, P. N., and McAdam, K. P. W. J., Heterogeneity of
     human serum amyloid A proteins, *J. Exp. Med.* **152:**641 (1980).
386. Hoffman, J. S., and Benditt, E. P., Secretion of serum amyloid protein and assembly
     of serum amyloid protein-rich high density lipoprotein in primary mouse hepatocyte
     culture, *J. Biol. Chem.* **257:**10518 (1982).

387. Eriksen, N., and Benditt, E. P., Isolation and characterization of the amyloid-related apoprotein (SAA) from human high density lipoprotein, *Proc. Natl. Acad. Sci. USA* **77**:6860 (1980).
388. Parmelee, D. C., Titani, K., Ericsson, L. H., Eriksen, N., Benditt, E. P., and Walsh, K. A., Amino acid sequence of amyloid-related apoprotein (apoSAA₁) from human high-density lipoprotein, *Biochemistry* **21**:3298 (1982).
389. Hoffman, J. S., Ericsson, L. H., Eriksen, N., Walsh, K. A., and Benditt, E. P., Evidence that murine amyloid protein AA is related to only one of two serum amyloid protein (ApoSAA) gene products, *Fed. Proc.* **42**:1817 (1983).
390. Fredrickson, D. S., and Levy, R. I., Familial hyperlipoproteinemia, in: *The Metabolic Basis of Inherited Disease,* 3rd ed. (J. B. Stanbury, J. B. Wyngaarden, and D. S. Fredrickson, eds.), p. 545, McGraw-Hill, New York (1972).
391. Khachadurian, A. K., and Uthman, S. M., Experiences with the homozygous cases of familial hypercholesterolemia. A report of 52 patients, *Nutr. Metab.* **15**:132 (1973).
392. Slack, J., Inheritance of familial hypercholesterolemia, *Atherosclerosis Rev.* **5**:35 (1979).
393. Goldstein, J. L., Dana, S. W. Brunschede, G. Y., and Brown, M. S., Genetic heterogeneity in familial hypercholesterolemia: Evidence for two different mutations affecting functions of low-density lipoprotein receptor, *Proc. Natl. Acad. Sci. USA* **72**:1092 (1975).
394. Brown, M. S., and Goldstein, J. L., Analysis of mutant strain of human fibroblasts with a defect in the internalization of receptor-bound low density lipoprotein, *Cell* **9**:663 (1976).
395. Goldstein, J. L., Brown, M. S., and Stone, N. J., Genetics of the LDL receptor: Evidence that the mutations affecting binding and internalization are allelic, *Cell* **12**:629 (1977).
396. Miyake, Y., Tajina, S., Yamamura, T., and Yamamoto, A., Homozygous familial hypercholesterolemia mutant with a defect in internalization of low density lipoprotein, *Proc. Natl. Acad. Sci. USA* **78**:5151 (1981).
397. Brown, M. S., and Goldstein, J. L., Familial hypercholesterolemia: A genetic defect in the low-density lipoprotein receptor, *N. Engl. J. Med.* **294**:1386 (1976).
398. Brown, M. S., and Goldstein, J. L., Expression of the familial hypercholesterolemia gene in heterozygotes: Mechanism for a dominant disorder in man, *Science* **185**:61 (1974).
399. Goldstein, J. L., Sobhani, M. K., Faust, J. R., and Brown, M. S., Heterozygous familial hypercholesterolemia: Failure of normal allele to compensate for mutant allele at a regulated genetic locus, *Cell* **9**:195 (1976).
400. Anderson, R. G. W., Goldstein, J. L., and Brown, M. S., A mutation that impairs the ability of lipoprotein receptors to localize in coated pits on the cell surface of human fibroblasts, *Nature* **270**:650 (1977).
401. Carpenter, J. L., Gorden, P., Goldstein, J. L., Anderson, R. G. W., Brown, M. S., and Orci, L., Binding and internalization of ¹²⁵I-LDL in normal and mutant human fibroblasts: A quantitative autoradiographic study, *Exp. Cell. Res.* **121**:135 (1979).
402. Fredrickson, D. S., Altrocchi, P. H., Avioli, L. V., Goodman, D. W. S., and Goodman, H. C., Tangier disease, *Ann. Intern. Med.* **55**:1016 (1961).
403. Heinen, R. J., Herbert, P. N., Fredrickson, D. S., Forte, T., and Lindgren, F. T., Properties of the plasma very low and low density lipoproteins in Tangier disease, *J. Clin. Invest.* **61**:120 (1978).
404. Kostner, G., Holasek, A., Schoenborn, W., and Fuhrmann, W., Immunochemische

untersuchung und analytische isoelektrische forussiereines patienten mit Tangier krankheit, *Clin. Chim. Acta* **38**:155 (1972).

405. Lux, S. E., Levy, R. I., Gotto, A. M., and Fredrickson, D. S., Studies on protein defect in Tangier disease. Isolation and characterization of an abnormal high density lipoprotein, *J. Clin. Invest.* **51**:2505 (1972).

406. Herbert, P. N., Henderson, L. O., Heinen, R. J., and Fredrickson, D. S., The anomalous distribution of apolipoprotein A-I in Tangier disease, *Circulation* **54**(Suppl. II):27 (1976).

407. Assmann, G., Smootz, E., Adler, K., Capurso, A., and Oette, K., The lipoprotein abnormality in Tangier disease, *J. Clin. Invest.* **59**:565 (1977).

408. Schaefer, E. J., Blum, C. B., Levy, R. I., Jenkins, L. L., Alaupovic, P., Foster, D. M., and Brewer, H. B., Jr., Metabolism of high-density lipoprotein apolipoproteins in Tangier disease, *N. Engl. J. Med.* **299**:905 (1978).

409. Henderson, L. O., Herbert, P. N., Fredrickson, D. S., Heinen, R. J., and Easterling, J. S., Abnormal concentration and anomalous distribution of apolipoprotein A-I in Tangier disease, *Metab. Clin. Exp.* **27**:165 (1978).

410. Assmann, G., Capurso, A., Smootz, E., and Wellner, U., Apoprotein A metabolism in Tangier disease, *Atherosclerosis* **30**:321 (1978).

411. Franceschini, G., Sirtori, C. R., Capurso, A., II, Weisgraber, K. H., and Mahley, R. W., Decreased high density lipoprotein cholesterol levels with significant lipoprotein modification and without clinical atherosclerosis in an Italian family, *J. Clin. Invest.* **66**:892 (1980).

412. Weisgraber, K. H., Bersot, T. P., Mahley, R. W., Franceschini, G., and Sirtori, C. R., Isolation and characterization of a cysteine-containing variant of the A-I apoprotein from human high density lipoproteins, *J. Clin. Invest.* **66**:901 (1980).

413. Utermann, G., Feussner, G., Franceschini, G., Haas, J., and Steinmetz, A., Genetic variants of group A apolipoproteins, *J. Biol. Chem.* **257**:501 (1982).

414. Weisgraber, K. H., Rall, S. C., Jr., Bersot, T. P., Mahley, R. W., Franceschini, G., and Sirtori, C. R., Detection of normal A-I in affected subjects and evidence for a cysteine for arginine substitution in the variant A-I, *J. Biol. Chem.* **258**:2508 (1983).

414a. Rall, S. C., Menzel, H. J., Assmann, G., Utermann, G., Haas, J., Harris, R. J., Weisgraber, K. H., Bersot, T. P., and Mahley, R. W., Identification of amino acid substitutions in five human apolipoprotein A-I variants, *Circulation* **68III**:290 (1983).

415. Zannis, V. I., Breslow, J. L., Uterman, G., Mahley, R. W., Weisgraber, K. H., Havel, R. J., Goldstein, J. L., Brown, M. S., Schonfeld, G., Hazzard, W. R., and Blum, C. B., Proposed nomenclature of apo E isoprotein genotypes and phenotypes, *J. Lipid Res.* **23**:911 (1982).

416. Norum, R. A., Lakier, J. B., Goldstein, S., Angel, A., Goldberg, R. B., Block, W. D., Noffze, D. K., Dolphin, P. J., Edelglass, J., Bogorad, D. D., and Alaupovic, P., Familial deficiency of apolipoprotein A-I and C-III and precocious coronary-artery disease, *N. Engl. J. Med.* **306**:1513 (1982).

417. Karathanasis, S. K., Norum, R. A., Zannis, V. I., and Breslow, J. L., A mutation in the human apo A-I gene locus related to the development of atherosclerosis, *Nature* **301**:718 (1983).

418. Karathanasis, S. K., Zannis, V. I., and Breslow, J. L., A DNA insertion has occurred in the apolipoprotein A-I gene of patients with premature atherosclerosis, *Nature,* **305**:823–825 (1983).

419. Lindeskog, G. R., Gustafson, A., and Enerbach, L., Serum lipoprotein deficiency in diffuse "normolipidemic" plane xanthoma, *Arch. Dermatol.* **106**:592 (1972).

420. Gustafson, A., McConathy, W. J., Alaupovic, P., Curry, M. D., and Persson, B., Iden-

tification of lipoprotein families in a variant of human plasma apolipoprotein A deficiency, *Scand. J. Clin. Lab. Invest.* **39**:377 (1979).

421. Carlson, L. A., and Philipson, B., Fish-eye disease. A new familial condition with massive corneal opacities and dyslipoproteinemia, *Lancet* **2**:921 (1979).

422. Schaefer, E. J., Zech, L. A., Schwartz, D. W., and Brewer, H. B., Jr., Coronary heart disease prevalence and other clinical features in familial high-density lipoprotein deficiency (Tangier disease), *Ann. Intern. Med.* **93**:261 (1980).

423. Schaefer, E. J., Heaton, W. H., Wetzel, M. G., and Brewer, H. B., Jr., Plasma apolipoprotein A-I absence associated with a marked reduction of high density lipoproteins and premature coronary artery disease, *Arteriosclerosis* **2**(1):16 (1982).

424. Montag, J., Flynn, M., Friedel, J., and Glueck, C. J., Familial hypoalphalipoproteinemia, *Circulation* **66**(II):160 (1982).

425. Glueck, C. J., Fallat, R. W., Millett, F., Gartside, P., Elston, R. C., and Go, R. C. P., Familial hyperalphalipoproteinemia: Studies in 18 kindreds, *Metabolism,* **24**:1243 (1975).

426. Glueck, C. J., Gartside, P., Fallat, R. W., Sielski, J., and Steiner, P. M., Longevity syndromes: Familial hypobeta- and familial hyperalpha-lipoproteinemia, *J. Lab. Clin. Med.* **88**:941 (1976).

427. Siervogel, R. M., Morrison, J. A., Kelly, K., Mellies, M., Gartside, P., and Glueck, C. J., Familial hyperalphalipoproteinemia in 26 kindreds, *Clin. Genet.* **17**:13 (1980).

428. Patsch, W., Kuisk, I., Glueck, C., and Schonfeld, G., Lipoproteins in familial hyperalphalipoproteinemia, *Arteriosclerosis* **1**(2):156 (1981).

429. Zannis, V. I., and Breslow, J. L., Characterization of a unique human apolipoprotein E variant associated with type III hyperlipoproteinemia, *J. Biol. Chem.* **255**:1759 (1980).

430. Utermann, G., Steinmetz, A., and Weber, W., Genetic control of human apolipoprotein-E polymorphism—Comparison of one-dimensional and 2-dimensional techniques of isoprotein analysis, *Hum. Genet.* **60**:344 (1982).

431. Wardell, M. R., Suckling, P. A., and Janus, E. D., Genetic variation in human apolipoprotein E, *J. Lipid Res.* **23**:1174 (1982).

432. Bouthillier, D., Tremblay, M., Mailloux, H., Sing, C. F., and Davignon, J., Determination of the six apolipoprotein E phenotypes with a single gel isoelectric focusing technique—Application to the study of informative matings, *J. Lipid Res.,* **24**:1060–1069 (1983).

433. Utermann, G., Jaeschke, M., and Menzel, J., Familial hyperlipoproteinemia type III: Deficiency of a specific apolipoprotein (apo E-III) in the very low density lipoproteins, *FEBS Lett.* **56**:352 (1975).

434. Utermann, G., Hees, M., and Steinmetz, A., Polymorphism of apolipoprotein E and occurrence of dysbetalipoproteinemia in man, *Nature* **269**:604 (1977).

435. Utermann, G., Langenback, U., Beisiegel, U., and Weber, W., Genetics of the apolipoprotein E system in man, *Am. J. Hum. Genet.* **32**:339 (1980).

436. Weisgraber, K. H., Rall, S. C., Jr., and Mahley, R. W., Human E apoprotein heterogeneity. Cysteine–arginine interchanges in the amino acid sequence of the apo E isoforms, *J. Biol. Chem.* **256**:9077 (1981).

437. Innerarity, T. L., Friedlander, E. J., Rall, S. C., Weisgraber, K. H., and Mahley, R. W., Identification of the region of apolipoprotein E responsible for lipoprotein receptor binding, *Circulation* **66**(II):11 (1982).

437a. Weisgraber, K. H., Rall, S. C., Jr., Innerarity, T. L., and Mahley, R. W., A novel electrophoretic variant of human apolipoprotein E: Identification and characterization of apolipoprotein E1, *J. Biol. Chem.* **83**:1059 (1984).

437b. Gregg, R. E., Ghiselli, G., and Brewer, H. B., Jr., Apolipoprotein $E_{Bethesda}$: A new variant of apolipoprotein E associated with type III hyperlipidemia, *J. Clin, Endocrinol. Metab.* **57**:969 (1983).

438. Breslow, J. L., Zannis, V. I., SanGiacomo, T. R., Third, J. L. H. C., Tracy, T., and Glueck, C. J., Studies of familial type III hyperlipoproteinemia using as a genetic marker the apo E phenotype E2/2, *J. Lipid Res.* **23**:1224 (1982).

439. Ghiselli, G., Schaefer, E. J., Gascon, P., and Brewer, H. B., Jr., Type III hyperlipoproteinemia associated with apolipoprotein E deficiency, *Science* **214**:1239 (1981).

440. Breslow, J. L., McPherson, J., Nussbaum, A. L., Williams, H. W., Lofquist-Kahl, F., Karathanasis, S. K., and Zannis, V. I., Identification and DNA sequence of a human apolipoprotein E cDNA clone, *J. Biol. Chem.* **257**:14639 (1982).

441. Fredrickson, D. S., Levy, R. I., and Lees, R. S., Fat transport in lipoproteins—An integrated approach to mechanisms and disorders, *N. Engl. J. Med.* **276**:34 (1967).

443. Fredrickson, D. S., Levy, R. I., and Lindgren, F. T., A comparison of heritable abnormal lipoprotein patterns as defined by two different techniques, *J. Clin. Invest.* **47**:2446 (1968).

443. Hazzard, W. R., Porte, D., Jr., and Bierman, E. L., Abnormal lipid composition of very low density lipoproteins in diagnosis of broad beta disease (type III hyperlipoproteinemia), *Metabolism* **21**:1009 (1972).

444. Fredrickson, D. S., Goldstein, J. L., and Brown, M. D., The familial hyperlipoproteinemias, in: *The Metabolic Basis of Inherited Disease* (J. B. Stanbury, J. D. Wyngaarden, and D. S. Fredrickson), pp. 604–655, McGraw-Hill, New York (1978).

445. Mishkel, M., Nazir, D. J., and Crother, S., A longitudinal assessment of lipid ratios in the diagnosis of type III hyperlipoproteinemia, *Clin. Chim. Acta* **58**:121 (1975).

446. Fredrickson, D. S., Morganroth, J., and Levy, R. I., Hyperlipoproteinemia: An analysis of two contemporary definitions, *Ann. Intern. Med.* **82**:150 (1975).

447. Morrison, J. A., Kelly, K., Horvitz, R., Khoury, P., Laskarzewski, P. M., Mellies, M. J., and Glueck, C. J., Parent–offspring and sib–sib lipid and lipoprotein associations during and after sharing of household environments; The Princeton school district family study, *Metabolism* **31**:158 (1982).

448. Morganroth, J., Levy, R. I., and Fredrickson, D. S., The biochemical, clinical, and genetic features of type III hyperlipoproteinemia, *Ann. Intern. Med.* **82**:158 (1975).

449. Hazzard, W. R., O'Donnell, T. F., and Lee, Y. L., Broad-beta disease (type III hyperlipoproteinemia) in a large kindred, *Ann. Intern. Med.* **82**:141 (1975).

450. Marien, J. J. C., Hulsmans, H. A. M., and vanGent, C. M., On a family with coexistence of phenotypes II and III hyperlipoproteinemia, *Acta Med. Scand.* **196**:149 (1974).

451. Kwiterovich, P. O., Neill, C., Margolis, S., Thamer, M., and Bachorik, P., Allelism, nonallelism, and genetic compounds in familial hypolipoproteinemia, *Clin. Res.* **23**:262A (1975).

452. Utermann, G., Pruin, N., and Steinmetz, A., Polymorphism of apolipoprotein E. 3. Effect of a single polymorphic gene locus on plasma lipid levels in man, *Clin. Genet,* **15**:63 (1979).

453. Utermann, G., Vogelberg, K. H., Steinmetz, A., Schoenborn, W., Pruin, N., Jaeschke, M., Hees, M., and Canzler, W., Polymorphism of apolipoprotein E. II. Genetics of hyperlipoproteinemia type III, *Clin. Genet.* **15**:37 (1979).

454. Hazzard, W. R., Warnick, G. R., Utermann, G., and Albers, J. J., Genetic transmission of isoapolipoprotein E phenotypes in a large kindred: Relationship to dysbetalipoproteinemias and hyperlipidemia, *Metabolism* **30**:79 (1981).

455. Rall, S. C., Jr., Weisgraber, K. H., Innerarity, T. L., and Mahley, R. W., Identical structural and receptor binding defects in apolipoprotein E2 in hypo-, normo-, and hypercholesterolemic dysbetalipoproteinemia, *J. Clin. Invest.* **71**:1023 (1983).

456. Breslow, J. L., and Zannis, V. I., Genetics of human apolipoprotein E and type III hyperlipoproteinemia, *Arteriosclerosis Rev.,* in press (1983).

457. Menzel, H. J., Kovary, P. M., and Assmann, G., Apolipoprotein A-IV polymorphism in man, *Hum. Genet.* **62**:349 (1982).

458. Herbert, P. N., and Fredrickson, D. S., The hypobetalipoproteinemias, in: *Handbuch der Inneren Medizin,* VII/4:*Fettstoffwechsel* (G. Schettler, H. Greten, G. Schlierf, and D. Seidel, eds.), p. 485, Springer-Verlag, Heidelberg (1976).

459. Cooper, R. A., and Gulbrandsen, C. L., The relationship between serum lipoproteins and red cell membranes in abetalipoproteins: Deficiency of lecithin:cholesterol acyl-transferase, *J. Lab. Clin. Med.* **78**:323 (1971).

460. Gotto, A. M., Levy, R. I., John, K., and Fredrickson, D. S., On the nature of the protein defect in abetalipoproteinemia, *N. Engl. J. Med.* **284**:813 (1971).

461. Scanu, A. M., Aggerbeck, L. P., Kruski, A. W., Lim, C. T., and Kayden, H. J., A study of the abnormal lipoproteins in abetalipoproteinemia, *J. Clin. Invest.* **53**:440 (1974).

462. Glickman, R. M., Green, P. H., Lees, R. S., Lux, S. E., and Kilgore, A., Immunofluorescence studies of apolipoprotein B in intestinal mucosa. Absence of abetalipoproteinemia, *Gastroenterology* **76**:288 (1979).

463. Mars, H., Lewis, L. A., Robertson, A. L., Jr., Butkus, A., and Williams, C. H., Jr., Familial hypo-B-lipoproteinemia: A genetic disorder of lipid metabolism with nervous system involvement, *Am. J. Med.* **46**:886 (1969).

464. Ricket, G., Durepaire, H., Hartmann, L., Ollier, M. P., Polonovski, J., and Maitrot, B., Hypolipoprotiemie familiale asymptomatique predominant sur les beta-lipoproteines, *Presse Med.* **77**:2045 (1969).

465. Levy, R. I., Langer, T., Gotto, A. M., and Fredrickson, D. S., Familial hypobetalipoproteinemia, a defect in lipoprotein synthesis, *Clin. Res.* **18**:539 (1970).

466. Fosbrooke, A., Choksey, S., and Wharton, B., Familial hypo-B-lipoproteinemia, *Arch. Dis. Child.* **48**:729 (1978).

467. Tamir, I., Levtow, O., Lotan, D., Lequin, C., Heldenberg, D., and Werbin, B., Further observations on familial hypobetalipoproteinemia, *Clin. Genet.* **9**:149 (1976).

468. Forsyth, C. C., Lloyd, J. K., and Fosbrooke, A. S., A-beta-Lipoproteinaemia, *Arch. Dis. Child.* **40**:47 (1965).

469. Khachadurian, A. K., Freyha, R., Shamma'a, M. M., and Baghdassarian, S. A., A-beta-Lipoproteinemia and colour blindness, *Arch. Dis. Child.* **46**:871 (1971).

470. Kostner, G., Holasek, A., Bohlmann, H. G., and Thiede, H., Investigation of serum lipoproteins and apoproteins in abetalipoproteinemia, *Clin. Sci. Mol. Med.* **46**:457 (1974).

471. Steinberg, D., Grundy, S. M., Mok, H. Y. I., Turner, J. D., Weinstein, J. J., Brown, W. V., and Albers, J. J., Metabolic studies in an unusual case of asymptomatic familial hypobetalipoproteinemia with hypoalphalipoproteinemia and fasting chylomicronemia, *J. Clin. Invest.* **64**:292 (1979).

472. Kannel, W. B., Castelli, W. P., Gordon, T., and McNamara, P. M., Serum cholesterol, lipoproteins, and the risk of coronary heart disease: The Framingham Study, *Ann. Intern. Med.* **74**:1 (1971).

473. Kannel, W. B., Castelli, W. P., and Gordon, T., Cholesterol in the prediction of atherosclerotic disease; New perspectives based on the Framingham Study, *Ann. Intern. Med.* **90**:85 (1979).

474. Sniderman, A., Shapiro, S., Marpole, D., Skinner, B., Teng, B., and Kwiterovich, P. O., Jr., Enhanced drug-metabolizing capacity within liver adjacent to human and rat liver tumors, *Proc. Natl. Acad. Sci. USA* **77**:601 (1980).

475. Yamamura, T., Dudo, H., Ishikawa, K., and Yamamoto, A., Familial type I hyperlipoproteinemia caused by apolipoprotein C-II deficiency, *Atherosclerosis* **34**:53 (1979).

476. Crepaldi, G., Fellin, R., Baggio, G., Augustin, J., and Gretan, H., Lipoprotein and apoprotein, adipose tissue and hepatic lipoprotein lipase levels in patients with familial hyperchylomicronemia and their immediate family members, in: *Atherosclerosis V* (A. M. Gotto, Jr., L. C. Smith, and B. Allen, eds.). p. 250, Springer-Verlag, New York (1980).

477. Miller, N. E., Rao, S. N., Alaupovic, P., Noble, N., Slack, J., Brunzell, J. D., and Lewis, B., Familial apolipoprotein CII deficiency: Plasma lipoproteins and apolipoproteins in heterozygous and homozygous subjects and the effects of plasma infusion, *Eur. J. Clin. Invest.* **11**:69 (1981).

478. Cox. P. W., Breckenridge, W. C., and Little, J. A., Inheritance of apolipoprotein C-II deficiency with hypertriglyceridemia and pancreatitis, *N. Engl. J. Med.* **299**:1421 (1978).

479. Menzel, H. J., Kane, J. P., and Havel, R. J., A variant primary structure of apolipoprotein C-II in hyperlipemic patients, personal communication.

480. Rees, A., Shoulders, C. C., Stocks, J., Galton, D. J., and Baralle, F. E., DNA polymorphism adjacent to human apoprotein A-I gene: Relation to hypertriglyceridemia, *Lancet* **1**(8322):444 (1983).

481. Kashyap, M. L., Hynd, B. A., Robinson, K., and Gartside, P. S., Abnormal preponderance of sialyated apolipoprotein CIII in triglyceride rich lipoproteins in type V hyperlipoproteinemia, *Metabolism* **30**:111 (1981).

482. Maeda, H., Uzawa, H., and Kamei, R., Unusual familial lipoprotein C-III associated with apolipoprotein C-III-0 preponderance, *Biochim. Biophys. Acta* **665**:578 (1981).

483. Klatskin, G., and Gordon M. D., Relationship between relapsing pancreatitis and essential hyperlipemia, *Am. J. Med.* **12**:3 (1952).

484. Ferrans, V. J., Buja, L. M., Roberts, W. C., and Fredrickson, D. S., The spleen in type I hyperlipoproteinemia. Histochemical, biochemical, microfluorometric and electron microscopic observations, *Am. J. Pathol.* **64**:67 (1971).

485. Lees, R. S., Wilson, D. E., Schonfeld, G., and Fleet, S., The familial dyslipoproteinemias, in: *Progress in Medical Genetics*, Vol. 9 (A. G. Steinberg and A. G. Bearn, eds.), p. 237, Grune & Stratton, New York (1973).

486. Brunznell, J. D., Chait, A., Nikkila, E. A., Ehnholm, C., Huttunen, J. K., and Steiner, G., Heterogeneity of primary lipoprotein lipase deficiency, *Metabolism* **29**:624 (1980).

487. Norum, K. R., and Gjone, E., The influence of plasma from patients with familial plasma lecithin:cholesterol acyltransferase deficiency on the lipid pattern of erythrocytes, *Scand. J. Clin. Lab. Invest.* **22**:94 (1968).

488. Nelson, G. J., Lipid composition and metabolism of erythrocytes, in: *Blood Lipids and Lipoproteins: Quantitation, Composition, and Metabolism* (G. J. Nelson, ed.), p. 317, Wiley-Interscience, New York (1972).

489. Hovig, T., and Gjone, E., Familial lecithin:cholesterol acyltransferase deficiency: Ultrastructural aspects of a new syndrome with particular reference to lesions in the kidneys and the spleen, *Acta Pathol. Microbiol. Scand.* **81**:681 (1973).

490. Gjone, E., Familial lecithin:cholesterol acyltransferase deficiency: A clinical survey, *Scand. J. Clin. Lab. Invest.* **33**(137):73 (1974).

491. Stokke, K. T., Bjerve, K. S., Blomhoff, J. P., Oystese, B., Flatmark, A., Norum, K. R., and Gjone, E., Familial lecithin:cholesterol acyltransferase deficiency: Studies on lipid composition and morphology of tissues, *Scand. J. Clin. Lab. Invest.* **33**(137):93 (1974).

492. Albers, J. J., Adolphson, J. L., and Chen, C. H., Radioimmunoassay of human plasma lecithin:cholesterol acyltransferase, *J. Clin. Invest.* **67**:141 (1981).

493. Albers, J. J., and Utermann, G., Genetic control of lecithin:cholesterol acyltransferase: Measurement of LCAT mass in a large kindred with LCAT deficiency, *Am. J. Hum. Genet.* **33**:702 (1981).

494. Glomset, J. A., Nichols, A. V., Norum, K. R., King, W., and Forte, T., Plasma lipoproteins in familial lecithin:cholesterol acyltransferase deficiency: Further studies of very low and low density lipoprotein abnormalities, *J. Clin. Invest.* **52**:1078 (1973).

495. Abramov, A., Schorr, S., and Wolman, M., Generalized xanthomatosis with calcified adrenals, *AMA J. Dis. Child.* **91**:282 (1956).

496. Fredrickson, D. S., Newly recognized disorders of cholesterol metabolism, *Ann. Intern. Med.* **58**:718 (1963).

497. Sloan, H. R., and Fredrickson, S. D., Rare familial diseases with neutral lipid storage: Wolman's disease, cholesteryl ester storage disease, and cerebrotendinous xanthomatosis, in: *The Metabolic Basis of Inherited Disease,* 3rd ed. (J. B. Stanbury, J. B. Wyngaarden, and D. S. Fredrickson, eds.), p. 808, McGraw-Hill, New York (1972).

498. Fredrickson, D. S., and Ferrans, V. J., Acid cholesteryl ester hydrolase deficiency, in: *The Metabolic Basis of Inherited Disease,* 4th ed. (J. B. Stanbury, J. B. Wyngaarden, and D. S. Fredrickson, eds.), p. 670, McGraw-Hill, New York (1978).

499. Young, E. P., and Patrick, A. D., Deficiency of acid esterase activity in Wolman's disease, *Arch, Dis. Child.* **45**:664 (1970).

500. Burke, J. A., and Schubert, W. K., Deficient activity of hepatic acid lipase in cholesterol ester storage disease, *Science* **176**:309 (1972).

501. Wolman, M., Histochemistry of lipids in pathology, in: *Handbuch der Histochemie* (W. Graumann and K. Heumann, eds.), Vol. V, Part 2, p. 228, Fisher Verlag, Stuttgart (1964).

502. Crocker, A. C., Vawter, G. F., Neuhauser, E. B. D., and Rosowsky, A., Wolman's disease: Three new patients with a recently described lipidosis, *Pediatrics* **35**:627 (1965).

503. Brown, M. S., Dana, S. E., and Goldstein, J. L., Receptor-dependent hydrolysis of cholesteryl esters contained in plasma low density lipoprotein, *Proc. Natl. Acad. Sci. USA* **72**:2925 (1975).

504. Warner, T. G., Dambach, L. M., Shin, J. H., and O'Brien, J. S., Purification of the lysosomal acid lipase from human liver and its role in lysosomal lipid hydrolysis, *J. Biol. Chem.* **256**:2952 (1981).

505. Chin, D. J., Luskey, K. L., Faust, J. R., MacDonald, R. J., Brown, M. S., and Goldstein, J. L., Molecular cloning of 3-hydroxy-3-methylglutaryl coenzyme A reductase and evidence of regulation of its mRNA, *Proc. Natl. Acad. Sci. USA* **79**:7704 (1982).

506. Cheung, P., and Chan, L., Nucleotide sequence of cloned cDNA of human apolipoprotein A-I, *Nucl. Acids Res.* **11**:3703 (1983).

507. Weatherall, D. J., and Clegg, J. B., Thalassemia revisited, *Cell* **29**:7 (1982).

508. Orkin, S. K., Antonarakis, S. E., and Kazazian, H. H., Jr., Polymorphism and molecular pathology of the human beta-globin gene, *Prog. Hematol.,* **13**:49 (1983).

Chapter 4

Glucose-6-Phosphate Dehydrogenase

L. Luzzatto and G. Battistuzzi

Department of Haematology
Royal Postgraduate Medical School
University of London, London, England

INTRODUCTION

Genetic systems have been of interest to human genetics mainly because they exhibit polymorphism in various populations, and therefore seem to be relevant to human evolution, or because they are associated with pathological manifestations. In addition, whereas frequently biological systems are easier to investigate in microorganisms or in experimental animals, from which one tries to extrapolate to humans, sometimes this species lends itself ideally to direct analysis, and features of general interest then emerge. Glucose-6-phosphate dehydrogenase (G6PD) exhibits all of these characteristics. G6PD is a ubiquitous enzyme, since it is found, as far as we know, in all contemporary organisms and in all tissues: it is certainly very ancient in evolution. The metabolic role of G6PD is well outlined. On the one hand, it catalyzes the first step of one pathway for producing pentose, a precursor of nucleic acids and of all nucleotide coenzymes. On the other hand, it provides the NADPH required for a variety of biosynthetic and detoxification reactions. In certain organisms and in certain circumstances it may also provide an alternative to the main glycolytic pathway for glucose utilization. Thus, it can be regarded legitimately as a typical and generally essential household or housekeeping enzyme. Whether by accident or by design, the gene for this protein is located in mammals on the X chromosome, and it has thus become subject to the unique phenomenon of X-chromosome inactivation. Because this feature is combined with those mentioned above, G6PD has become one of the most useful markers for investigating this phenomenon and the resulting mosaicism in somatic cells and tissues. In particular, it has been employed to investigate the clonal nature of proliferative processes, whether developmental or pathological, including a variety of human tumors.

G6PD was reviewed in this series over a decade ago (Kirkman, 1971). The justification for doing so again must lie with the progress made since. In the meantime, several other reviews have covered, in different combinations, the genetic, biochemical, and clinical aspects of this topic (Luzzatto, 1975; Beutler, 1978; Luzzatto and Testa, 1978; Levy, 1979; Bienzle, 1981; Panich, 1981 and 1982; Beutler, 1983). Therefore, here we will try to concentrate selectively on developments that are either new, or less explored in previous reviews, or both. The literature survey has been carried out comprehensively up to June 1983, but a number of papers that have appeared subsequently have also been consulted.

GLUCOSE-6-PHOSPHATE DEHYDROGENASE IN EVOLUTION

Evolution of Enzyme Structure and Function

Subunit Structure

Since the amino acid composition of G6PD has been determined in only very few species, we are limited for the moment, in a comparative analysis of G6PD, to relatively gross features or to indirect methods.

Subunits within the oligomeric molecule are usually identical, with one exception. In *Neurospora crassa* genetic evidence suggests that G6PD is coded by at least three structural gene loci (Scott and Mahoney, 1976). The monomer molecular weight is lower, on the average, in bacteria and in lower prokaryotes than in mammals. Monomers aggregate to form oligomeric structures. The smallest oligomeric structure that has catalytic activity is invariably the dimer. The common structures are dimeric and tetrameric, but in *Bacillus subtilis* and in some mammals larger oligomeric molecules have also been found (Table I). In the large majority of

Table I. Molecular Features of G6PD and Evolution[a]

	Average molecular weight of monomer	Oligomeric composition			Average K_m for G6P, μM	Average K_m for NADP+, μM	Average K_i for NADPH, μM
		Dimer	Tetramer	Multimer			
Bacteria	56,800	+	+	+[b]	1500	55	40
Lower eukaryotes	54,700	+	+[b]	—	212	30	21
Plants	55,000	+	—	—	307	48	10–200
Drosophila	55,000[c]	—	+	—	300; 170[d]	23; 58[d]	—
Mammals	61,300	+	+	+[b]	56	19	36

[a] Data are compiled from Levy (1979), Kato *et al.* (1979), Lee *et al.* (1978, 1979), Ben-Bassat and Goldberg (1980), and Steinbach *et al.* (1978).
[b] In different species either one or more oligomeric forms have been found.
[c] Although this is a current estimate, the size of the *Drosophila* enzyme on side-by-side comparison in SDS-PAGE was larger than mouse G6PD (Lee *et al.*, 1979).
[d] For allelic forms of G6PD A and B, respectively.

cases the coenzyme is essential either for the formation or for the stabilization of the quaternary structure.

Kinetics

G6PD is defined as a dehydrogenase highly specific for glucose 6-phosphate (G6P). A few exceptions have been reported: for instance, in humans the G6PD variant called Kobe has approximately 1000-fold higher activity with galactose 6-phosphate than with G6P (Fujii *et al.*, 1981), and a hamster cell mutant is much more active on 2dG6P than on G6P (see p. 250). However, even in these cases the physiological substrate is certainly G6P. The pattern of coenzyme specificity is more complex. The great majority of G6PD types can use both NADP+ and NAD+, albeit not indifferently. However, various combinations of coenzyme specificities are seen in various groups of organisms (see Table II). Preferential binding of NAD+ or NADP+ must obviously depend on differences in structure of the active center, and these in turn have likely evolved in relation to different physiological roles of the enzyme. This is especially clear in *Pseudomonas,* where a NAD-preferring G6PD is part of the catabolic Entner-Doudoroff pathway, whereas a NADP-preferring G6PD supplies NADPH for biosynthetic processes. Accordingly, the lat-

Table II. Evolution of Coenzyme Specificity of G6PD

Group	Specificity parameter[a]	Specificity class[b]				
		I	II	III	IV	V
Bacteria[c]	n	3	2	18	1	1
	$\bar{r}_v$	—	ND[d]	1.17	1.29	—
	$\bar{r}_k$	—	110	14	0.42	—
Mycetes	n	8	—	—	—	—
Mammals	n	—	21[e]	—	—	—
	$\bar{r}_v$	—	.01	—	—	—
	$\bar{r}_k$	—	1400	—	—	—

[a] n, Number in each class; $\bar{r}_v$ ratio of V_{max} with NAD as substrate to V_{max} with NADP substrate; $\bar{r}_k = K_m^{NAD}/K_m^{NADP}$.

[b] According to Levy (1979). Class I: exclusive use of NADP; class II: negligible activity with NAD compared to NADP; class III: no marked preference for either coenzyme; class IV: reverse of class II; class V: reverse of class I. Thus $\bar{r}_v$ values would be, by definition, infinity and zero in class I and class V, respectively.

[c] Data from a total of 22 organisms, three of which have two G6PD species each.

[d] Not determined.

[e] Enzyme preparations obtained from different tissues from seven different species.

ter but not the former is sensitive to feedback inhibition by fatty acids and acyl-CoA, suggesting that lipid synthesis is one of its main functions (Cacciapuoti and Lessie, 1977). As an extreme situation, *Acetobacter xylinum* has one unique type of G6PD that functions only with NAD and another that functions only with NADP. In *Thiobacillus ferrooxidans* a single G6PD species with intermediate properties fulfills instead, under different growth conditions, the catabolic or the anabolic role, respectively. In *Leuconostoc mesenteroides* NAD and NADP are associated with different conformations of the enzyme (Haghighi and Levy, 1982a,b), and the same is true for rat mammary gland G6PD. By contrast, G6PD from *Bacillus cereus*, *Vibrio alginolyticus,* yeasts, and fungi have been uniformly strictly NADP-specific.

Because sequence data are so scarce and other data are fragmentary a meaningful evolutionary history of G6PD cannot be traced yet. However, from the comparative data that are available a few general features do emerge (Table I). From the point of view of kinetics, the most striking trend when comparing bacteria, lower eukaryotes, and mammals is the decrease in K_m for both G6P and NADP, suggesting that the fit of these ligands has been perfected, while the affinity for the product-inhibitor NADPH changes much less.

Hexose 6-Phosphate Dehydrogenase

The discovery of a true isozyme of G6PD was first reported in the deer mouse, *Peromiscus maculatus* (Shaw and Barto, 1965), in which two enzyme species with G6PD activity were designated A and B. Subsequently, a similar situation was also observed in other vertebrates, such as various fishes, birds, and mammals, including humans (Shaw, 1966). Recently a similar enzyme activity has been reported also in echinoderms (Matsuoka and Hori, 1980) but not in lower invertebrates (Ohnishi and Hori, 1977).* In mammals the gene for the A enzyme is located on the X chromosome, while the B enzyme is autosomal (Shaw and Barto, 1965). Since the B enzyme, compared to A, displays a much broader substrate specificity (it is active on galactose 6-P, 2 deoxy-G6P, and even glucose), it was renamed hexose-6-phosphate dehydrogenase (H6PD) (Ohno *et al.,* 1966). H6PD can use as coenzyme both NAD and NADP, with an activity ratio of 0.22 (Yoshida, 1975): thus, it fits into Levy's class III (see Table II). In contrast to G6PD, which is a cytosol enzyme in all tissues, H6PD is associated with the microsomal fraction in various tissues, and it is not found in RBC [see Hori *et al.* (1975) for detailed references].

Since structural data are lacking, the evolutionary relationship between H6PD and G6PD is as yet problematic. At first sight, the two enzymes are quite different, but the dual coenzyme specificity of H6PD is reminiscent of class III or IV bacterial G6PD (see Table II), and the broad substrate specificity does not necessarily rule out homology with G6PD, since we have evidence that point mutations can affect substrate specificity quite dramatically. From the functional point of view, since 2dG6P and Gal6P are unlikely to be physiological substrates, H6PD is a candidate for a true G6PD activity, whether vestigial or otherwise. Indeed, because H6PD is not very sensitive—if at all—to inhibition by NADPH, Oka *et al.* (1981) have estimated that *in vivo* H6PD activity in some tissues may be as high as 1.6 times that of G6PD. From the evidence of pathology associated with G6PD deficiency, it is clear that H6PD cannot effectively be a surrogate for the role of G6PD. However, since H6PD is not inhibited by steroids and by fatty acids and it is not affected by diet (Hori *et al.,* 1975), it might provide an alternative source

---

* However, Silva-Pando *et al.* (1978) have found in mussel hepatopancreas, at a level much lower than G6PD, a noncytosolic enzyme with properties similar to H6PD.

of reductive potential in a cellular compartment different from that occupied by G6PD itself.

Evolution of Genetic Variability*

Electrophoretic analysis of G6PD has been performed on a wide variety of organisms. In *Escherichia coli,* Bowman *et al.* (1967) found G6PD to be polymorphic and observed eight electrophoretic variants in 14 different strains, meaning that the average number of variants per strain is $n = 0.57$. More recently, Milkman (1975) analyzed 829 independent isolates from a wide variety of hosts. He found in each isolate up to four electrophoretic classes, with one and the same among them uniformly having the highest frequency (0.90–1.00). Genetic variation has also been described in *Pasteurella pseudotuberculosis* ($n = 0.43$) (Bowman *et al.,* 1967) and in *Vibrio cholerae* ($n = 0.11$) (Momen and Salles, 1981), but not in *V. parahaemolyticus* and in *V. fluvialis,* although for these latter species the number of isolates was very low (Momen and Salles, 1981).

In plants and animals G6PD is generally found among the least polymorphic genes, as measured by the fraction of polymorphic populations within a given species, by the percent of species exhibiting polymorphism, and by the rate of heterozygosity (Table III). The degree of heterozygosity is higher in invertebrates (groups 2 + 3 in Table III), 0.0271, compared to vertebrates, 0.0059, which is in agreement with the average trend obtained for electrophoretic variation (0.1123 versus 0.0494) as reported by Nevo (1978). Among mammals, G6PD is abundantly polymorphic only in the human species. However, a few other examples of polymorphism have been reported in the apes of the genera *Cercopithicus* and *Macaca* (Palmour *et al.,* 1980), in *Pan troglodytes* (Lucotte, 1980), in the red-necked wallaby, *Macropus rufogriseus banksianus* (Cooper *et al.,* 1975), and in the pika, *Ochotona rufescens rufescens* (Vergnes *et al.,* 1974), although no precise quantitative data are available. The regularly lower than average polymorphism and heterozygosity shown by G6PD compared to other enzymes in populations and species of widely different

---

* The abbreviation used for the G6PD gene is not uniform. It is *zwf* (from the old German name *Zwischenferment*) in *E. coli, gpd* in *Neurospora,* and *Zw* in *Drosophila.* We have mostly retained the nomenclature used by the individual authors, but for the human species and in general we have used *Gd,* as recommended by the WHO (Betke *et al.,* 1967).

Table III. Extent of Genetic Variation of G6PD in a Variety of Organisms

Grouping	Approximate number of extant species	Number of species studied for G6PD	Percent of species polymorphic for G6PD	Average rate of heterozygosity for G6PD	General rate of heterozygosity[a]	Ref.[b]
1. Plants	295,000	15	13	0.0123	0.0706	c
2. Invertebrates (excluding insects)	288,000	34[d]	6	0.0164	0.1001	e
3. Insects	743,000	62	29	0.0329	0.0743	f
4. Fishes	20,000	16	6	0.0005	0.0513	g
5. Amphibia	2,500	4	25	0.0315	0.0788	h
6. Reptiles	6,300	6	50	0.0720	0.0471	i
7. Birds	8,600	None			0.0473	—
8. Mammals	3,700	86	1	0.001	0.0359	j

[a] Data in this column are based on at least 14 enzyme loci as compiled by Nevo (1978).

[b] These references concern the study of G6PD.

[c] Guries and Ledig (1982), Levin (1977, 1978), Roose and Gottlieb (1976), Ledig and Conkle (1983), Mashburn et al. (1978).

[d] G6PD polytypic in one species.

[e] Ritte and Pashtan (1982), McCracken and Brussard (1980), M. S. Johnson et al. (1977), L. Bullini (personal communication, 1983).

[f] Zera (1981), Halliday (1981), Bryant et al. (1981), Cabrera et al. (1980), Ward (1980), Metcalf et al. (1975), Brittnacher et al. (1978), Prakash (1977), Barker and Mulley (1976), Varvio Aho and Pamilo (1979), Snyder (1974), L. Bullini (personal communication, 1983); Lester and Selander (1979), Wagner and Briscoe (1983), Gill (1981).

[g] Graves and Somero (1982), Winans (1980), M. S. Johnson and Mickevich (1977), Anderson et al. (1981), Shaklee and Tamaru (1981), Sidell et al. (1978), Taggart et al. (1981).

[h] Wright (1975), Wright et al. (1980), Larson (1980), Bullini et al. (personal communication, 1983).

[i] Sites and Greenbaum (1983), Gartside et al. (1977), Bullini et al. (personal communication, 1983).

[j] Schmitt (1978), Bruce and Ayala (1978), Simonsen (1982), Simonsen et al. (1982a, b); Allendorf et al. (1979), Ryman et al. (1977), Mathai et al. (1966), Trujillo et al. (1965), Richardson et al. (1971), Ohno et al. (1965), Chapman and Shaws (1976), Eriksson et al. (1976), Bullini et al. (personal communication, 1983), Bonnell and Selander (1974), Serov et al. (1976) Fisher et al. (1976), Cameron and Vyse (1978), Greembaum and Baker (1976), Patton et al. (1975), Avise et al. (1974), Cooper et al. (1975), Nozawa et al. (1975), Vergnes et al. (1974), Laudenslager (1978), Anderson and Giblett (1975), Lucotte (1979), Turner (1981), Buettner-Janusch et al. (1974), Saha et al. (1983a); Nobrega et al. (1970).

taxa suggests that some form of selection may be operating at the *Gd* locus. Milkman (1975) reports that in *E. coli* the results of electrophoretic analysis are incompatible with the hypothesis that electrophoretic variation is due mainly to random genetic drift of adaptively neutral alleles.

In *Drosophila melanogaster* two common alleles are present at the G6PD locus, Zw^A and Zw^B (Young *et al.*, 1964; Young, 1966), specifying, respectively, a fast and a slow electrophoretic form of the enzyme. The gene frequencies in natural populations are approximately 0.80 and 0.20, respectively. When cage populations of *D. melanogaster* were allowed to evolve starting from different frequencies of Zw^A and Zw^B, the frequency of Zw^A invariably ended up at 0.8, suggesting some sort of balanced polymorphism at or near the *Zw* locus (Bijlsma and Van Delden, 1977). However, specific tests on differential hatchability in normal and modified media, rate of wastage in development from larva to adult, and adult survival have not yet identified the nature of selective phenomena (Bijlsma, 1978). Moreover, an analysis of the geographic distribution of Zw^A has revealed a significant cline of the frequency of this gene with latitude and longitude (decreasing eastward and southward), but no association with any climatic variable or with altitude (Oakeshott *et al.*, 1983).

Evolution of Expression

Mutations within the Gd Gene

G6PD mutants affecting the level of enzyme activity *in vitro, in vivo,* or both have been described in *E. coli* (Banerjee and Fraenkel, 1972), *N. crassa* (Scott and Mahoney, 1976), *D. melanogaster* (Cavener and Clegg, 1981; W. J. Young, quoted in Geer *et al.*, 1974; Gvozdev *et al.*, 1976; Hughes and Lucchesi, 1977), rat (Werth and Müller, 1967), dog (Smith *et al.*, 1976), chimpanzee (Beutler and West, 1978), *Cercopithecus* and *Macaca* (Palmour *et al.*, 1980), and in humans (see below).

Neurospora Crassa (Scott and Mahoney, 1976). Mutants so far described in this organism are characterized by normal activity *in vitro* but severely altered kinetic and/or physical properties of the molecule. The genes *bal, col-2,* and *fr* map in linkage groups II, VII, and I, respectively. From both genetic and biochemical evidence it appears that each of these nonallelic genes is a structural gene for G6PD. Phenotypically, mutants are prototrophic, but they grow at a reduced rate and show developmental abnormalities, abnormal mycelial growth pattern, and abnormal hyphal morphology, resulting in a colonial or spreading-colonial morphology. They complement in heterokaryons, and double mutants are more restricted in terms of morphology and growth rate. From a metabolic point of view mutants are characterized by accumulation of G6P and reduction of steady state NADPH to 50–58% of wild type. Growth on pentose has no effect on morphology or growth rate of mutants, indicating that these strains are not deficient in pentose and that the prime function of the hexose monophosphate shunt (HMS) is NADPH production. Apparently the lack of NADPH due to G6PD deficiency is not compensated by the two other NADPH-producing enzymes (NADP-linked isocitric dehydrogenase and malic enzyme). G6PD deficiency affects lipid synthesis in that there is accumulation (1.7- to 3-fold) of neutral lipids, and lower content (3–43%) of linolenic acid, which is directly related to short supply of NADPH. Thus, the phenotypic effects of G6PD deficiency in *Neurospora* are mainly related to the role of G6PD in lipid synthesis and consequently in producing a competent plasma membrane. In keeping with this notion, in the *fr* mutant linolenic or arachidonic acid supplementation corrects morphology and growth rate.*

Drosophila Melanogaster.   In this organism, as already mentioned, the two common forms of G6PD differ in electrophoretic mobility. It turns out that this is not due to a difference in charge, but rather to differences in subunit structure, and hence in molecular weight. Apparently the A type moves in the electric field predominantly as a dissociated molecule, while type B is predominantly undissociated (Steele *et al.,* 1968). Thus, the mutation responsible for the difference between A and B in *Drosophila* is unique in affecting the association between G6PD subunits.† The B molecules can be forced to dissociate *in vitro* by lowering pH and increasing the ionic strength of the medium. The A and B forms have similar enzyme activity in larval extracts; however, G6PD A causes a 5% greater flow through the pentose pathway (Cavener and Clegg, 1981). A number of deficient mutants have been produced by feeding

---

* A recently reported curious nongenetic phenomenon is that when *Neurospora* is grown in a higher phosphate medium, G6PD becomes undetectable in extracts, due to the presence of an inhibitor (Savant *et al.,* 1982). The significance of this is unknown.

† The A(−) variant of G6PD was identified in humans on the grounds of enzyme deficiency and altered electrophoretic mobility, but it has been found subsequently to also have changes in quaternary structure (Babalola *et al.,* 1976).

ethyl methanesulfonate (EMS) to adult male flies (Young *et al.,* 1964; Gvozdev *et al.,* 1976; Hughes and Lucchesi, 1977) and some of the mutant proteins have been partially purified (Hori and Tanda, 1980). They are characterized by a more or less severely reduced to totally abolished activity. The analysis of pentose shunt activity under various experimental conditions of larvae and adult flies carrying the Zw^{lol} mutation of Young, which causes a mild deficiency, reveals that the shunt is effectively blocked. As a consequence NADPH concentration is reduced by 40% compared to normal, resulting in a sixfold reduction of the NADPH/NADP ratio. On optimal medium G6PD($-$) flies grow as well as their normal counterparts, but the length of their growth period and survival are affected on minimal amino acid diet (Geer *et al.,* 1974). They also synthesize triglycerides less efficiently (73% of wild type) on a high sucrose diet (Geer *et al.,* 1979).

An interesting feature of Zw^- mutants is their intergenic complementation with Pgd^- mutants of 6PGD. Lethal Pgd^- mutants can be efficiently rescued by inducing a Zw^- mutation (Gvozdev *et al.,* 1976, 1977; Hughes and Lucchesi, 1977). It has been suggested that suppression of lethality occurs because block of the pentose phosphate shunt at the G6PD level prevents the toxic effects of 6PG accumulation (Gvozdev *et al.,* 1976).

Control of G6PD by Other Genes

Genetic variation at the G6PD locus accounts for only a portion of the total phenotypic variation in the level of G6PD activity. In very limited numbers of species efforts have been made to identify genes whose variable expression could account for at least some of the remaining extent of variation (Table IV). The classical genetic approach, based on the study of mutants, has been used to identify suppressor genes in *Neurospora* (Scott and Mahoney, 1976) and modifier genes in *Drosophila* (Komma, 1968a,b; Belote and Lucchesi, 1980). Other genes have been identified, also in *Drosophila,* by the use of regional trisomies (Rawls and Lucchesi, 1974a,b) or by outcrossing experiments (Lawrie-Ahlberg *et al.,* 1980, 1982; Steele *et al.,* 1969; Erickson and Harper, 1980). Some of these genes (Table IV) affect G6PD specifically; the majority, however, seem to have a rather more general action, since other enzymes are affected as well.

Table IV. Changes in G6PD Determined by Genes Other Than the G6PD Structural Gene

Species	Modifier	Chromosomal location	Effect	Specificity of effect	Reference
Neurospora crassa	*su*-B	Lg. I	Restores normal G6P affinity of *bal* mutant	Acts on *bal* only	Scott and Mahoney (1976)
	su-C	Lg. I (13 mU from *su*-B)	Restores physical properties and probably function of *col-2* mutants	Acts on *col-2* only	
Drosophila melanogaster	Various genes[a]	2.21A 2.41–43A	Decreases G6PD 16% Increases G6PD 7%	Other enzymes also affected	Rawls and Lucchesi (1974a,b)
		2.45F–50C 2.54F–57B 3.94C–100A	Decreases G6PD 21% Decreases G6PD 8% Increases G6PD 8%	G6PD only affected	
	msl-2[b]	2.9.0	Decreases G6PD	Acts on X-linked genes	Belote and Lucchesi (1980)
	mle[s]	2.56.8	Decreases G6PD; decreases RNA synthesis on X chromosome	Acts on X-linked genes	Belote and Lucchesi (1980)
	M^{Zw}	X, 2 cM from *Zw*	Alters electrophoretic mobility of G6PD in males only	Unknown	Komma (1968a,b)
Mus musculus	Unnamed gene	4(?)	Increases G6PD activity in erythrocytes	—	Erickson and Harper (1980)

[a] These effects were detected by the study of regional trisomies; the genes involved might be the same as those postulated by Lawrie-Ahlberg et al. (1980, 1981) based on analysis of flies with chromosome 2 or 3 obtained from the wild, but otherwise isogenic. In at least some cases the variation in G6PD was shown to be in the amount of protein present.

[b] Similar loci, *msl-1* and *msl-1*[b], have also been reported by the same authors.

Developmental Changes. The ontogenetic profile of G6PD activity has been studied in several organisms, such as *D. melanogaster* (Wright and Shaw, 1970; Bijlsma and Van der Meulen-Bruijns, 1979), sea urchins (Krahl *et al.,* 1955; Backstrom, 1959), fishes (Yamauchi and Goldberg, 1974; Champion *et al.,* 1975), *Rana pipiens* (Wallace, 1961), chicks (Burt, 1965), and mammals (Brinster, 1966, 1970; Bittner *et al.,* 1978; Madvig and Abraham, 1980; Dovrat and Gershon, 1981). In general, variations in G6PD activity correlate well with the pattern of carbohydrate and lipid metabolism during development.

In *Drosophila,* for example, the level of G6PD is constant until hatching, and then it increases gradually during the larval stages to reach a maximum in third instar larvae, followed by a drop during pupation and again a rise in the adult (Bijlsma and Van der Meulen-Bruijns, 1979). This correlates well with the main source of nutrients being lipids in the embryo and in the pupa, and carbohydrate in the larva and in the adult. In fishes the major sources of energy during development are protein and fat. Carbohydrate as energy source is limited to the period of blood system development, to hatching, and to the time after completion of yolk resorption. G6PD activity increases during the same periods (Yamauchi and Goldberg, 1974). In the mammalian embryo, whose major nutrient is maternal blood glucose throughout fetal life, G6PD activity stays high until birth. After birth, the pattern of G6PD activity becomes diversified in various organs, but it is still related to changes in calorie source. Thus, in the suckling, fatty acid synthesis in liver falls rapidly in response to the high-fat, low-carbohydrate content of milk, and so does the level of G6PD. After weaning, the diet is again composed mainly of carbohydrate and the G6PD level rises (Madvig and Abraham, 1980). Is this close correlation between source of energy supply and G6PD activity achieved by the ability of the developing organism to respond at each stage to the nutritional environment, or is it dictated by a built-in ontogenetic program? The evidence from experiments on the trout, in which artificial changes in the environment were affected at the period of starvation onset (Yamauchi and Goldberg, 1974), support the latter view. Indeed, it appears that responses to hormones physiologically taking place in the adult rat are precluded in the perinatal period (Bittner *et al.,* 1978). These data, admittedly fragmentary, suggest that the ontogenetic control is strictly predetermined, and that the ability to respond to environmental changes is acquired with maturity.

In mammals it is generally observed that G6PD activity (per gram of tissue or per milligram of protein) is higher in fetal than in adult organs (see, for instance, Madvig and Abraham, 1980), and we have confirmed this for humans (G. Battistuzzi *et al.*, 1985). However, we have also found that the amount of G6PD activity *per cell* is similar in adults and fetal organs, with the notable exception of the brain. It has been suggested that in the brain a special G6PD isozyme is expressed during development only (Toncheva *et al.*, 1982).

A remarkable phenomenon in early development is the delayed expression of the paternally derived G6PD gene. In *Drosophila* the delay is about 24 hr (Wright and Shaw, 1970), and because the G6PD gene is X-linked, this phenomenon may be somehow related to dosage compensation. However, in the splake trout the G6PD gene is autosomal, and why the paternal gene should be expressed only after yolk resorption, at 20 weeks from fertilization (Yamauchi and Goldberg, 1974), remains entirely a puzzle.

Dosage Compensation. A special effect of other genes in the control of G6PD activity takes place in those species in which sexes have different chromosomal constitution and the locus for G6PD is located on one of the sex chromosomes. This is true in *Drosophila* (T. R. F. Wright, quoted by Young, 1966; Stewart and Merriam, 1974; Gvozdev *et al.*, 1976) and in mammals (Beutler *et al.*, 1962). Nevertheless, in these species G6PD activity is similar in males (with one X chromosome and therefore only one dose of the gene) and in females (with two X chromosomes and therefore two doses of the gene) (Seecof *et al.*, 1969; Komma, 1966; Bowman and Simmons, 1973; Lucchesi and Rawls, 1973; Steele *et al.*, 1969; Maroni and Plaut, 1973; Davidson *et al.*, 1963). How the phenomenon of X-chromosome inactivation, characteristic of mammals, relates to G6PD expression will be discussed later (see p. 240ff).

In *Drosophila*, dosage compensation (Muller *et al.*, 1931) is effected without X-inactivation (Kazazian *et al.*, 1965; Steele *et al.*, 1968). It is seen to operate with respect to G6PD (Table V) in adult flies differing in the numbers of X chromosomes and of autosome sets: diploid males and females and triploid females (Seecof *et al.*, 1969; Maroni and Plaut, 1973; Lucchesi and Rawls, 1973), triploid intersexes (Lucchesi *et al.*, 1977), metafemales (Lucchesi *et al.*, 1974; Stewart and Merriam, 1975), and metamales (Lucchesi *et al.*, 1977); although Maroni and Plaut (1973) found that, by comparison to diploid females, G6PD activity in meta-

Table V. Complete and Incomplete Dosage Compensation for the G6PD Gene in *D. melanogaster*

Type	Autosomes	X chromosomes	Zw copies	Relative G6PD activity[a]		
				Per fresh weight	Per cell[b]	Per gene copy
Wild type female	2n	2	2	1	1	0.5
Wild type male	2n	1	1	1	1	1.0
Metafemale	2n	3	3	1	1	0.33
Metamale	3n	1	1	0.87–1	1.3–1.5	1.3–1.5
Triploid intersex	3n	2	2	1–1.13	1.5–1.7	0.75–0.85
Triploid	3n	3	3	1	1.5	0.5
Duplication	2n	2	3	1.40–1.43	1.40–1.43	0.47–0.48
Duplication	2n	1	2	1.52–1.72	1.52–1.72	0.76–0.86
Deletion	2n	3	2	0.82	0.82	0.41

[a] Due to differences from strain to strain and laboratory to laboratory, all activity data were expressed relative to normal female. Where disagreement between different authors exists, extreme values are reported. For reference to original papers see text.

[b] In order to correct for larger cell volumes, activity values in triploids were multiplied by 1.5 (Maroni and Plaut, 1973).

males and in triploid intersexes is slightly lower and slightly higher, respectively. On the other hand, dosage compensation is only partial in duplication and deletion individuals (Table V), suggesting that it operates basically at the level of the individual gene, but that the chromosome as a whole plays some role as well. Dosage compensation is already seen in larvae (Lucchesi *et al.*, 1974), and it appears to regulate the activity of *Zw* and other X-linked genes in all Drosophilidae (Abraham and Lucchesi, 1974). The exact mechanism and the genes involved in dosage compensation are not known. It is not clear, for example, if the genes described in Table V that show differential effects in males and females are involved in the process. Some evidence that the process of sex differentiation may also affect G6PD levels has been produced by Komma (1966), who showed that at 20°C, but not at 29°C, G6PD activity in intersexes is higher in males than in females, and thought this finding could be related to a previously known masculinizing effect of low temperature (Dobzhansky, 1930). For a more general discussion on dosage compensation see the review by Stewart and Merriam (1980).

Other Examples. A very peculiar increase in G6PD activity has been observed upon infection of the cyanobacterium *Anacystis nidulans* by cyanophage (Balogh *et al.*, 1979). This is apparently not due to *de novo* protein synthesis, but rather to a phage-conditioned molecular reorganization of preexisting G6PD.

Cell growth and cell division may be by themselves associated with higher levels of G6PD activity, as found in *E. coli*, where the increase is very likely due to new synthesis of protein (Wolf *et al.*, 1979), in some human cancers (Zampella *et al.*, 1982), and possibly in developing human brain (Toncheva *et al.*, 1982; G. Battistuzzi and L. Luzzatto, unpublished).

Physiological Adaptive Phenomena

Given a certain genetic constitution and a specific developmental stage of the organism and the differentiated state of a particular tissue, there is still scope for further changes in the basal level of enzyme activity. Such temporary changes, or modulation, take place generally in response to changes in metabolic requirements determined by internal or environmental changes. Modulation phenomena can be of two types: a coarse modulation involving relatively major adjustments in the cell's metabolic machinery, which will therefore display some time lag, as after a change in the nutritional environment; and a fine modulation, requiring very rapid changes, as in response to an oxidative stress.

Response to Physical Environment. During cold acclimation in poikilotherms considerable restructuring of cellular and tissue components takes place, and lipids play an important role. It has been observed in the brook trout that when the animal lives at 5°C the levels of G6PD, H6PD, and 6PGD are higher in the liver than when it lives at 10 or 15°C (Yamauchi *et al.*, 1975). Since hepatic dehydrogenases supply NADPH for lipid synthesis, their increase can be viewed as related to the restructuring process. This physiological response seems to have general significance, because increased G6PD and increased lipogenesis in cold acclimation is observed also in invertebrates [*Mythilus edulis* (Livingstone, 1981)] and even in homeotherms [rat (Goubern and Portet, 1981)].

Responses to Nutrients. These have been observed in a wide range of organisms and experimental conditions. G6PD activity increases in *E. coli* in a high-carbohydrate medium (Wolf *et al.*, 1979). In *Drosophila*, increasing concentrations of sucrose in the medium induce proportionally higher levels of G6PD and 6PGD activities (Geer *et al.*, 1976, 1979). Concomitantly, tissue concentrations of glycolytic intermediates also increase, and so does lipid biosynthesis. On the other hand, lipids reduce the level of G6PD and 6PGD, and of malic enzyme and NADP-isocitric dehydrogenase as well, suggesting that the four NADP-linked dehydrogenases all contribute to the NADPH pool that is needed for lipid synthesis. The relationship between increased G6PD activity and increased lipogenesis is not straightforward, since, for instance, larvae fed on fat-free acetate diet have active shunt activity and lipid synthesis but unaffected levels of shunt enzymes (Geer *et al.*, 1976), whereas with D-glycerate the reverse is true (Geer *et al.*, 1978). Thus, it seems that hexose monophosphate shunt (HMS) activity certainly correlates with lipid synthesis, but it is sensitive to a variety of effectors and it can increase either by enzyme induction or by activation of preexisting enzymes.

Interestingly, induction by carbohydrates and repression by lipids of G6PD occur irrespective of the number of copies and types of G6PD genes present, i.e., they are independent of the basal level of G6PD (Geer *et al.*, 1979). On the other hand, lipid composition does depend on a G6PD(−) or G6PD(+) phenotype, since it is a direct function of the NADPH supply.

Characteristic dietary effects have been well outlined in rodents. In a typical experiment an animal is subjected to fasting and subsequently refed on a high-carbohydrate, fat-free diet or on a fat-rich, carbohydrate-free diet. In the rat liver G6PD decreases by approximately 50% upon acute starvation. When the animal is refed a high-carbohydrate diet G6PD increases by approximately tenfold, i.e., fivefold the original normal level. This overshoot phenomenon does not take place if the refeeding diet is low in protein. If, after starvation, the animal is placed on a diet in which all of the energy is supplied as fat, the animal recovers, but liver G6PD remains at the levels observed during starvation. If the rat is maintained on a high-fat diet without previous starvation, liver G6PD decreases to levels identical to those observed on a starvation regimen. Upon switching to a high-carbohydrate diet, G6PD returns to normal without overshooting (Tepperman and Tepperman, 1963 and 1965; B. C. Johnson and Sassoon, 1967). This phenomenon can also be reproduced in primary hepatocyte cultures (Kurtz and Wells, 1981). Basically similar changes have also been seen in the mouse (Yagil *et al.*, 1974; Hizi and Yagil, 1974*a,b*), although experimental conditions (diet, age of the animals) were somewhat different.

Changes in diet are likely to affect G6PD activity not only in the liver, but in other organs as well, although to a lesser extent. Accordingly,

Madvig and Abraham (1980) have observed increased G6PD levels in brain, kidney, and small intestine in weaning rats compared to sucklings.

Decreased G6PD activity upon starvation and recovery to normal levels upon refeeding has been reported also in the brook trout (Yamauchi *et al.*, 1975). Here the time course is longer (several weeks), recovery to normal level of liver G6PD is slow, and overshoot does not occur, possibly because the metabolic rate in fishes is much lower than in mammals.

Action of Hormones.   It has been suggested that some of the dietary effects summarized in the previous section are mediated by hormones, but the evidence is somewhat controversial. For instance, it seems that insulin is required for induction of G6PD by carbohydrates both *in vivo* and in isolated hepatocytes (Nakamura *et al.*, 1982); however, other authors favor the hypothesis that insulin promotes induction by increasing appetite, while others deny a role of insulin altogether (Kurtz and Wells, 1981; Kukulansky and Yagil, 1979). Evidence has also been produced that glucagon inhibits rat liver G6PD (Rudack Garcia and Holten, 1974); and that adrenal glucocorticoids are involved in causing the overshoot response to starvation–refeeding (Wurdeman *et al.*, 1978). Estradiol plays a role in inducing G6PD in the rat levator ani muscle (Max and Knudsen, 1980) and in rat uterus (Donohue and Barker, 1983), and it mediates neural control of muscle G6PD (Schaerf *et al.*, 1982). Indeed, G6PD activity increases after denervation of muscle more rapidly in females than in males, and estrogen administration to males tends to abolish this difference to an extent that is dose-related. Estradiol modulation has been invoked also to explain the different levels of G6PD in male and female rat liver (Hori *et al.*, 1975). Progesterone behaves as an antagonist of estradiol (Swanson and Barker, 1983).*

The most impressive physiological variation of G6PD activity in mammals is, appropriately, that observed in the lactating mammary gland. In the rat, for example, G6PD (and 6PGD) activity increases from the end of pregnancy to reach, during lactation, a peak of approximately 60-fold the basal level. At the end of lactation, involution of parenchymal tissue is associated with a rapid decrease of dehydrogenase activity to a

---

* Different levels of G6PD activity in males and females have been found in mammalian lung cells (Steele and Migeon, 1973) and in liver (Glock and McLean, 1953, 1954; Teutsch and Rieder, 1979). Hori and Matsui (1967) have shown that in rat liver the difference is under hormonal control by estradiol and dehydroepiandrosterone.

level lower than in pregnancy (Glock and McLean, 1954).It is quite clear that this increase in G6PD and 6PGD activity is related to increased rate of HMS operation and increased lipogenesis. In organ cultures it has been shown that this induction is mediated probably by increased glucose uptake in mammary tissue during lactation (Green *et al.,* 1971).

Molecular Basis of Adaptive Changes. The main question regarding the changes in G6PD levels discussed in the previous section is whether they are effected at the level of transcription, at the level of translation, or after translation. In intact animals and in organ cultures agents such as actinomycin D or cycloheximide have been shown to interfere with induction, suggesting that *de novo* synthesis of enzyme molecules was involved (Yagil *et al.,* 1974). However, it is well known that such experiments must be interpreted with caution, because these inhibitors, while specific in cell-free systems for RNA polymerase and ribosome function, respectively, may have a multitude of secondary complicating effects when used in intact cells or intact animals. A more direct and presumably more specific test is the immunochemical assay of G6PD by using heterologous antibodies. Since this assay is not based on the catalytic activity of the enzyme, it should be possible to measure, for instance, whether the G6PD increase observed after starvation–refeeding is due to an increased number of enzyme molecules or to activation of preformed molecules. Unfortunately, this approach has yielded conflicting data. Thus, Hizi and Yagil (1974*b*) and Kelley *et al.* (1975) have failed to detect any increase in the concentration or rate of synthesis of G6PD. Winberry and Holten (1977) found instead that, under a variety of experimental conditions, there was good correlation between G6PD assayed by activity and by immunochemical reactivity, and dietary induction of G6PD was associated with a marked increase in polysome-bound G6PD. Subsequently, doubt has been cast on previous immunotitration experiments by the finding that a mouse antiserum raised against highly purified rat liver G6PD cannot recognize palmitoyl-CoA-inactivated G6PD (Dao *et al.,* 1979), which may be present in substantial amounts in animals on a fat-rich diet. Even more recently, Dao *et al.* (1982) have developed a monoclonal antibody that recognizes a G6PD epitope other than the active center, and that does cross-react with palmitoyl-CoA-inactivated G6PD. By using this antibody, they have found similar amounts of immunochemically reactive protein in previously starved rats refed a high-carbohydrate or a high-fat diet. These data favor the view that at least the majority of the diet-induced changes in G6PD described above (p. 232) are actually post-translational.

Is G6PD an Indispensable Protein?

This question could be refuted by finding mutants that lack G6PD, and this has been done in a few cases. A G6PD-deficient strain of *E. coli* was isolated by Fraenkel (1968) among derivatives of a strain already deficient in glucose-6-phosphate isomerase that was unable to grow on glucose, but able to grow reasonably well on glycerol. Since the mutation was shown to consist of a μ insertion in the *Zwf* gene (the code for *Gd* in the language of bacterial genetics), gene expression must be totally abrogated and we must conclude that *E. coli* can do without G6PD under certain environmental conditions.

The case of *Pasteurella pestis* is so far unique, in that absence of G6PD activity seems to be the wild-type condition (Bowman *et al.*, 1967). Apparently pentose phosphate synthesis via transketolase–transaldolase is adequate at 5°C, a temperature at which the organism behaves upon assay in mouse as having low virulence (Naylor *et al.*, 1961). Change in temperature to 37°C quickly restores virulence, but only in the presence of xylose and gluconate, suggesting that higher pentose phosphate is required for the production of "virulence factors" (Mortlock, 1962). Thus, *P. pestis* clearly does grow without G6PD. In this case, however, the biological importance of the enzyme seems to be vindicated by the evolution of a mechanism for the control of virulence that is based on its absence. More recently, a G6PD-deficient mutant of the lower eukaryote, *Saccharomyces cerevisiae,* has also been isolated (Lobo and Maitra, 1982): its phenotype is inconspicuous under ordinary laboratory conditions. However, when we come to higher organisms, we do not find any comparable evidence. The earlier literature on spontaneously occurring human G6PD deficiency included several reports of "complete absence" of G6PD in red cells. In routine assays of hemolysates enzyme activity may be indeed quite frequently undetectable. However, when the undetectable activity is purified away from hemoglobin, which limits the amount of preparation that can be added to the reaction mixture in a spectrophotometer, residual G6PD activity, no matter how low, is invariably recovered (Testa *et al.*, 1980). In addition, G6PD attributable to the same gene is found in leukocytes (Morelli *et al.,* 1981, see also p. 287). It is also noteworthy that G6PD-deficient mutants isolated from cultured cells have never been proven to involve gene deletion. Thus, it may well be that total absence of G6PD, and therefore a *Gd* deletion, is lethal in animal cells. This might be an example of a general pattern that will reflect on our ability to investigate household genes in general. Indeed, a differentiation gene can afford to be deleted, because all cells in which it is not expressed are unaffected, even when the cells in which it is normally expressed suffer severely, as erythroid cells do in the homozygous state for α-thalassemia. By contrast, deletion of an ubiquitously expressed gene is going to affect to a greater or lesser extent all somatic cells. If the gene is autosomal and the product is an enzyme, homozygotes would be extremely rare, and ascertainment of heterozygotes would require a specific search by appropriate nucleic acid probes in very large population samples. If the gene is X-linked, like G6PD, a deletion is likely to be lethal in males but detectable in their heterozygous mothers. Thus, to find in the human species household gene mutants that are totally inactive, whether by deletion or otherwise, will be quite difficult, and perhaps feasible in practice only for X-linked genes, and by specially aimed selection of samples.

THE G6PD GENE IN HUMANS

It is clear that the role of G6PD has become firmly established in the course of evolution as that of a housekeeping gene with a major role in metabolism, particularly at the interface between carbohydrate and lipid metabolism. Because several effectors of regulatory phenomena have been discovered, the obvious remaining task is to identify the structural domains within the protein that enable it to respond to them. On the other hand, the thrust of the work in humans has been on the identification of mutants that compromise to a greater or lesser degree the function of G6PD in preventing cell damage that could accrue from the generation of both endogenous and exogenous toxic oxidants. These mutants could potentially explain in detail which residues within the enzyme molecule are crucial for binding of both substrates and specific inhibitors. Thus, from both ends the elucidation of primary structure seems clearly a crucial bottleneck. At the same time, with the increasing amount of information becoming available on the organization of genes by direct sequencing, one wonders how the functional distinction between house-hold genes and specific differentiation genes will be reflected in differences at the DNA level: indeed, most of the information thus far has been derived from the latter rather than from the former. The recent developments in this respect have been the publication of a nearly complete amino acid sequence of human erythrocyte G6PD worked out by A. Yoshida (Beutler, 1983), and the isolation of a human cDNA clone.

Cloning of cDNA

The main limiting factor in cloning of household genes as opposed to differentiation genes has been the shortage of specific mRNA. In the case of G6PD, one might have considered using as a source an organ in which enzyme activity is high, such as the adrenal gland, but this is not very practical in the human species, and besides there is no certainty as yet that higher levels of enzyme are matched by higher levels of mRNA. After considering several alternatives, cultured fibroblasts from primary explants were selected. These cells, although more laborious to obtain, do have a much higher G6PD specific activity than any solid tissue. A prerequisite for cloning was enrichment in G6PD-specific mRNA, and a prerequisite for that was the development of a specific assay. Persico *et al.* (1981) have shown that, after translation of fibroblast mRNA in a reticulocyte cell-free system, a polypeptide with the molecular weight of G6PD could be identified on SDS gels of the translation product immunoprecipitated with an anti-G6PD antiserum. The identity of the product was confirmed by comparison with authentic G6PD by peptide mapping (Toniolo *et al.*, 1984a). By using this assay, G6PD-specific mRNA was purified about 50-fold, and the resulting preparation cloned in pBR 322 (Fig. 1). The major subsequent task was the identification of the desired clones, since the G6PD mRNA abundance in the cloned preparation was estimated to be only between 0.1% and 1%. An ideal screening procedure might have been one making use of mRNA from a G6PD-free cell line or tissue. Interestingly, despite the large number of available mutants, such a biological material has not yet been discovered in mammals (see p. 236). As an alternative, a variety of preliminary screening devices were applied, and over 200 clones were in the end tested directly by positive

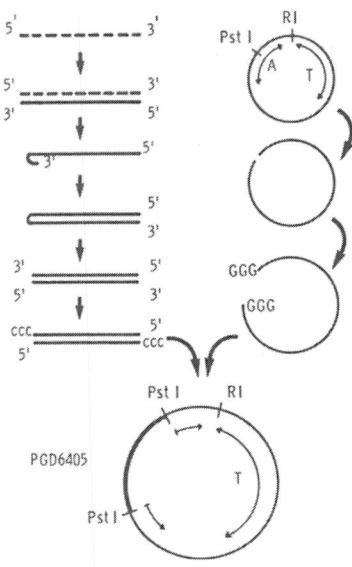

Fig. 1. Construction of a cDNA library enriched in G6PD sequences. On the left, from top to bottom: mRNA; RNA-cDNA hybrid molecule after reverse transcription step; cDNA with 3' end loop after alkaline digestion of RNA; double-stranded cDNA after DNA polymerase step, with hairpin structure; double-stranded linear cDNA molecule after SI nuclease step; double-stranded cDNA molecule after "poly-C tailing." On the right, from top to bottom: a diagram of the circular plasmid pBR 322, showing the positions of two unique restriction sites and of the genes conferring to the bacterial host cells resistance to ampicillin (A) and tetracycline (T); pBR 322 after cleavage ("linearization") with endodeoxyribonuclease Pst I; same after "poly-G tailing." Bottom center: recombinant plasmid (pGD 6405) containing G6PD-specific DNA insert (thick line). Two Pst I sites are regenerated by this method, so that the insert can be conveniently recovered by digestion with this enzyme. For details and references to methodology see Persico et al. (1981).

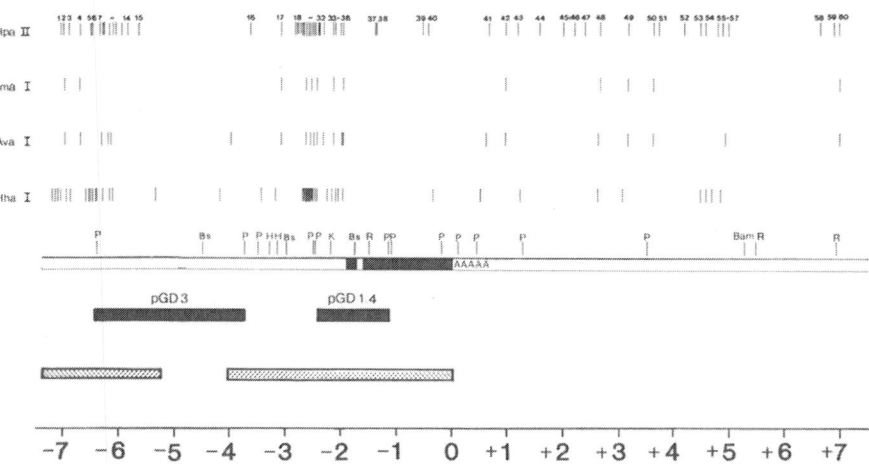

Fig. 2. Diagram of 3' end of human Gd gene, from bottom to top. The scale on the abscissa is marked in kilobases, with the origin at the end of the transcript. The dotted segments indicate DNA that has been sequenced. The dark segments indicate the two probes used in this work. The double line is genomic DNA, which is blacked in for known exons. The length of the intron on the 5' side of −1.9 kb is not known. On this double line a partial restriction map is shown, with the following symbols: P: pst I; BS: Bst EII; H: Hind III; K: Kpn I; R: Eco RI; Bam: Bam H1. The four lines above give a detailed map of the four methylation sensitive restriction enzymes, as shown. The Hpa II sites have been numbered from left to right in order to ease reference to them in the text.

mRNA hybridization followed by translation in a cell-free system and immunoprecipitation. One of the clones identified by this approach, pGd 6405, was shown in Southern blots by dosage effect to be X-chromosome-specific (Persico *et al.*, 1981), and it was also mapped to the Xq26–Xqter region by using appropriate somatic cell hybrids (De Leon *et al.*, 1984—see addendum).

The cDNA clone obtained has been used to screen a human genomic library, and a number of homologous phages have been isolated (Fig. 2). At the same time, sequencing of the 600-bp-long insert in plasmid pGd 6405 has revealed that it does have a poly-A tail but it does not have any open reading frame, indicating that it constitutes the 3′ end of G6PD mRNA. Hybridization of genomic clones with mRNA has identified an intron at about 1000 bp proximally to the poly-A tail. Elucidation of the remaining structure of the gene and search for DNA polymorphisms are in progress.

The Gd *Gene and the X Chromosome*

Mapping Data

More than 100 genetic loci have been mapped on the human X chromosome (McKusick, 1981), and extensive meiotic recombination data based on family studies have helped to identify two major clusters of closely linked genes on this chromosome (Race and Sanger, 1975). One is defined, on the short arm (Xp), by close linkage to the Xg blood group; the other is referred to as the G6PD–color-blindness cluster and is located in the subtelomeric region of the long arm (Xq). Recently, the G6PD gene locus has been more precisely assigned, by using somatic cell hybrids with various X-autosomal translocations, to the Xq28 band (Pai *et al.*, 1980). The genes for adrenal leukodystrophy (ALD) (Migeon *et al.*, 1982b), hemophilia A (HA) (Boyer and Graham, 1965), and protan and deutan color-blindness (Siniscalco *et al.*, 1964) are estimated to be within a distance of 6 cM on either side of the G6PD gene. The Xm locus is not as close, but is still within measurable linkage to *Gd* [6–22 cM (Berg and Bearn, 1968)]. That protan and deutan were located on opposite sides with respect to *Gd* had been proposed long ago (Siniscalco *et al.*, 1964), and has been recently confirmed (Purrello *et al.*, 1984). ALD seems to be closer to G6PD than to HA, since no recombinants have been found among the 18 progeny in the two kindreds examined by Migeon *et al.*

(1982b). Because a form of X-linked mental retardation has been found to be closely linked (6 cM) to *Gd* (Filippi *et al.,* 1983), and this form is associated cytologically with a fragile site at Xq28, we can infer that it is also very near deutan. By reviewing all available physical and family data, Keats (1983) has proposed that the relative position of the genes within the G6PD cluster is: Xm–deutan–G6PD–hemophilia A–protan–qter (see Fig. 3). From this map, it would appear that band Xq28 may be smaller in genetic terms than one might have thought from inspection of metaphase chromosomes. One wonders whether this is related to a relatively higher rate of crossing over at or near the adjacent fragile site. Recent data support this concept (Szabo *et al.,* 1984, Purrello *et al.,*1984).

G6PD and X-Chromosome Inactivation

As mentioned earlier, G6PD was the tool for the first validation of the Lyon phenomenon at the cellular level. Fibroblast clones from heterozygotes Gd^A/Gd^B express only one *Gd* allele (Davidson *et al.,* 1963), and it was subsequently realized that even in extracts from uncloned cells the haploid expression in individual cells can be inferred from the absence of a heterodimeric enzyme band on electrophoresis. G6PD has been used to establish the timing of X-inactivation in early embryonic life and of its reactivation in maturing oocytes, and to follow events involving the X chromosome that take place during the differentiation of teratocarcinoma cells (Martin, 1982). A full discussion of X-chromosome inactivation, the mechanism of which remains elusive, is clearly outside the scope of this review (Gartler and Andina, 1976; Gartler and Cole, 1981). The original (though not strictly necessary) concept was that X-inactivation (1) involves the whole chromosome and (2) is totally irreversible (for instance, it is stable in cultured cells even after transformation with SV40—Romeo and Migeon, 1975). However, the study of the

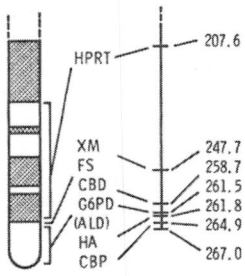

Fig. 3. Diagram of a portion of the long arm of the human X chromosome. On the left, the bottom clear band is Xq28 and the top hatched band is Xq23. The abbreviations not defined elsewhere are as follows: XM, a plasma protein group; FS, fragile site; CBD, color-blindness, deutan; ALD, adrenal leukodystrophy; HA, hemophilia A; CBP, color-blindness, protan. The figures on the right are best estimates of genetic distance, in centimorgans, from the tip of the short arm. On this scale the centromere is at 106 cM. [Modified by kind permission from Keats (1983).]

Xg blood group system shed considerable doubt on the first concept in the early 1970s (Race and Sanger, 1975). It is accepted now that at least part of the short arm partially escapes the ban on gene expression (Mohandas *et al.*, 1980) but this can hardly concern *Gd*, firmly based as it is at the opposite end of the chromosome. The axiom of irreversibility was put to a stringent test when Kahan and De Mars (1975) successfully obtained expression in mouse–human hybrids of a human HGPRT gene that must have been on the inactive X, because the active X carried at the corresponding locus a mutation associated with HGPRT deficiency. These findings remained unconfirmed for several years, and there may have been an unexpressed feeling (in a field where expression can be characteristically switched off!) that they were somehow related to the strong selection procedure employed. However, those results were entirely vindicated when Mohandas *et al.* (1981) and De Mars's group itself (Lester *et al.*, 1982) reported systematic work on reactivation of several X-linked genes, including *Gd*, by the use of the pyrimidine analogue 5-azacytidine (5AC). These experiments were still carried out on mouse–human hybrids, but at about the same time Migeon *et al.* (1982a) described a totally unexpected event of *Gd* reactivation in a human diploid fibroblast clone after thawing from prolonged storage in liquid nitrogen.

The reactivation phenomenon, whether spontaneous or 5AC induced, provides a much needed handle for understanding X-chromosome inactivation at the molecular level. To cover this topic is outside the scope of this review, and summaries of current thought have been recently published (Martin, 1982; Luzzatto and Gartler, 1983; Blasi and Toniolo, 1983). In principle, the primary chromosomal change associated with X-inactivation might reside (1) in chromosomal proteins; (2) in the DNA sequence; (3) in a DNA modification not affecting its sequence. The finding by Liskay and Evans (1980) and by Venolia and Gartler (1982) that transformation of HGPRT(−) cells to HGPRT(+) cells can be effected at significant frequencies only by active X-DNA but not by inactive X-DNA has virtually eliminated the first possibility. On the other hand, because 5AC is a methylase inhibitor, the reactivation mediated by this agent has been interpreted as supporting the notion (Riggs, 1975) that DNA methylation is crucial in X-chromosome inactivation, in keeping with the third alternative listed above. Indeed, DNA from cells so reactivated regains competence for transfection (Lester *et al.*, 1982). Of course it is still possible that 5AC acts by some mechanism other than demethylation, and sequence changes have not been formally ruled out. But the features of the reactivation phenomenon do convey the important message that, although X-inactivation characteristically takes place *en bloc,* a particular gene can be reexpressed individually, while the rest remain silent. This suggests that, whatever the mechanism that turns off the X chromosome, its continued inactivity is maintained by a different mechanism, which operates at the level of individual genes. At least the latter should become accessible through the study of reactivants. A spontaneous reactivant, like the Migeon clone, may turn out to be more informative than the induced ones, since it is more certain that reactivation is due to a single (mutational?) event.

Mosaicism

G6PD is closely associated with the history of X-linked inactivation mosaicism, since it was used as just mentioned for the first, classical, proof of the then recently formulated Lyon hypothesis (Lyon, 1961). (One wonders why this well-established fact in developmental biology is still so frequently referred to as a "hypothesis.") The features of G6PD-linked mosaicism have been reviewed (Gartler and Andina, 1976; Gartler and Cole, 1981). Here we discuss only a few special aspects.

How Does This Mosaicism Relate to Phenotypic Expression? That G6PD deficiency heterozygotes can develop hemolysis is only to be expected, since a proportion of their cells are as deficient as in hemizygous males. In this respect, a G6PD-deficient allele could be regarded formally as dominant. This is of some practical importance, since the laboratory identification of heterozygotes is not straightforward even by quantitative assay, because of overlap with normal homozygotes (Bienzle *et al.,* 1981); a rather delicate cytochemical test may be required. However, not surprisingly, the likelihood and severity of hemolysis are directly related to the proportion of G6PD(−) cells (Panizon *et al.,* 1970). Therefore, from the practical point of view those heterozygotes who have total hemolysate levels within the normal range are not going to experience severe manifestations, whereas those who are most at risk will be detected as abnormal by a quantitative assay, and often even by screening tests set at the appropriate threshold of sensitivity.

What Determines and How Stable Is the Proportion of G6PD(+) and G6PD(−) Cells in a Heterozygote? There are limited data on this question. It is generally assumed, and probably true in most cases, that the ratio is determined by chance at the time of X-chromosome inactivation, and that deviations from a 1:1 ratio could be attributed to statistical fluctuations, which in extreme cases could yield an extreme ("pseudohomozygote") phenotype. However, in a series of $Gd^B/Gd^{Mediterranean}$ heterozygotes (Rinaldi et al., 1976) it was observed that there were more pseudonormal than pseudodeficient extreme phenotypes, suggesting some measure of selection against G6PD($-$) cells within the mosaic. That this selection may be age-related is suggested by a study of G6PD heterozygous Bantu women carried out by Hitzeroth and Bender (1981), who observed that among teenage girls the proportion of those who were certainly heterozygotes on grounds of their G6PD electrophoretic pattern (either Gd^A/Gd^B or Gd^{A-}/Gd^B) was about 30%. This proportion decreased gradually with age and became about 17% for women in their 30s. Although, unfortunately, the authors did not fully determine the genotype of these subjects by either quantitation or a cytochemical test, they point out that, on grounds of the known gene frequencies in the population studied, these data would fit with ongoing somatic selection only in Gd^{A-}/Gd^B subjects and not in Gd^A/Gd^B subjects. Of course other explanations are conceivable, and formal proof of this suggestion will need a longitudinal rather than a cross-sectional study.

Independent evidence for somatic selection can be obtained by formal genetic analysis.* The concordance in expression of Gd alleles is higher in monozygotic than in dizygotic twins (Brewer et al., 1967), and this again is in favor of selection favoring cells with a certain one of the two X chromosomes active. The gene involved may not be Gd, but another syntenic gene. In extreme cases G6PD was indeed used as a marker to show, in doubly heterozygous women, that blood cells with the active X chromosome carrying the normal gene were overwhelmingly predominant in number over those with the active X chromosome carrying a Lesch–Nyhan (Nyhan et al., 1970) or a Wiskott–Aldrich [(Gealy et al., 1980; Carroll et al., 1980; Prchal et al., (1980)] mutant gene. Evidently hemopoietic cells with these mutations were at a disadvantage in growth.

An extremely imbalanced mosaic phenotype was also observed, and shown to be inherited, in all female members of a three-generation family without any apparent X-linked pathological condition (Fig. 4) (Luzzatto

---

* By contrast, little or no evidence of selection was found when the expression of parental Gd genes was analyzed in blood cells of interspecific hybrids [mules (Serov et al., 1978b)] or intergeneric hybrids [foxes from *Alopex lagopus* $\times$ *Vulpes vulpes* crosses (Serov et al., 1978a)].

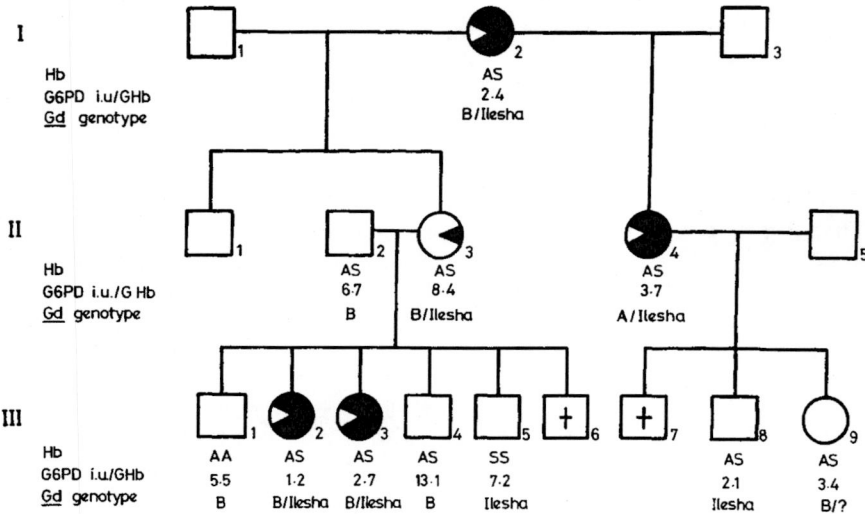

Fig. 4. Extreme mosaic phenotypes presumably attributable to somatic selection after X-chromosome inactivation. This family was ascertained through the propositus III-5, who had sickle-cell anemia. All other live members of the family were clinically and hematologically normal. Subjects III-6 and III-7 had died at the time of the study, the latter from severe neonatal jaundice. Under each symbol are given the hemoglobin electrophoretic pattern, the G6PD activity, and the *Gd* genotype, determined from quantitation and electrophoresis. The wedge-shaped shading in the heterozygotes who were fully investigated indicates the predominance (over 90%) of G6PD Ilesha (in black) or G6PD A or B (in white). The hemolysate of subject III-9 on starch-gel electrophoresis showed only a single band of G6PD B. However, on the basis of her mother's genotype, she cannot be a Gd^B homozygote: rather, her genotype must be either Gd^B/Gd^A or Gd^B/Gd^{Ilesha}. Therefore, her phenotype also consists of an unbalanced mosaic in favor of the cells with Gd^B on the active X chromosome. The low values of G6PD activity in the hemizygous Gd^{Ilesha} subject III-8 and in the phenotypically similar subjects I-2, II-4, III-2, and III-3 are explained by the fact that G6PD Ilesha is a mildly deficient variant (Usanga *et al.*, 1977). The normality of the enzyme activity value in the case of III-5, who is also a Gd^{Ilesha} hemizygote, is easily explained by the association of his younger red cell population with sickle-cell anemia (Bienzle *et al.*, 1975). [Reprinted with permission from Luzzatto *et al.*, (1979a).]

et al., 1979). This finding suggested the existence of a polymorphic X-linked gene that affects the proliferation of hemopoietic cells. The difference in proliferation rate must be slight, since males in which either allele segregates do not show evidence of hemopoietic failure. In a similar family (Williams *et al.*, 1983) it was conclusively proven by testing skin fibroblasts that the extremely imbalanced phenotype was not generalized (Williams, *et al.*, 1984). Interestingly, the proband of this family had polycythaemia rubra vera, a disorder in which hemopoietic cell proliferation is indeed pathologically increased. These data illustrate how, especially in rapidly turning over cell populations, mosaicism offers the potential for selective processes at the somatic level, even when differences in "somatic cell fitness" values between two alleles are small.*

G6PD As a Marker of Monoclonal Disorders

Somatic cell mosaicism constitutes a unique opportunity to trace the origin of any multicellular structure in the body. If such a structure consists of the progeny of a single cell, it will no longer be a mosaic, since all of its cells will have the same X chromosome active (Fig. 5). On the other hand, if the structure consists of the progeny of several cells, it is likely still to be a mosaic. This test has been used abundantly in order to prove the monoclonal origin of a variety of human tumours.† In principle, it can be applied whenever an affected female is heterozygous for any X-linked gene. In practice, because *Gd* is the only known gene expressed in all somatic cells and with common allelic variants, G6PD has been used almost exclusively. Not all variants lend themselves equally well to this kind of study, because quantitative expression of the enzyme may be affected by abnormal growth. It is much preferable to rely on qualitative differences, and the easiest and most widely used has been the electrophoretic difference between G6PD B and G6PD A. This of course limits the applicability of this approach to conditions arising in women who

---

* It is tempting to draw an analogy between genetic selection in populations and genetic selection in somatic cell populations within an organism. The mathematical theory of the former is well developed (Cavalli-Sforza and Bodmer, 1971). The latter is much simpler, at least in the case in question, since we are dealing with a functionally haploid system. If we start from a 1:1 ratio between Gd^+ and Gd^- cells, and the fitness of Gd^+ cells relative to that of Gd^- cells is w^+, it is easy to see that the number of cell divisions required for the ratio to become 2 is $n = \log 2/\log w^+$. For example, with $w^+ = 1.01$ (1% growth advantage), $n = 70$; with $w^+ = 1.05$, $n = 14$.

† Of course it must be accepted that if a structure derives from more than one but just very few cells, it might still be homogeneous by statistical fluctuation alone. If the cells are two, there is a 50% chance that they are identical by chance; if the cells are three, the chance of homogeneity will be 25%; if the cells are n, the chance will be $(1/2)^{n-1}$. Thus the strength of the "proof" is subject to this limitation. However, when several cases are examined, the chance that this situation will happen to apply to each of them becomes negligibly small.

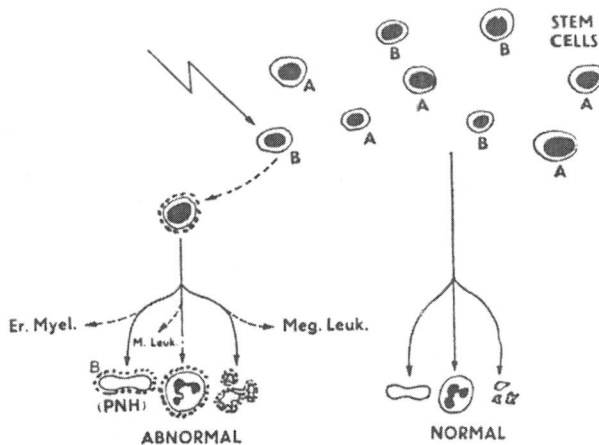

Fig. 5. G6PD mosaicism and monoclonal disorders. This diagram regards the condition paroxysmal nocturnal hemoglobinuria (PNH). The patient is heterozygous for two G6PD electrophoretic variants (genotype Gd^A/Gd^B). Letters A and B indicate cells in which the X chromosome carrying the respective Gd allele is active. A single somatic mutational event (represented by the arrow) is assumed to have hit one of the hemopoietic stem cells. The mutated cell will give rise to an abnormal "clone" comprising erythroid, myeloid, and mega-karyocytic cells (all the abnormal elements are circled by a broken line), while normal cells continue to arise from the nonmutated stem cells. Since the stem cell hit was labeled B, all PNH cells will have G6PD B, while remaining normal cells exhibit mosaicism (Oni *et al.*, 1970). The diagram further shows that in some cases PNH can evolve into acute leukaemia, with the leukemic cell population presumably arising from within the PNH clone (see Luz-zatto *et al.*, 1979*b*). [This diagram is reproduced, with permission, from Luzzatto and Lewis, (1972).]

happen to be Gd^B/Gd^A or Gd^B/Gd^{A-} heterozygotes, who in turn will be found only among people in Africa or of African descent. However, recently Gaetani's group have elegantly shown that a known clearcut difference between the electrophoretically identical G6PD B and G6PD Mediterranean can be similarly made use of in the large number of heterozygotes for this and similar variants present in southern Europe, North Africa, and the Middle East. The difference is in the relative utilization of the substrate analogue 2dG6P (Ferraris *et al.*, 1981). Since this is also significantly altered compared to normal in other high-frequency variants (for instance, Mahidol in Thailand), there is no reason why the same trick could not be used elsewhere.

From a list of various tumors (Table VI) it is apparent that in some cases the proof of monoclonal origin comes only from the use of G6PD

Table VI. G6PD As a Marker of Monoclonal Disorders[a]

Condition	Cells found to have single allelic form of G6PD	Independent evidence of monoclonal origin	Reference
Uterine fibroids	Smooth muscle	—	Linder and Gartler (1965)
Chronic myeloid leukemia	Granulocytes, erythrocytes, platelets, monocytes	Ph[1] chromosome	Fialkow et al. (1967, 1977)
Paroxysmal nocturnal hemoglobinuria	Erythrocytes	—	Omi et al. (1970)
Polycythemia vera	Erythrocytes, granulocytes, platelets	—	Adamson et al. (1976)
Thrombocythemia	As above	—	Gaetani et al. (1982)
Erythroleukemia	As above	—	Ferraris et al. (1983)
Burkitt tumor	B cells	Homogeneous surface Ig	Fialkow et al. (1973)
Chronic lymphocytic leukemia	B cells	Homogeneous surface Ig	Fialkow et al. (1978), Solanki et al. (1982)

[a] The list is not exhaustive. Further references in Fialkow (1979).

as a marker,* whereas in others independent evidence comes from a marker chromosome (e.g., Ph[1]) or a special gene product, like a particular immunoglobulin. On the other hand, a cell population homogeneous with respect to G6PD cannot be automatically regarded as monoclonal, because somatic selection may occur (see above and Williams et al., 1984).

Gd *Mutants in Cultured Cells*

Fibroblasts

Most of what we know about the biochemistry of human G6PD stems from work on erythrocytes. While these cells have proven a suita-

---

* Because this word has become widely used in the study of neoplasms, especially leukemias and lymphomas, it seems pertinent to point out that the term "marker" has been used with different meanings. Surface components recognized by an antibody and regarded as specific for a particular cell type are "expression markers," whose presence may or may not be permanent. A chromosomal marker in a certain cell population can be regarded as a witness of its monoclonal origin, and may or may not play a role in the pathogenesis of its abnormal proliferation. G6PD as a marker is only a strong evidence of monoclonality, since it is most unlikely to be in any way involved in oncogenesis, but it does mark which X chromosome is active.

ble, if not very generous, source for enzyme purification, and an excellent system for investigating the *in vivo* function of the enzyme, they have the major drawback that they do not synthesize it. From this point of view fibroblasts grown from skin explants are ideal. First, they could be used as a potential source for purification and characterization of enzyme variants for indefinite periods of time. Indeed, some *Gd* mutant strains are included in the Genetic Mutant Repository (Camden, New Jersey), and it is only regrettable that their number is so much smaller than that of known G6PD variants: evidently it is easier to obtain samples of blood than fragments of skin from donors and patients. Second, fibroblasts can be used to analyze under well-controlled experimental conditions the synthesis and turnover of G6PD, and possibly its regulation both in the case of the normal enzyme and with mutants. While this will soon be undertaken by using molecular probes, it has already been observed by a semi-quantitative cytochemical method that considerable variation of G6PD activity occurs among cells in individual explants from male subjects, despite the fact that they must all have the same *Gd* gene (Terzi *et al.*, 1978). This has been confirmed by quantitative assay on individual clones (M. D'Urso and L. Luzzatto, unpublished). The basis for this variability is thus far entirely obscure, but it suggests some modulation mechanism that can be somatically inherited. Fibroblast cultures have also been used to measure G6PD turnover (Table VII). The half-life of the normal enzyme is about 2 days, as compared to 60 days in erythro-

Table VII. Molecular Data on Human G6PD

	In erythrocytes	In fibroblasts
Protein[a]		
Subunit molecular weight, kd	59	59
Amino acids, number	495	—
Percent of total cell protein	0.001	0.07
Molecules per cells, $\times 10^3$	2.2	2000
Half-life of protein, days	60	1.9
Rate of synthesis, molecules/sec	0	6.1
G6PD mRNA[b]		
Size, nucleotides	—	3000
Percent of total mRNA	—	0.016
Molecules per cell	0	55

[a] For source of data see text.
[b] Data from Persico *et al.* (1981) and Toniolo *et al.* (1983).

cytes. In addition, mutants with decreased *in vivo* stability in erythrocytes have normal half-life in fibroblasts, suggesting that different mechanisms are responsible for G6PD breakdown in the two types of cells (C. Mareni, M. D'Urso, and L. Luzzatto, unpublished results). From these data a quantitative pattern of G6PD at the molecular level can be evinced (Table VII).

Cell Hybrids

The key enzyme in cell hybrids has been hypoxanthine-guanine phosphoribosyltransferase (HGPRT), because it is one of the few genetic markers in animal cells that lends itself to both selection in HAT medium and back-selection in thioguanine (Littlefield, 1964). However, since *Gd* shares with the HGPRT gene the prerogative of being on the X chromosome, whenever this is retained in a hybrid under HAT selection *Gd* is also retained. Siniscalco *et al.* (1969) first showed that in mouse–human cell hybrids both parental *Gd* genes are expressed: in these cells, in contrast to normal female somatic cells, both X chromosomes remain active. As a result mouse and human G6PD subunits are produced in the same cytoplasm, giving rise to mouse homodimers and heterodimers and human homodimers in approximately 1:2:1 ratios. Similar findings have been obtained in other (see Silagi *et al.*, 1969) systems, and by constructing hybrids from human cells carrying X-autosomal translocations it was possible to map *Gd* to near the tip of the X chromosome (band Xq28). G6PD was also used in order to demonstrate successful human–human hybridization between lymphoblastoid cells and fibroblasts (Migeon *et al.*, 1974).

The cell hybrid approach also has another potential. Human fibroblasts have a limited life span, and sometimes they are difficult to grow for a variety of reasons. Although we cannot conclusively state that this is related to G6PD activity, we have noticed that this was true in the case of two variants with very severe enzyme deficiency: G6PD New York (strain GM 412 of the Genetic Mutant Cell Repository, Camden, New Jersey) and G6PD Barcelona (for which a skin fragment was received in our laboratory through the kindness of Dr. J. L. Vives Corrons). Slow-growing fibroblasts can be fused with one of the currently available permanent rodent cell lines, such as mouse A9 or hamster HGPRT(−) CHO, and after selection, hybrid clones are obtained in which the respective human *Gd* gene has been "immortalized" and is expressed. Since human autosomes will be lost in steps from the hybrids, this approach also offers a handle for tackling the question of whether and which factors extraneous to the *Gd* gene can affect its function. Thus far, it has been clearly shown that the level of human G6PD activity in the hybrids is much lower than in the parental fibroblasts (D'Urso *et al.*, 1983), but it is not yet known whether this is due to factors affecting transcription, translation, or post-translational events, for instance, the rate of degradation of the enzyme. Immortalized *Gd* genes also lend themselves to characterizing the gene product, should this be impossible by conventional approaches.

Artificial Mutants

With Decreased Activity.   The isolation of eukaryotic cell mutants is notoriously rather difficult, largely because only few strong selective conditions are available, because true minimal media can rarely be used, and because these cells are diploid. At least the last difficulty is relieved in the case of G6PD, and Rosenstraus and Chasin (1975) have been able to isolate, by an elegant sib-selection technique, after mutagenesis with ethyl methanesulfonate (EMS) a G6PD-deficient derivative (YH-21) from a CHO line that was already HGPRT-deficient. The mutant has extremely low G6PD activity, but revertants have been obtained (Rosenstraus and Chasin, 1977), indicating that the *Gd* gene was not deleted, and it was shown subsequently that YH-21 in fact produces substantial amounts of enzyme subunits with a markedly abnormal substrate specificity [2dG6P is preferred to G6P (D'Urso *et al.*, 1983)]. The mutant has no gross phenotypic abnormality in conventional media, but it is extremely sensitive to concentrations of diamide (a GSH-oxidizing compound) that are completely harmless to the parental cells. More recently, Stamato *et al.* (1982) have also subjected CHO cells to EMS mutagenesis and have obtained G6PD-deficient mutants at a frequency of about one in 1000 colonies. By omitting the conventional step of subculturing before plating, these authors have shown that colonies containing G6PD-deficient cells are often sectored, thus elegantly proving postreplicative segregation of normal and mutant cells from mutational events that presumably had affected only one DNA strand. This result is reminiscent of the sectoring phenomenon well characterized in fungi (Fincham *et al.*,

1979), although we ignore whether the underlying mechanism is the same. G6PD from the mutants has not been qualitatively characterized, but the level of activity, when assayed, was always very low (2–10% of the parent line activity), and it is interesting to relate this relatively high frequency of rather severely deficient variants obtained *in vitro* with what is found in human populations in nature (see below).

With Increased Activity. Not surprisingly, G6PD activity is easier to lose than to gain. This is again quite obvious when looking at spontaneous human mutants (see Table VIII), although it is true that mutants with increased activity might be unlikely to be ascertained, except by chance. *In vitro,* the demands on the cell's G6PD activity can be artificially increased, for instance, by using the aforementioned agent diamide. By EMS mutagenesis of a line obtained by hybridizing YH-21 with normal human fibroblasts, D'Urso *et al.* (1983) have obtained diamide-resistant mutants, some of which had increased G6PD activity. This was shown to be due not to a reversion in the hamster *Gd* gene, but to an increase in human G6PD activity, which displayed unchanged electrophoretic and kinetic behavior. Thus, diamide seems a useful addition to our armamentarium of selective media for cells in culture, and diamide-resistant strains may be regulatory mutants, or they might have amplified the *Gd* gene (Town and Luzzatto, unpublished results).

GENETIC VARIABILITY OF HUMAN G6PD

General Patterns of Variation

Since a comprehensive list of human G6PD variants was first compiled (Betke *et al.,* 1967) their number has been gradually increasing. Several updated tables have been published (Yoshida *et al.,* 1971; Beutler and Yoshida, 1973; Yoshida and Beutler, 1978, 1983). By combining these with a few additional original data, we come to an estimated total of 279 variants published through 1982, 87 of which are polymorphic. Their distribution according to a widely accepted classification is shown in Table VIII.

Analysis of biochemical characteristics of protein variants and of the effects of genetically determined changes upon cell metabolism has often provided insights into the molecular mechanisms and physiological role of the protein itself in normal subjects. The vast number of biochemically

Table VIII. Data on G6PD Variants: Extent of Polymorphism[a]

	Class	Sporadic	Polymorphic		Total
			Number	Percent	
I	Severe enzyme deficiency with CNSHD[b]	79	0	0	79
II	Severe enzyme deficiency[c]	54	46	46	100
III	Moderate to mild deficiency[c]	40	25	38	65
IV	Normal enzyme activity[c]	17	16	48	33
V	Increased enzyme activity	2	0	0	2
	Total	192	87		279

[a] Tabulation based on Betke et al. (1967), Yoshida et al. (1971), Beutler and Yoshida (1973), and Yoshida and Beutler (1978, 1983). In addition, we have included those variants reported by Usanga et al. 1980, Modiano et al. (1979), and Perona et al. (1983) that had not been covered in the above references.

[b] Some variants included in this class show only moderate deficiency in RBC lysates, which could, however, be explained by marked reticulocytosis (Luzzatto and Testa, 1978).

[c] Classification in classes II–IV is based on residual G6PD activity in RBC as follows: class II, ≤ 10%; class III, from 10% to 60%; class IV, from 60% to 130%.

characterized G6PD variants has allowed detailed analyses of various characteristics of G6PD (Kirkman, 1971; Rattazzi et al., 1971; Luzzatto, 1973a,b; Yoshida, 1973; Luzzatto and Testa, 1978; Vergnes et al., 1982; Panich, 1981, 1982; Bienzle, 1981; Persico et al., 1982). Here we will briefly review the results of previous studies that we have been able to confirm by the analysis of all the presently known variants and discuss in detail some aspects not covered in previous reviews.

Most genetic variants are thought to have arisen through point mutations leading to single amino acid replacements (but see p. 275). A direct proof has been obtained only for variants G6PD A, a replacement of aspartic acid for asparagine (Yoshida, 1967), and G6PD Hektoen, a replacement of tyrosine for histidine (Yoshida, 1970).

Electrophoretic Variants

On the basis of amino acid composition, an estimate of the expected relative proportion of variants with altered (electrophoretic) and unaltered (nonelectrophoretic) electrical net charge (resulting from single amino acid substitutions) can be obtained. Given the pH at which electrophoresis is usually performed, the expected proportion of G6PD electrophoretic variants (EV) is 0.30. The observed proportion is in fact

Table IX. Data on G6PD Variants: Extent of Electrophoretic Changes

Class of variant	Electrophoretic mobility		Total variants	Percent electrophoretic variants
	Slow	Fast		
I	23	22	78	57.7
II	32	34	100	67.0
III	33	22	64	85.9
IV + V	21	12	35	97.1
Total	109	90	277[a]	72.6

[a] This figure differs from the total in Table VIII because for one variant in class I and for one variant in class III electrophoretic mobility was not recorded.

much higher, 0.73 (Table IX). Is this discrepancy real or is it related to some sort of bias in the identification of G6PD variants? In practice, G6PD samples with normal activity will not be detected as variants unless they are EV. The G6PD-deficient samples are more often more fully investigated. However, even when this is done, electrophoresis is still one of the most convincing tests for identifying a variant as new. This may well explain why the percentage of EV decreases from class IV to class I (see Table IX), but EV are still in excess even in class I. We have noticed an empirical relationship between percentage of EV and average enzyme activity of variants in classes II–IV (see Fig. 6; class I variants have been excluded because they are ascertained from pathological cases and therefore the true average activity cannot be calculated). This relationship extrapolates to the theoretical 30% of EV only for an average

Fig. 6. The excess of electrophoretic variants of G6PD is accounted for by ascertainment bias. The three points reflect data on variants in classes II, III, and IV (see Tables VIII and IX). For each class the mean activity and the proportion of electrophoretic versus nonelectrophoretic variants were calculated. The horizontal broken line indicates the theoretical overall percentage of electrophoretic variants expected based on the amino acid composition of G6PD.

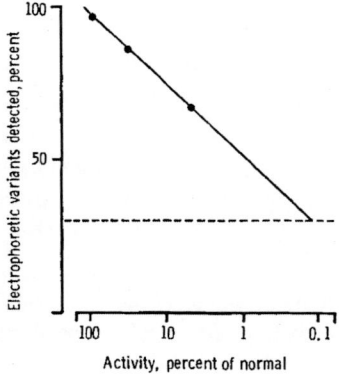

Table X. Altered Kinetic Parameters in G6PD Variants[a]

Class of variant	K_m for G6P[b]			K_m for NADP[c]		
	Low	Normal	High	Low	Normal	High
I	52	27	21	13	21	66
II	70	19	11	25	30	45
III + IV	70	22	8	24	30	46
Total	65	22	13	21	27	52

[a] Figures given are percentages of total in each class.
[b] Distribution of K_m values analyzed by χ^2 on a 3 × 3 table has shown no significant differences among classes.
[c] Frequency of high values in class I is significantly higher ($X^2 = 6.05$; df = 2; $p < 0.05$).

activity as low as 0.1%; thus, an experimental test cannot be entertained by this approach. On the other hand, one could analyze in detail any defined set of variants by totally independent criteria and see whether the expected proportion of EV is now found. Until then, we feel it is safer to assume that the excess of EV is probably due to ascertainment bias.

Variation and Covariation of Enzymic Properties

The availability of quantitative parameters in a large number of G6PD variants makes it possible to analyze not only how the parameters vary among and within variant classes, but also if and how they correlate. We have considered the following seven properties: activity,* K_m^{G6P}, K_m^{NADP}, K_i^{NADPH}, utilization of 2dG6P, utilization of dNADP, and heat stability. For each of these properties we first looked at the distribution of the data and then we tested them for correlation with each of the other six properties. Analysis of distributions confirmed patterns that had already been recognized on a smaller number of variants (see Tables X and XI) and no new significant patterns have emerged. Correlation anal-

---

* Any analysis involving G6PD activity variations and the conclusions drawn therefrom should be taken very cautiously, for several reasons. Usually the activity in red cell lysates is not corrected for heterogeneity between individuals in mean red cell age. It is known that G6PD activity decreases with increasing age of erythrocytes and G6PD variants can affect the age composition of the RBC population. Moreover, there is a wide variation in normal values reported in controls. To overcome this problem all our analyses involving activity levels have been performed using activities expressed as percent of normal as reported by the author.

Table XI. Enzymic Properties of G6PD Variants Related to Clinical Expression and to Each Other

Property	Deviation from randomness in distribution of values among the classes of variants	Correlation[a]	
		With what other property	Within what subset of variants
K_m^{G6P}	High in class I, low in classes II and III[b]	Activity[c]	Polymorphic variants only*
K_m^{NADP}	Higher in class I[d] than in classes II and III	K_m^{G6P}[e]	Class II only*
K_i^{NADPH}	High in class I[f]	K_m^{NADP}[g]	Entire set†
Reaction rate with 2dG6P	—	Reaction rate with dNADP	Entire set*
Heat stability	Very low in class I[h]; Low in class II	K_m^{NADP}[i]	Entire set†

[a] Asterisk, direct correlation; dagger, inverse correlation.
[b] See Luzzatto and Testa (1978) and Table X.
[c] See Persico et al. (1982).
[d] See Yoshida (1973), Luzzatto and Testa (1978), and Table X.
[e] See Table X.
[f] See Yoshida (1973); Luzzatto and Testa (1978).
[g] An inverse correlation between these two parameters was previously noticed (Luzzatto, 1973b). This still holds true for 34 variants, an analysis of which shows that the correlation can be attributed mainly to the unique distribution of values pertaining to variants in class I (see also Fig. 7 and Table XII).
[h] See Table XIII.
[i] See Table XIV.

yses were mostly new. Most of them were not significant and here we will summarize the few that are (see Tables X–XIV).

From the point of view of pathophysiology the striking difference in K_m^{G6P} values between class I and classes II and III argues strongly for the crucial importance of this parameter. Moreover, the correlation between K_m^{G6P} and K_m^{NADP} (Table XI) suggests an interaction between the two sub-

Table XII. Coordinate Changes in Substrate and Product Binding Affinity in G6PD Variants

Affinity for		Number of variants of	
NADPH	NADP+	Class I	Other classes
Increased	Decreased or normal	15	7
All other variations		0	11

Table XIII. Correlation between Heat Stability of G6PD and Severity of G6PD Deficiency

	Number of variants having *in vitro* stability[a]		
Class of variants	Normal	Low	Very low
I	8	16	24
	(16.1)	(21.8)	(10.1)
II	20	40	7
	(22.5)	(30.4)	(14.1)
III	26	17	3
	(15.4)	(20.8)	(9.8)

[a] Values in parentheses are expected number of variants. The χ^2 value for heterogeneity (df = 4) = 44.34, $p < 0.001$.

strate ligands, which would be most likely mediated by the protein itself. We must be very cautious in proposing specific enzymic features from a tabulation of variants. However, the suggestion we make certainly seems in keeping with the G6P relief of NADPH inhibition observed by Shreve and Levy (1980) in rat mammary gland G6PD and it is also supported by the direct correlation between 2dG6P and dNADP utilization. That heat stability should increase monotonically from class I to class V (Table XIII) is not surprising. On the other hand, an unexpected finding was that the least stable variants are also those with the lowest affinity for NADP$^+$ (Table XIV). One possible interpretation is that greater heat stability is the result of firmer NADP binding. Indeed, independent evidence that NADP stabilizes the quaternary structure of the enzyme is quite abundant.

An inverse correlation between K_m^{NADP} and K_i^{NADPH} has been previously noticed (Luzzatto, 1973a). We have now observed that, when

Table XIV. Association between K_m^{NADP} and Heat Stability in G6PD Variants[a]

		K_m^{NADP}	
		Lower than normal	Higher than normal
Heat stability	Normal	16 (11.4)	27 (31.6)
	Lower than normal	2 (6.6)	23 (18.4)

[a] Expected number of variants in parentheses; χ^2 was calculated applying the Yates correction; $\sigma^2 = 5.46$; df = 1; $p < 0.025$.

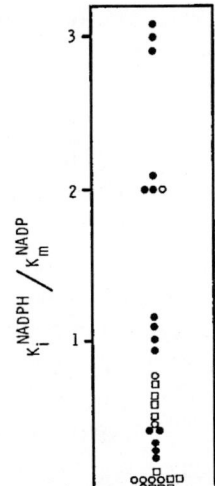

Fig. 7. Relative affinities for NADP and NADPH are not randomly distributed in a range of G6PD variants. (●) Class I variants (see Table VIII); (○) class II; (□) classes III and IV.

numerous variants are considered, the ratio between these two parameters tends to cluster around discrete integer values more often than would be expected by chance (Fig. 7). This finding is in keeping with the partially competitive character of NADPH inhibition and it corroborates the notion that a particular amino acid replacement shifts both the relative affinities for NADP and NADPH of the same binding site.

A Note on Techniques

The standardization of methods for characterizing G6PD proposed by a WHO Scientific Group in 1966 (Betke *et al.*, 1967) has been extremely valuable. Most authors have adhered to the recommendations and this has greatly facilitated comparison among variants worldwide. Not surprisingly, some of the parameters chosen have turned out to be more useful than others in having a high resolving power for differentiating variants. In practice, most variants can be recognized by a combination of electrophoretic mobility, K_m^{G6P}, and utilization of substrate analogues. Differences in level of activity are useful only when they are considerable, since they are markedy affected by the mean red cell age. Variants that do not differ with respect to any of these parameters can hardly be stated confidently to be different. Indeed, K_m^{NADP} tends to be always very low, while differences in thermostability and in pH dependence are difficult to quantitate and, in our experience, not very informative except in extreme cases.

With nearly two decades of hindsight, some changes in methodology would probably be desirable. The main deterrent to introducing any, apart from likely differences in opinion among investigators as to what is best, is the fear that comparison with the 279 variants already characterized might become difficult. In fact, this would not be a serious problem if the techniques for the most discriminating parameters listed above were left unchanged. We think that the K_m^{NADP} would be more usefully measured in the absence of Mg^{2+}, since this ion decreases the K_m to a very low level, which makes its determination experimentally difficult and yields uniform values for most variants: without Mg^{2+}, differences in K_m^{NADP} become apparent (Afolayan and Luzzatto, 1971). As for pH dependence of enzyme activity, the technique recommended (Betke et al., 1967) has turned out not to be ideal, because the five components of the buffers used (tris, glycine, phosphate, Na^+, Cl^-) vary in concentration over the pH range covered and affect markedly the enzyme activity by effects other than pH itself (Luzzatto, 1973b; Babalola et al., 1976). The elution profile from DEAE-Sephadex columns (Luzzatto and Allan, 1965) has been shown to have a very high resolving power (Luzzatto and Testa, 1978), but it has relatively limited popularity (see, however, for instance, Rattazzi et al., 1969; McCurdy et al., 1973; Usanga et al., 1977; Testa et al., 1980; Fenu et al., 1982) probably because it is regarded as too laborious, although it lends itself to automation (D'Urso et al., 1980).

Our hope regarding comparative compilations of analytical data on G6PD variants, such as Tables XV–XVII, is that they will soon be largely obsolete as the amino acid replacements for each individual variant become known. In the meantime, and pending possible changes in recommended characterization procedures, we think a very informative analysis, in addition to the usual parameters, would be the determination of the in vivo half-life of G6PD, which can be estimated by assaying several fractions of erythrocytes separated by centrifugation, i.e., on grounds of age. Such data are available for only very few variants, but they are enough to indicate that they do not necessarily correlate with conventional in vitro heat stability. For the purpose of estimating frequencies in populations it would also be very useful if the basis for ascertainment of a new variant (from random samples, from hospital patients, from jaundiced babies, etc.) was explained in greater detail than it sometimes is in the relevant publications.

Polymorphic Nondeficient Variants

A full survey of the geographic distribution of G6PD variants and G6PD deficiency is outside the scope of this review. Most data have been compiled by Mourant *et al.* (1976) and Livingstone (1967; 1973). Here we discuss selected data concerning populations in which biochemical characterization of samples (deficient or otherwise) has been sufficient for identification of individual polymorphic variants.*

The extensive study of many human populations has led to the discovery of a considerable number of polymorphic variants with normal or nearly normal enzyme activity in RBC. At present 19 are in this category (Table XV) and all are in tropical areas. Seventeen of 19 have been discovered because of altered electrophoretic mobility.

Only three such variants appear to be widely distributed. The wild type G6PD B is found worldwide. [Interestingly, it is indistinguishable from G6PD of chimpanzee and gorilla (Lucotte and Ruffié, 1982)]. G6PD A is common in populations of African ancestry, where it is present at frequencies ranging from 0% to nearly 40% [in the Balundu Ekondo Kiti in Cameroon (Bernstein *et al.*, 1980*a*)]. G6PD Karthoum is found in northeast Africa and in Arabia (Saha *et al.*, 1983*b*; Bayoumi *et al.*, 1979). All other variants appear to be examples of local or "private" polymorphisms, each confined to a single or a few populations living within a limited area. For instance, in their analysis of G6PD distribution in the Bantu populations of Mozambique, Reys *et al.* (1970) observed, besides the usual B, A, and A(−), four additional variants, three of which have normal activity in RBC lysates: these were G6PD Lourenzo Marques and G6PD Inhambane in Thonga and G6PD Manjacaze in Chopi.

Although it is clear from the above that electrophoretic analysis has been effective in outlining the genetic variation of G6PD, it was to be expected that other approaches would detect additional variants. Bernstein *et al.* (1980*b*) attempted to detect non-electrophoretic genetic variants in Cameroon by thermostability studies, an approach that had already been successfully employed for other enzymes in *Drosophila* (Bernstein *et al.*, 1973) and in humans (Scozzari *et al.*, 1981). The authors suggested the existence of several thermostability variants within all three

---

* Ford's classical definition of a polymorphic allele is one that has a frequency higher than can be accounted for by recurrent mutation. We have classified as polymorphic any variant with a population frequency higher than 0.1%.

Table XV. Biochemical Characteristics of Polymorphic G6PD Variants with Normal or Slightly Reduced Activity[a]

Name[b]	Population	Activity in RBC, percent of normal	Electrophoretic mobility, (percent of normal)			K_m^{G6P}, µM	K_m^{NADP+}, µM	Percent utilization		References
			TEB	Ph	T			2d G6P	dNADP	
B	Worldwide	100	100	100	100	$50-70$	$2.9-4.4$	<4	55–60	Betke et al. (1967)
B2[c]	Nigerians	?	100	—	—	80 ± 5[d]	$21, 12$[d]	4–8	71 ± 5	Modiano et al. (1979)
A	Black ancestry	90	110	115	110	57 ± 5[d]; $50-70$[d]	12[d]; $2.9-4.4$	<4	50–60	Betke et al. (1967)
A2[e]	Nigerians	?	110	—	—	47[d]; 70 ± 5[d]	12[d]; $45, 13$[d]	5	53	Modiano et al. (1979)
Takoma-like[f]	Niokolonko, Bedik	100	91	81	93	62	$9-11$	<6	70	Vergnes et al. (1975)
Gambia[f]	Mandinka	78	—	85	—	58	5.3	3.9	69	Welch et al. (1978a,b)
Bali[g]	Balinese	100	105	125	—	$56.6-64.8$	16.6	1.5–2.7	44.9–50.4	Breguet et al. (1982), Chokkalingam et al. (1982a)
Kiwa[h]	Japanese	64	103	105	102	42	6.1	5.7	68	Miwa, (1980), Nakatsuji and Miwa (1979)
Chao Phya	Japanese	130	109	—	—	70	5.6	0	54.2	Miwa (1980), Nakatsuji and Miwa (1979)
S-Sakorn	Thai	68	107	—	—	236	5.0	1.6	40.8	Panich (1980)
Ayutthay[i]	Thai	66.74	95	—	—	28	$2.5-2.6$	12.1–12.5	114–122	Panich (1980)
Karthoum	Sudanese, Saudi Arabian	123	"Slow"	—	—	—	—	—	—	Saha et al. (1983b), Bayoumi et al. (1979)

Variant	Population									Reference
Ibadan	Aka Pygmies, Saharians, Egypt	90	92	93	85	48	12.7	4	73	Vergnes et al. (1979a,b), McCurdy et al. (1979)
Madrona	Saharians, Mali, Senegal, Egypt	100	—	80	—	39	5	<6	50	Vergnes et al. (1979b), McCurdy et al. (1979), Kahn et al. (1973)
Martinique	Martinique	89	—	100	—	54	6	<6	—	Kahn et al. (1973)
Lourenzo Marques	Ronga, Thonga, Chopi	100	106	106	—	66	4.3	<4	55	Reys et al. (1970)
Inhambane[j]	Thonga	100	112	112	—	38	4.7	<4	50	Reys et al. (1970)
Manjacaze	Chopi	100	90	90	—	141	3.8	<4	52	Reys et al. (1970)

[a] These variants correspond to class IV (see Table VIII), and characterization has been almost uniformly according to the WHO (Betke et al., 1967). The customary thermostability ahd pH optimum columns have been omitted because these parameters were normal unless otherwise indicated. The following variants have been found at polymorphic frequencies but have not been characterized: G6PD Baltimore (see next footnote for the explanation of the underlining) in Mauretania (Kahn et al., 1973); a G6PD C in the Sara Majingay of Chad (Hiernaux, 1976); an unnamed variant in Mofau in Cameroon (Bernstein et al., 1980a); possibly two variants, one with electrophoretic mobility of G6PD A and one slower than B, in the Aymara Indians of Bolivia and Northern Chile (Ferrell et al., 1978, 1980); one unnamed variant in Kurds and several in Surinam (Mourant et al., 1976). The Karthoum variant is listed because both activity and electrophoretic mobility have been quantitated.

[b] Names underlined indicate variant known to have frequency ≥1% in at least one population.

[c] Elution peak from DEAE-Sephadex column (Luzzatto and Allan, 1965; D'Urso et al., 1980) was 252 mM KCl, compared with 230 for normal G6PD B.

[d] Determined according to Afolayan and Luzzatto (1971).

[e] Elution peak (see footnote c) at 242 mM KCl, compared with 220 for G6PD A.

[f] In view of the rather slight difference in the properties of these two variants, one wonders whether side-by-side comparison might not ultimately reveal that they are the same.

[g] Slightly reduced thermostability.

[h] K_i^{NADPH} = 8.6 μM compared with 40 for normal G6PD B.

[i] Biphasic pH dependence.

[j] Thermostability markedly reduced.

Table XVI. Biochemical Characteristics of Polymorphic G6PD(−) Variants in the Mediterranean Populations[a]

Name	Population	Activity in RBC, percent of normal	Electrophoretic mobility, percent of normal			$K_m^{G6P}, \mu M$	$K_m^{NADP}, \mu M$	Percent utilization			Thermostability[b]	pH optimum[c]	Reference
			TEB	Ph	T			2dG6P	Gal6P	dNADP			
Mediterranean[d]	Various	<10	98–99	—	—	11 ± 1	2.1 ± 0.3	50 ± 6	42 ± 5	313 ± 27	VL	6.5, 9.5	Stamatoyanno-poulos et al. (1971)
Athens-like[e]	Various	1–10	98–99	—	—	17 ± 2	3.3 ± 0.3	15 ± 4	22 ± 3	153 ± 12	—	—	
Orchomenos	Greek	<7	92–94	—	—	10 ± 1	2.1 ± 0.2	105 ± 9	58 ± 5	350 ± 34	—	6.0, 9.5	
Union-Markham	Greek, Spanish	<4	102–104	—	—	7 ± 1	1.7 ± 0.3	200 ± 25	113 ± 2	397 ± 23	—	6.0, 9.5	
Corinth	Greek, Rumanian, Bulgarian	<7	100	—	100	19 ± 6	1.2–1.6	20–32	—	55–60	—	—	Shatskaya et al. (1980[f]), McCurdy et al. (1972)
Seattle-like	Greek, Sardinian	8–21	80	—	90	15–25	2.4–2.8	7–11	—	—	N	Biphasic	Rattazzi et al. (1969), Lenzerini et al. (1969)
Cagliari[e]	Sardinian	6–11	100	—	—	19 ± 1	—	11 ± 1	16 ± 2	154 ± 28	—	—	Fenu et al. (1982)
Sassari[f]	Sardinian	6–10	100	—	—	(23–25)	—	12–20	24	152	—	—	Testa et al. (1980)
Betica	Southern Spanish	2–13	112	111	—	59 ± 9	7.8 ± 1.6	3 ± 1	—	50 ± 9	N	Normal	Vives Corrons and Pujades (1982)
Menorca[g]	Spanish (Jewish origin)	2	94	92	—	15	1.9	26	—	261	VL	6.5, 9.5	
Kabyle[h]	Berber (Algeria)	5–25	—	104	104	32–75	—	5	5	48–75	N	Normal	Benabadji et al. (1978)
Laghouat	North-Saharian (Algeria)	7–18	—	107	107	35–60	—	7–24	12–17	30–60	N	Normal	Benabadji et al. (1978)
Blida	Arabo-Berber (Algeria)	7	—	100	100	15	—	25	16	45	L	7	Benabadji et al. (1978)

Site	Population												Reference
Thenia	Berber (Algeria)	25	—	90	90	60	—	2	3	18	N	Biphasic	Benabadji et al. (1978)
Titteri	Arab (Algeria)	10	—	92	92	34	—	7	7	50	N	6.5–9.0	Benabadji et al. (1978)
Alger	Arab (Algeria)	0	—	92	85	45	—	12	5	40	VL	Biphasic	Benabadji et al. (1978)
Debrousse	Egyptian (Siwa and Cairo), Algeria	15	—	110	110	48 ± 4	—	6 ± 4	—	64 ± 3	L	8.5–9.5	McCurdy et al. (1974)
Ramat-Gan[i]	Egyptian	3	—	80–90	80–90	21 ± 10	—	23 ± 9	—	161 ± 66	L	6.5, 9.0	McCurdy et al. (1974)
Kabyle[h]	Egyptian (Nile Delta and El-Fayoum)	9	—	100	—	61	—	3	—	39	L	8.5–9.0	McCurdy et al. (1974)
Tel-Hashomer	Egyptian	6	—	50–60	50–70	65 ± 12	—	4 ± 0.5	—	58 ± 12	L	8.5–9.0	McCurdy et al. (1974)
Columbus	Egyptian (Bani Suef)	9	—	100	100	96	—	4	—	89	N	8.5–9.0	McCurdy et al. (1974)
Chicago	Egyptian (Cairo)	7	—	100	100	90	—	4	—	63	VL	8.5	McCurdy et al. (1974)
West Bengal	Egyptian, Bulgarian	4	—	80–90	80–90	55	—	4	—	61	N	—	McCurdy et al. (1974)
Ohio	Egyptian (Siwa)	19	—	110	110	53	—	9	—	68	L	7, 9	McCurdy et al. (1974)
Tahta	Egyptian (Tahta)	15	—	103	103	39	—	6	—	78	L	7, 8.5	McCurdy et al. (1974)
Siwa	Egyptian (Siwa)	7	—	98–100	98–100	17	—	26	—	201	L	5.5, 9.0	McCurdy et al. (1974)
El-Kharga	Egyptian (El-Kharga)	11	—	100	100	61 ± 4	—	6	—	51	L	8.5–9.0	McCurdy et al. (1974)
El-Fayoum	Egyptian (El-Fayoum), Bulgarian	5	—	100	100	41 ± 1	—	26	—	229	L	7, 9	McCurdy et al. (1974)
Ohut II	Bulgarian	5–22	90–95	—	—	53	—	9	6	75	L	Normal	Shatskaya et al. (1980)[o]

Table XVI. (Continued)

Name	Population	Activity in RBC, percent of normal	Electrophoretic mobility, percent of normal			$K_m^{G6P}, \mu M$	$K_m^{NADP}, \mu M$	Percent utilization			Thermostability[b]	pH optimum[c]	Reference
			TEB	Ph	T			2dG6P	Gal6P	dNADP			
Mediterranean[d]	Various	<10	98–99	—	—	11 ± 1	2.1 ± 0.3	50 ± 6	42 ± 5	313 ± 27	VL	6.5, 9.5	Stamatoyanno-poulos et al. (1971) (1980[a])
Poznan	Bulgarian	3	90	—	—	26	—	45		245	L	Biphasic	Shatskaya et al. (1980[a])
Panay	Bulgarian	7	90	—	—	24	—	11	10	137	L	Biphasic	Shatskaya et al. (1980[a])
Petrich	Bulgarian	5	100	—	—	17	—	6	8	75	L	Biphasic	Shatskaya et al. (1980[a])
Gotze-Delchev	Bulgarian	2	100	—	—	16	—	14	20	96	L	Biphasic	Shatskaya et al. (1980[a])

[a] These variants belong to classes II and III and have been almost uniformly characterized according to the recommendations of the WHO (Betke et al., 1967).

[b] N, Normal; L, lower than normal; VL, very low; H, higher than normal.

[c] Whenever pH optima stated, these have been shown.

[d] Elution peak from DEAE-Sephadex column (Luzzatto and Allen, 1965; D'Urso et al., 1980) was 232.

[e] Elution peak (see footnote d) at 214. In view of the very similar properties of these two variants, side-by-side comparison could reveal that they are the same.

[f] Elution peak (see footnote d) at 251.

[g] $K_i^{NADPH} = 118 \mu M$.

[h] These two variants are said by Benabadji et al. (1978) to be different, although, unfortunately, the same name has been used.

[i] This variant is different from G6PD Ramat-Gan reported in a patient with CNSDH by

suggested the existence of several thermostability variants within all three groups of G6PD, B, A, and A(−). In some families inheritance of thermostability behavior was shown.

Another approach is to test for (even modest) quantitative variation as a probe for the existence of structural variants. This was validated by the knowledge that polymorphic electrophoretic variants have modal values of activity different from G6PD B: for instance, 20% lower for G6PD A (Nance, 1967, 1977; Battistuzzi *et al.*, 1977*a,b*) and approximately 23% higher for G6PD Karthoum (Samuel *et al.*, 1981). On these grounds it can be estimated that about 10–40% of the enzyme activity variation has a genetic basis, as indeed has been discussed in detail for several other enzyme systems by Modiano (1976). That different structural alleles might underlie quantitative variation was further suggested in the case of G6PD by the finding that the mean enzyme activity of the same electrophoretic type in Caucasoids, Amerindians, and Blacks, compared side by side, were different (Tashian *et al.*, 1967; Saldanha *et al.*, 1976). Moreover, Davidson *et al.* (1964) had already shown that intrasibship variance of G6PD activity among Gd^+ sons of Gd^+/Gd^- mothers, who have necessarily received the same Gd^+ allele, was less than the variance in a random sample of Gd^+ males. These results were confirmed in a larger study carried out in 213 sons of 84 Nigerian mothers with known Gd genotype (Modiano *et al.*, 1979). More important, full biochemical characterization of selected samples indeed proved the existence of two G6PD B variants, B1 and B2, and two G6PD A variants, A1 and A2 (see Table XV). One wonders whether this structural nonelectrophoretic polymorphism is related to the other known polymorphism in Nigeria, since a similar study carried out in a population nonpolymorphic for G6PD has failed thus far to yield similar results in Rome, Italy (G. Modiano *et al.*, unpublished).

Polymorphic Deficient Variants

Mediterranean Populations

In the early 1960s several studies converged to give the impression that G6PD deficiency in Mediterranean and related populations was associated with a variant having very low activity and B-like electrophoretic mobility, as opposed to the variant characteristic of Black popula-

Table XVII. Biochemical Characteristics of Polymorphic G6PD($\rightleftharpoons$) Variants in the Southeast Asia–Pacific Region[a]

Name	Population	Activity in RBC, percent of normal	Electrophoretic mobility, percent of normal TEB	pH	T	K_m^{G6P}, μM	K_m^{NADP}, μM	Percent utilization 2dG6P	Gal6P	dNADP	Heat stability[b]	pH optimum[c]	Reference
Mahidol	Southeast Asian	11	—	100	100	41	3.7	2.7	2.6	62.6	N	Normal	Panich and Na-Nakorn (1980[a])
Taiwan-Hakka	Chinese	<9	—	110	105	11	—	15	—	—	N	7, 9.5	McCurdy et al. (1970)
Canton	Southeast Asian	8	106–108	—	—	29	4.3	13.5	10.3	144.8	N	6.5–7, 9.5	Chan and Todd (1972)
Dhon	Chinese, Thai	10	105	—	—	39	3.2	3.2	2.9	75.5	N	Normal	Panich and Na-Nakorn (1980[a])
Haad Yai	Chinese	9	106	—	—	73	—	18	18	82	L	Normal	Panich et al. (1980[a])
Hong Kong	Chinese, Thai	7	92	—	—	42	3.8	6.6	6.0	78.3	N	Normal	Panich et al. (1980[a])
Tenganan	Balinese	13	99	75	64	11	6.9	18.3	—	109	L	Normal	Chockkalingam et al. (1982[a])
Übe	Japanese	39	107–108	112–115	107–109	53	5.6	2.8	—	55	N	Normal	Nakatsuji and Miwa (1979), Miwa (1980)
Konan[d]	Japanese	60	105–109	109–114	105–109	41	5.6	4.3	—	61	N	Normal	Nakatsuji and Miwa (1979), Miwa (1980)
Kamiube[e]	Japanese	46	100	100	100	37	3.9	3.5	—	53	N	Normal	Nakatsuji and Miwa (1979), Miwa (1980)
Long Xuyen	South Vietnamese	3	106	—	—	12	—	109	80	389	L	5.5, 10	Panich et al. (1980[b])
Union	Southeast Asian	2	103–106	—	—	13	1.2	134.9	101.7	469.0	VL	5.5–6.5, 9.5–10	Panich and Na-Nakorn (1980[a])
N-Pathom	Lao, Thai	18	110	—	—	59	3.4	1.3	1.2	57	N	Normal	Panich and Na-Nakorn (1980[a])
Songkhla	Thai	2	100	—	—	14	—	48.8	26.3	297.8	L	7, 9.5–10	Panich and Na-Nakorn (1980[a])
Siriraj	Thai	11	100	—	—	21	—	9.1	7.0	137	L	7, 9.5	Panich and Na-Nakorn (1980[a])
Chainat	Thai	1	98	—	—	68	5.0	1.2	1.9	72	H	Normal	Panich and Na-Nakorn (1980[a])
Kan	Thai	10	102	—	—	—	—	36	41	149	VL	—	Panich and Na-Nakorn (1980[a])
Anant	Thai	18	100	—	—	42	—	19	18	97	N	Normal	Panich and Na-Nakorn (1980[a])
Padrew	Thai	2	109	—	—	27	5.3	19	—	132	L	6, 10	Panich and Na-Nakorn (1980[a])
N-Sawan	Thai	4	110	—	—	9	1.5	0	1.6	141	VL	7, 9.5	Panich and Na-Nakorn (1980[a])
Goodenough	Papua New Guinea	<2	101	100	—	8	7.0	68.5	—	365.0	L	Biphasic	Chockkalingam and Board (1980)
Markham	Papau New Guinea	<10	103–104	106	—	11	2.2	152	—	376	L	Biphasic	Chockkalingam et al. (1982[b])
Kalnan	Papau New Guinea	<10	98	97	—	161	11.4	4.4	—	20.0	L	Normal	Chockkalingam et al. (1982[b])

Variant	Origin											pH optima	Reference
Bogia	Papua New Guinea	<10	96	95	—	56	7.0	8.6	—	63.3	N	Normal	Chockkalingam et al. (1982)[b]
Bukitu	Papua New Guinea	<10	103	100	—	75	11.0	12.0	—	64.6	L	Normal	Chockkalingam et al. (1982)[b]
Wewak	Papua New Guinea	<2	97	95	91	35	1.0	23.9	—	83.5	L	Normal	Chockkalingam et al. (1982)[b]
Amboin	Papua New Guinea	5	103	—	104	30	10.6	9.9	—	73.7	L	Normal	Chockkalingam et al. (1982)[b]
Angoram	Papua New Guinea	8	96	—	87	15	3.2	9.7	—	71.6	N	Normal	Chockkalingam et al. (1982)[b]
Yangoru	Papua New Guinea	11	94	90	96	20	5.9	15.2	—	73.1	L	5.5, 7, 9	Chockkalingam et al. (1982)[b]
Castilla-like	Papua New Guinea	9	105	105	—	31	4.7	10.6	—	87.9	L	Normal	Chockkalingam et al. (1982)[b]
Swit	Papua, New Guinea	<2	101	98	86	6	0.8	106.0	—	344.0	L	Biphasic	Chockkalingam et al. (1982)[b]
Madang	Papua New Guinea	<2	95	96	95	45	3.9	52.8	—	62.3	L	Normal	Chockkalingam et al. (1982)[b]
Kar Kar	Papua New Guinea	<2	94	92	87	24	1.0	19.0	—	83.0	N	Normal	Chockkalingam et al. (1982)[b]
Manus	Papua New Guinea	4	97	95	96	17	1.3	12.1	—	79.0	L	Biphasic	Chockkalingam et al. (1982)[b]
Palaukau	Papua New Guinea	4	100	95	88	51	8.0	18.9	—	46.7	L	Normal	Chockkalingam et al. (1982)[b]
Mainoki	Papua New Guinea	<2	96	93	89	26	3.5	4.3	—	85.3	L	Normal	Chockkalingam et al. (1982)[b]
Popondetta	Papua New Guinea	<2	95	87	67	5	1.0	66.7	—	295.3	L	Biphasic	Chockkalingam et al. (1982)[b]

[a] See Table XV, footnote b, for the significance of the underlining. The variants in the present table belong to classes II and III, and their characterization has been according to the WHO (Betke et al., 1967). Variants Mediterranean-like, Corinth-like, Union-like, and Manum found in Markham Valley, Papua New Guinea, by Yoshida et al. (1973) have not been included because they were incompletely characterized.

[b] N, Normal; L, lower than normal; VL, very low; H, higher than normal.

[c] Whenever pH optima have been stated, these are shown.

[d] $K_i^{NADPH} = 9.7$.

[e] $K_i^{NADPH} = 7.9$.

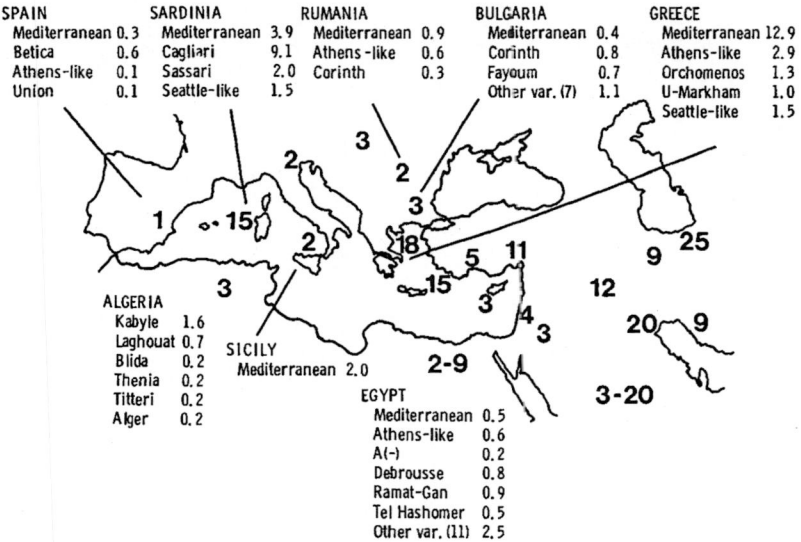

SPAIN		SARDINIA		RUMANIA		BULGARIA		GREECE	
Mediterranean	0.3	Mediterranean	3.9	Mediterranean	0.9	Mediterranean	0.4	Mediterranean	12.9
Betica	0.6	Cagliari	9.1	Athens-like	0.6	Corinth	0.8	Athens-like	2.9
Athens-like	0.1	Sassari	2.0	Corinth	0.3	Fayoum	0.7	Orchomenos	1.3
Union	0.1	Seattle-like	1.5			Other var. (7)	1.1	U-Markham	1.0
								Seattle-like	1.5

ALGERIA	
Kabyle	1.6
Laghouat	0.7
Blida	0.2
Thenia	0.2
Titteri	0.2
Alger	0.2

SICILY	
Mediterranean	2.0

EGYPT	
Mediterranean	0.5
Athens-like	0.6
A(-)	0.2
Debrousse	0.8
Ramat-Gan	0.9
Tel Hashomer	0.5
Other var. (11)	2.5

Fig. 8. Map of G6PD polymorphism in the Mediterranean and Middle East. Bold figures indicate overall frequencies (%) of male G6PD deficiency in the respective locations. When sufficient data were available, individual variants with respective gene frequencies are given. Data are from the references listed in Table XVI and from Grech and Vicatou (1973), Tzoneva et al. (1975), Mourant et al. (1976), Schilirò et al. (1979), Aksoy et al. (1980), and Corbo et al. (1981).

tions, which was less severely deficient and electrophoretically fast (A-like). The distribution of this phenotype is shown in Fig. 8. The highest frequency is found in Greece (mainland and islands). The frequency declines westward (Italy and Spain, with the exception of Sardinia), northward (Bulgaria and Rumania), eastward (Turkey, Lebanon), and on the southern shores, in Egypt and Algeria. Thus, at first sight this distribution could fit a simple diffusion model.

However, over the years more detailed work in various countries has identified numerous new variants and concomitantly eroded the uniformity of G6PD "Mediterranean" in this part of the world. Kirkman et al. (1965) had observed a considerable and coordinate variation of kinetic properties of the enzyme samples purified from G6PD-deficient Greek children: "At one end, moderate hemolysate activity, normal relative 2dG6P utilization, slightly low Km values and nearly normal pH optimum curve; at the other end, very low hemolysate activity, high relative 2dG6P utilization, very low Km values and a highly bimodal pH optimum curve" were seen (Kirkman *et al.*, 1965). Subsequently, Stamatoy-annopoulos *et al.* (1971) identified in the Greek populations of Karditza and Orchomenos four G6PD-deficient polymorphic variants: G6PD Mediterranean (the name was retained for the most frequent of the four), Athens-like, Orchomenos, and Union-Markham (Fig. 8).

Differences among the four variants were quite subtle with respect to degree of deficiency and substrate affinities, but quite marked with respect to substrate analogue utilization and pH dependence of the activity. Moreover, two of them differed from B in electrophoretic mobility (Table XVI). A variant characterized by less severe deficiency and altered electrophoretic mobility, G6PD Seattle-like, had already been reported to occur at a polymorphic frequency (1.5%) in the Greek districts of Kephalonia and Athens (Rattazzi *et al.*, 1969).

A heterogeneity perhaps even greater has been discovered in other Mediterranean populations. Three G6PD(−) variants were found in Rumania (McCurdy *et al.*, 1972); as many as 15 in Egypt (McCurdy *et al.*, 1974); six in Algeria (Benabadji *et al.*, 1978); at least four have polymorphic frequencies in Sardinia (Lenzerini *et al.*, 1969; Testa *et al.*, 1980; Fiorelli *et al.*, 1982; Fenu *et al.*, 1982); ten in Bulgaria (Shatskaya *et al.*, 1980a); and five in Spain (Vives Corrons and Pujades, 1982). Evidence for heterogeneity was also suggested in Israelis (Ramot *et al.*, 1964; Testa *et al.*, 1980).

This considerable "fragmentation" of the Mediterranean variant is clearly incompatible with diffusion *alone* explaining the complex pattern of G6PD deficiency now seen (Fig. 8). There are clearly two groups of variants. On the one hand, four variants, Mediterranean, Athens-like, Seattle, and Union, have frequencies compatible with their having radiated from Greece, perhaps concomitantly with the rise and spreading east and west of Greek civilization. On the other hand, various peoples seem to have evolved one or more autochthonous G6PD(−) variants of their own.

The relative contributions of these two components to the overall frequency of the G6PD(−) phenotype vary in different places. The second component is especially prominent in North Africa. In Egypt, for instance, the indigenous variants account for about 80% of the total, and in Algeria G6PD Mediterranean is absent altogether. Perhaps because of the more endogamic habits of North African populations the observed heterogeneity from deme to deme is much greater than that observed in southern European populations. At the other extreme, a large majority of

G6PD deficiency in Rumania is accounted for by the two (presumably immigrated) variants Mediterranean and Athens-like.

Finally, some special aspects of geographic distribution are undoubtedly the result of very recent migration phenomena. For instance, the cases of G6PD deficiency described in France by Gherardi *et al.* (1976) were in people from North Africa and southern Italy. In the major industrial cities of northern Italy G6PD deficiency, which was probably nonexistent, has recently reached the value of approximately 1%, obviously as a result of recent immigration from the South and from Sardinia. These changes obviously have important public health implications.

The Middle East and Indian Populations

G6PD deficiency is very high in the Middle East (Fig. 8). Indeed, in some ethnic groups, like the Shi'a of Al Hasa and Al Qatif in Saudi Arabia and in Kurdish Jews, the frequency of G6PD($-$) is the highest in the world (up to 60% of males). However, qualitative data are very scanty. Daneshbod (1975) has tested in Tehran, Iran, 370 patients of both sexes, of which 158 (42.7%) were reported to have "varying degrees of deficiency" (0–82.5% of normal). Of 26 samples further characterized from male subjects, 18 showed B electrophoretic mobility, four had a fast variant (105–110%), and four a slow variant (85–93%). Each of these three groups of subjects had approximately the same average activity (20–25% of normal) and an extremely wide range of variation (0–60%), suggesting further heterogeneity within each group. Banerjee *et al.* (1981) in Jordanians and Gelpi and King (1977) in Saudi Arabia have observed by electrophoresis samples with no visible G6PD band [designated by them "G6PD($-$)"] and samples with a deficient band in the B position [designated by them "G6PD B($-$)"]. Clearly the former group might be G6PD Mediterranean, whereas the latter cannot. Recently, several new variants have been described from Azerbaijan (Shatskaya *et al.,* 1980*b*); some of these have been subsequently observed also in Bulgaria (Shatskaya *et al.,* 1980*a*).

Further characterization of G6PD variants in the Middle East would be highly desirable. Indeed, this area combines the unique geographic and historical features of being at the crossroads of three continents with that of having the world's highest overall prevalence of G6PD deficiency. Therefore, it would be especially important to establish the presence or otherwise of any of the variants that are common in the Mediterranean, in Asia, or in Africa. If any of them were found at relatively high frequency, this could shed some light on the difficult problem of the origin and spread of G6PD deficiency.

In the Indian subcontinent there are again numerous scattered prevalence data, but ony very few variants have been identified: G6PD Campbellpore in Pakistan (McCurdy and Mahmood, 1970), and G6PD Kerala and West Bengal in these regions of India, respectively (Azevedo et al., 1968). In the latter paper the occurrence of G6PD Mediterranean in these regions and in Punjab, Pakistan, was also reported (however, it should be noted that at the time the heterogeneity of G6PD "Mediterranean" had not yet been fully appreciated).

Southeast Asia and the Pacific

The description of G6PD Canton in five Chinese male subjects living in North America by McCurdy et al. (1966), followed by the discovery of the same variant in a Thai and in four Chinese males from Hong Kong (McCurdy et al., 1970), led to the widespread assumption that G6PD deficiency in Orientals was mostly due to this variant (Beutler, 1971). Extensive screening and characterization performed in this area by numerous authors in recent years has shown instead an impressive multiplicity of genetic variants associated with G6PD deficiency in Orientals. The degree of genetic heterogeneity within each population and in the whole of Southeast Asia and the Pacific (Fig. 9 and Table XVII) is similar to or even greater than that found in Mediterranean populations.

G6PD Mahidol has the highest prevalence in Cambodians ($\sim$14%), where all G6PD($-$) subjects tested had this variant (Everett et al., 1977). It is still the most frequent variant, though at a lower rate, in Laotians (5%), Thais (7.3%), and possibly South Vietnamese (0.65%) (Panich et al., 1980a; Panich, 1973; Panich and Sungnate, 1973; Panich and Na-Nakorn, 1980a; Sicard et al., 1978; Panich, 1974). Chan et al. (1972) and Chan and Todd (1972) described a G6PD B($-$) Chinese in southern China that has very similar properties to G6PD Mahidol and indeed could be the same variant. G6PD Mahidol is also found in Thai Muslims of southern Thailand, which share a common ethnic origin with the people of the northern part of Malaysia, and in the Mon population, which is considered one of the most ancient ethnic groups of the area. Because

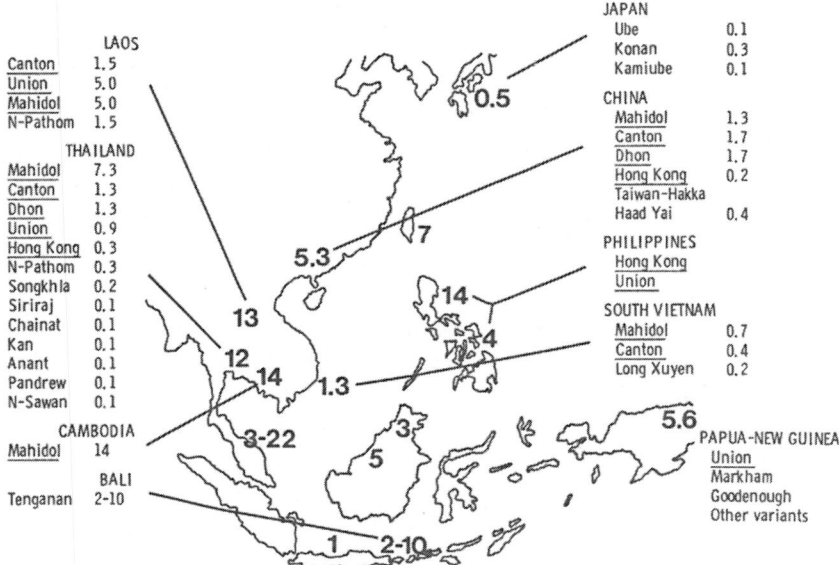

Fig. 9. Map of G6PD polymorphism in the Southeast Asia and Pacific region. Explanations as in Fig. 8. Data are from the references listed in Table XVII and from Lie-Injo (1969), Mourant *et al.* (1976), Baer *et al.* (1976), and Sicard *et al.* (1978).

Thai Muslims for many generations have intermarried more with Malay Muslims than with the predominantly Buddhist people of the rest of Thailand (Panich and Na-Nakorn, 1980*a*), it is possible that it has spread to Malaysia, and it has also been proposed that G6PD Mahidol and G6PD Indonesia described by Kirkman and Lie-Injo (1969) are the same variant. If this is true, then G6PD Mahidol would be definitely the most common variant in South East Asia.

By contrast, G6PD Canton is probably the most common variant in southern China (McCurdy *et al.*, 1966, 1970; Chan and Todd, 1972; Panich *et al.*, 1980*a*), together with G6PD Dhon (Panich *et al.*, 1980), which very likely is identical to the previously described Taipei-Hakka variant (McCurdy *et al.*, 1970; Chan and Todd, 1972). G6PD Hong Kong also has its highest frequency in China (Chan and Todd, 1972), and it is probably the same as the variant described by McCurdy *et al.* (1970) as similar to G6PD Panay, which had previously been characterized in the Philippines (Fernandez and Fairbanks, 1968). All these variants are found also in the neighboring populations of Indochina, but at a much lower frequency. G6PD Union was originally found in the Philippines (Yoshida *et al.* 1970), but its highest frequency may be in Laos (Panich, 1974). It is found also in Thailand (Panich, 1973) and in Papua New Guinea (Yoshida *et al.*, 1973). Estimates of its distribution and origin are not possible due to the lack of relevant information.

Papua New Guinea offers a striking example of a very high degree of genetic heterogeneity for G6PD within a very short range of distance. G6PD deficiency is totally absent in the eastern and western highlands, whereas it is common in coastal districts (McLoughlin *et al.*, 1982; Mourant *et al.*, 1981; Mourant *et al.*, 1982; Booth *et al.*, 1982). Here the degree of genetic heterogeneity is such that very few variants reach a level of 1% in the general population (see Fig. 10). However, within one or very few isolates each variant is in fact polymorphic (Booth *et al.*, 1982; Chockkalingam and Board, 1980; Chockkalingam *et al.*, 1982*a,b*).

Although any model in population genetics must be proposed as merely speculative, the overall pattern of G6PD deficiency in the Asian–Pacific area is quite distinctive. Whereas in the Mediterranean we saw that a set of variants seem to have radiated from a single center and local variants have remained local, here several variants seem to have spread

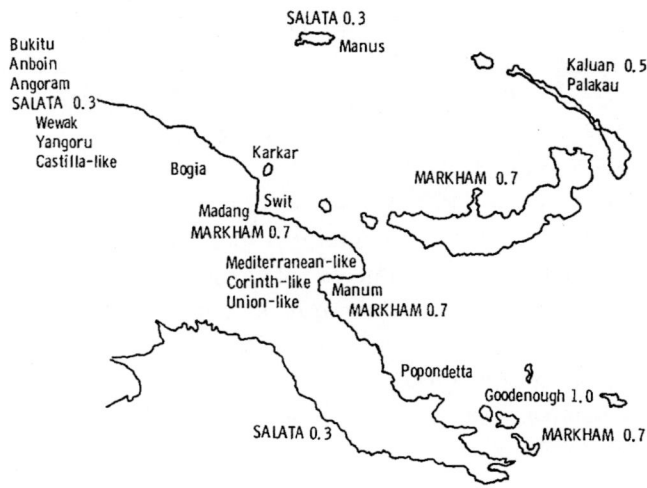

Fig. 10. Map of G6PD polymorphism in Papua New Guinea. Individual variants are shown in the approximate locations where they were found. Variants in all-capital letters are the more widely spread. Figures give approximate gene frequencies (%), calculated for the entire population shown on the map (i.e., local gene frequencies are often much higher). Where no figure is shown, it can be extimated that the overall gene frequency is of the order of 0.1%. For references see text.

from as many centers. This intermingling of frequency clines of various G6PD(−) variants, which is the main characteristic of G6PD deficiency in this part of the world, is evidence of active bidirectional gene flow between populations, and it deserves a deeper analysis at the microgeographic level in order to identify the migrational paths. However, here, too, almost all populations so far examined present one or more autochthonous variants (see Fig. 10 and Table XVII). In some cases, as in the Tenganam isolate of Bali (Breguet *et al.*, 1982; Chockkalingam *et al.*, 1982*a*) and in various parts of Papua New Guinea, these account for most of the prevalence of G6PD deficiency.

Africa South of the Sahara

G6PD deficiency in Africa is classically considered to be mostly of the A(−) type. Pertinent early data on 50 different population samples were compiled by Luzzatto (1973*a*). Indeed, *Gd* A⁻ is present in a large number of major ethnic groupings; for instance, Mandinka (Welch *et al.*, 1978*a,b*); Aka and Babinga Pygmies (Vergnes *et al.*, 1979*a,b*; Bernstein *et al.*, 1980*a,b*); Khoisan (Nurse *et al.*, 1977; Jenkins *et al.*, 1975, 1971); Yoruba (Luzzatto and Allan, 1968); Tutsi (le Gall *et al.*, 1982); Niokolonko and Bedik of Senegal (Vergnes *et al.*, 1975; Bouloux *et al.*, 1972); Bassa of Liberia (Willcox and Beckman, 1981); Gagu (Vergnes and Cabannes, 1976); Bantu (le Gall *et al.*, 1982; Bernstein *et al.*, 1980*a,b*; Hitzeroth and Bender, 1980; Nurse and Jenkins, 1975; Balinsky and Jenkins, 1967; Reys *et al.*, 1970); and the Creoles living in the Seychelle Islands (Welch *et al.*, 1975). By looking at this wealth of data as a whole in comparison with what is found in other parts of the world, one finds that G6PD A(−) emerges as unique in its continent-wide distribution. Quantitatively, its frequency varies considerably, more as a function of geography than of ethnic group.

Genetic heterogeneity of the G6PD(−) phenotype in Africa has been systematically explored in very few cases. Whereas in western Nigeria no polymorphic variant other than A(−) was found among over 5000 blood samples (Luzzatto, 1975), in the Shangana Bantu of Mozambique one "private" variant was found, with a low frequency of about 0.1% (Reys *et al.*, 1970). Kahn *et al.* (1973) have reported the occurrence of G6PD Mali in 12.5% and 4.5% of the Mali and Senegal populations, respectively, and of G6PD Dakar and G6PD Matam in 3% and 2%, respectively, of the population of Senegal. Since G6PD Mali is severely deficient (activity of 1–5% of normal) and its electrophoretic mobility is normal, it could well account for the G6PD(−) phenotype subsequently observed in Mali by Duflo *et al.* (1979). However, none of the variants described by Kahn *et al.* (1973) fits the B(−) phenotype observed in the Bedik of Senegal (Bouloux *et al.,* 1972).

These polymorphic G6PD(−) variants, other than A(−), are undoubtedly autochthonous to Africa. In addition, a number of electrophoretic studies have revealed the existence of "G6PD B(−)" and "undetectable activity" phenotypes in populations living immediately south of the Sahara: 3% in Sudan (Saha *et al.,* 1983*b*) in a population of "negroid" origin, 7% in the Sara Majingay of Chad (Hiernaux, 1976), 10% in Ghana (Owusu and Opare-Manta, 1972); 10% in Mali (Duflo *et al.,* 1979), and 1% in the Bedik of Senegal (Bouloux *et al.,* 1972). These data have been interpreted as indicating gene flow from Arabic people. However, in view of the present awareness about the enormous genetic heterogeneity underlying the G6PD(−) phenotype, and in the absence of biochemical analysis (of both these and the Arabic samples), any such inference based on electrophoretic data alone should be regarded as strictly hypothetical.

Finally, how much, if any, gene flow could have taken place across the Sahara in the opposite direction? The nondeficient variant G6PD A has been found at respectable frequencies in several North African populations: 5% in the Sinai peninsula and 2.4% in Aswan (Egypt) (Azim *et al.,* 1974; see also Bertin *et al.,* 1978); 3.5% in Tripoli, 4.9% in Benghazi, and 16.4% in Sabbah (Libya) (Kamel *et al.,* 1975); and 9–12% in two regions of Mali and Algeria (Lefèvre-Witier and Vergnes, 1977). On the other hand, G6PD A(−) has been found very rarely, if at all, in the same populations. These strikingly contrasting data raise a serious question as to whether G6PD A north and south of the Sahara are really one and the same thing.

Are Some G6PD Mutants Double Mutants?

The number of *Gd* mutants is larger than that known for any other single genetic locus in humans. Whether this is due merely to ease of ascertainment and selective pressure by malaria, or whether the *Gd* locus may also be a mutational hot spot (Luzzatto and Testa, 1978), has not been tested yet, and any discussion of this matter would have to be only speculative; we refrain from it here. A related question is whether the known mutations are totally independent of each other or whether they may be related at least in some cases; specifically, it has been proposed on grounds of circumstantial evidence that Gd^{A-} may be the result of a second mutation arising from Gd^A (Luzzatto, 1973*b*; Babalola *et al.*, 1976). Now that so many more variants have been identified and geographically mapped, a more general test of this notion can be carried out. Considering that in each broad area where G6PD deficiency is prevalent some mutant or mutants seem to dominate, we can ask whether enzymic properties of the other mutants found in the same area are randomly or nonrandomly distributed with respect to those of the predominant one(s). We have chosen the Michaelis constant for G6P (K_m^{G6P}) because this parameter has a number of desirable properties: (1) it is available for a large number of variants; (2) it is distributed over a wide range of values (from 2 to >100 μM); (3) the standard error of the measurement can be very low (Babalola *et al.*, 1976); and (4) K_m^{G6P} measures the affinity of G6PD for its substrate, and this can be expected and has been shown to be a physiologically important feature of the enzyme. The answer to our question is quite clearcut (see Fig. 11) in that the distributions of K_m^{G6P}

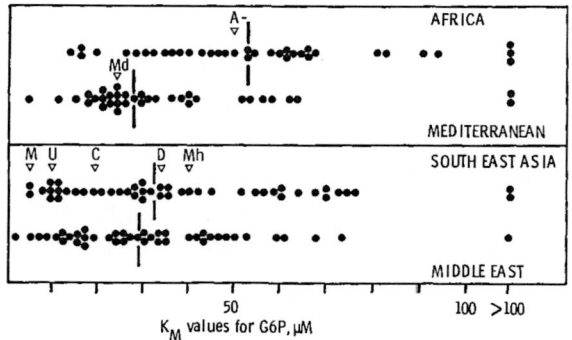

Fig. 11. G6PD variants within a geographic area are biochemically more closely related than would be expected by chance. The Km^{G6P} values, measuring substrate affinity, are shown in the form of scattergrams for all variants reported from each respective area. Vertical bars indicate the median value for each area. Letter symbols indicate the most common G6PD variants in the respective areas, as follows: G6PD A(−); Md, Mediterranean; M, Markham; U, Union; C, Canton; D, Dhon; Mh, Mahidol. The data are from references quoted in Table VIII. Close agreement between the median values and common variants is especially striking for A− and Md. The pattern observed is obviously nonrandom, and it remains so even if class I variants are left out.

values are different in different parts of the world. It is difficult to interpret this nonrandomness for Southeast Asia, because there are several widely distributed variants there, and in the Middle East, because we ignore the nature of the most common variants (Fig. 11, bottom). On the other hand, the data for the African continent and for the Mediterranean area are very informative (Fig. 11, top). In the first place, the two groups are distributed differently: there would be no reason for this to be so if these variants all arose by independent mutations from the wild-type gene Gd^B. Moreover, the median of the K_m^{G6P} values for all African variants is very close to that of the most common deficient variant, G6PD A($-$); and the median of the values for all variants in the Mediterranean is very close to that of the most common deficient variant, G6PD Mediterranean. We think it is not unreasonable to surmise that a significant fraction (by no means all) of these variants are derived not directly from Gd^B, but from Gd^{A-} and from $Gd^{Mediterranean}$, respectively. The underlying genetic event could either be a second mutation or intragenic recombination with a polymorphic site in the normal gene [which is known to exist in Africa (Modiano et al., 1979), and has been proposed to explain the nonrandom distribution of sporadic variants in Italy (Persico et al., 1982)]. In either case, the specific prediction of this model is that a number of these variants differ from G6PD B by at least two rather than one amino acid. Thus, the prediction is testable by sequencing of either the G6PD protein or the Gd DNA, which should be forthcoming.

EXPRESSION OF G6PD AND G6PD DEFICIENCY

G6PD Deficiency in Erythrocytes

The discovery of G6PD deficiency in red cells (Carson, 1956) has been a landmark in hematology because it provided at once a long-sought explanation for the previous clinical observations that primaquine or fava beans could trigger acute hemolytic anemia in some people and not in others. In addition, G6PD deficiency became a model system for exploring the way in which a genetically determined intracorpuscular factor and environmental extracorpuscular factors interact in causing hemolysis. Finally, G6PD deficiency became a prototype for what is now a whole group of red cell "enzymopathies," which account for a sizable fraction of congenital hemolytic anemias [reviewed by Beutler (1978) and Miwa (1981); see also Stanbury et al. (1983)].*

The molecular basis for enzyme deficiency in red blood cells might be, as in other systems, (1) decreased synthesis, (2) accelerated breakdown, (3) decreased catalytic activity, or any combination thereof. If we consider, among the many G6PD-deficient variants, the few that have been fully characterized from this point of view, we find that factor 2 is probably the commonest, factor 3 or a combination of 2 plus 3 occur, but 1 has not yet turned up. This is in striking contrast to the hemoglobin system, where decreased synthesis is found, by definition, in the many thalassemia syndromes. This topic has been fully discussed elsewhere (Luzzatto and Testa, 1978; Khan, 1978; De Flora, 1981).

Clinical Problems†

The clinical manifestations and pathophysiology of G6PD deficiency have been previously reviewed (Luzzatto, 1975; Luzzatto and Testa, 1978; Bienzle, 1981; Panich, 1981, 1982; Beutler, 1983), and will not be discussed here in detail, since we are concentrating on the genetic aspects. In contrast to other red cell enzymopathies, in which chronic hemolysis is the rule and acute exacerbations are often seen in concomitance with intercurrent conditions, in G6PD deficiency the reverse is true. In most subjects the clinical and hematological phenotype is practically normal, and acute hemolysis, which can be severe and even life-threatening, is only seen in response to an exogenous trigger (see Table XVIII).

In many cases the fact that a particular variant gives only episodic rather than chronic expression can be rationalized in terms of either the

---

* Among mammals, sheep and goats have very low red cell G6PD activity (<15%) compared to others (Cheun, 1966). However, they are not subject to oxidant-induced hemolysis (Beutler and West, 1978).

† It is still a common misconception that hemolytic anemia associated with G6PD deficiency is limited to people whose ancestry is from one of the areas where this abnormality is highly prevalent. This is of course true if any of the common variants is involved, and since these in turn are not associated with chronic hemolysis it applies to patients presenting, for instance, with drug-induced hemolysis. On the other hand, patients affected by CNSHD in most cases have a "private" variant, arisen by a unique mutation that has not and probably never will become polymorphic. The chance of this happening is simply a function of mutation rate, and therefore its a priori probability is uniform throughout the world. In a G6PD-deficient patient with CNSHD there is no reason to expect or suspect a Mediterranean or African ancestor.

Table XVIII. Clinical Manifestations of G6PD Deficiency

Common
  Acute hemolytic anemia
    Drug-induced
    Triggered by infection
    Favism
  Neonatal jaundice
Rare
  Chronic non spherocytic hemolytic anemia
  Proneness to infection associated with granulocyte dysfunction
  Interaction with sickle cell anemia

---

degree of deficiency or enzyme kinetics. Whenever this is not so, it seems reasonable to postulate that the *in vivo* rate of operation of the enzyme is affected, even if this is not reflected in the parameters that are routinely measured.

On the other hand, a persistently unsolved problem with clinical manifestations of the common forms of G6PD deficiency is their erratic character. This has been classically known with respect to favism [reviewed by Battistuzzi *et al.* (1982) and Arese (1982)], whereby only about 25% of G6PD-deficient individuals develop hemolysis upon eating the beans and no gross difference in bean consumption is apparent in G6PD-deficient children who have developed favism from those who have not (Hedayat *et al.,* 1981). Drug-induced and infection-induced hemolysis are more predictable, but not entirely so. Attempts to identify additional genetic factors other than G6PD deficiency required for a hemolytic attack have failed to yield significant results. At the moment, it would seem more likely that the decisive factors may be acquired, and that they appear erratic because they are variable and difficult to quantitate. For instance, an infection may cause hemolysis or not depending on the extent of on-going phagocytosis by neutrophils, which in turn will be a function of the level of leukocytosis and of the promptness of treatment. In areas where G6PD deficiency is prevalent, it may be the single most common cause of severe neonatal jaundice. For some time there has been an apparent discrepancy between data from Africa (Bienzle, 1981; Roux *et al.,* 1982) and Jamaica (Gibbs *et al.,* 1979) supporting this association, and lack of it in American Blacks, in spite of their having the same G6PD-deficient variant, A−; however, G6PD deficiency as a cause of neonatal hyperbilirubinemia is now recognized also in the United States

(Karayalcin *et al.,* 1979). As far as babies with G6PD Mediterranean are concerned, the suggestion has been made (Meloni *et al.,* 1973) that neonatal jaundice in many cases is nonhemolytic, and it might be related to the extent of expression of G6PD deficiency in hepatocytes and to the varying degree of liver "maturity" in newborns.

Thus, the study of the clinical expression of the common types of G6PD deficiency has not yet fully answered the questions of why and when this syndrome arises and how severe it is when it does occur. This topic ought to be singled out for further investigation by a specifically targeted approach, i.e., by a direct comparison of groups of G6PD-deficient individuals who have developed hemolysis or have not developed hemolysis upon comparable exposure to a particular triggering agent.

Membrane Abnormalities

The reason why some G6PD individuals are only susceptible to induced hemolysis and others have chronic nonspherocytic hemolytic disease (CNSHD) must reside primarily in the properties of each individual G6PD variant. Some of the most relevant properties have been previously identified (Kirkman, 1971; Luzzatto and Afolayan, 1971; Yoshida, 1973; Luzzatto and Testa, 1978) and some were discussed above. The sequence of events leading to induced hemolysis undoubtedly is related to the cell's inability to keep up with GSH consumption under oxidative stress. On the other hand, the sequence of events leading to chronic hemolysis has only begun to be elucidated. Afolayan (1979) first analyzed on SDS gels the membrane proteins of G6PD A(−) red cells (no CNSHD) and found them to be normal. This was confirmed by G. J. Johnson *et al.* (1979), who also found that red cells with four different G6PD(−) variants associated with CNSHD had instead unusual high-molecular weight-polypeptide aggregates: two distinct species were observed at 440 and at >50,000 kd. The former consists of spectrin and the latter contains spectrin as well as other proteins but not globins (therefore they are not related to Heinz bodies). Since both species of aggregates could be destroyed by mercaptoethanol, it was suggested that they arose *in vitro* through formation of intermolecular disulfide bridges, which would normally be prevented by GSH. These membrane protein changes may be responsible for altered physical properties of erythrocytes (reduced filterability) independently reported with other variants (Schro-

ter and Tillman, 1977) and for increased membrane fluidity observed in
G6PD($-$) cells with CNSHD (Jansson *et al.,* 1980) and to a lesser extent
in G6PD($-$) cells without CNSHD (Rice-Evans *et al.,* 1981).

Mechanism of Hemolysis

From the clinical point of view, the demarcation between patients
who have rare G6PD-deficient variants and chronic, mainly extravascu-
lar hemolysis (CNSHD), and those who have common variants and experience episodes of acute, mainly intravascular hemolysis, is quite sharp.*
The former run a prolonged course, with a varying degree of anemia,
which is usually fairly well tolerated, but can be disabling. The latter are,
in most cases, totally unaware of their genetic abnormality, but one of
their attacks, if not promptly treated, could be fatal. One would anticipate
that the biochemical mechanism of hemolysis must also be different, and
perhaps some confusion in the literature has sometimes arisen by insufficient appreciation of the difference between these two situations.

Although we lack formal proof that the membrane protein changes
previously mentioned are sufficient to account for the considerable shortening in red cell life span observed in patients with CNSHD, we would
regard this as a reasonable working hypothesis. By contrast, when trying
to investigate the mechanism of acute hemolysis we immediately encoun-
ter a practical difficulty: namely, that during the attack damaged cells are
destroyed, by definition, very rapidly; therefore, red cells drawn from the
patient before the attack may not yet exhibit the changes we are looking
for, and red cells drawn after the attack are those that have actually
escaped hemolysis, rather than those that have been irreparably damaged. The situation is further complicated by the rapid release into the
blood, in response to acute hemolysis, of reticulocytes with higher G6PD
activity. Attempts to circumvent these difficulties have been made by
obtaining blood samples very early during the attacks, for instance, less
than 72 hr from the ingestion of fava beans. At this time it was possible
to document a fall in NADPH and in GSH (Gaetani *et al.,* 1979), and

---

* G6PD Mediterranean and G6PD A($-$) red cells have slightly reduced *in vivo* survival [90–
100 days (Piomelli *et al.,* 1968)]. Thus, by definition, it is not strictly true that they are not
associated with CNSHD. This red-cell life span shortening is negligible from the hematological point of view, and therefore we have adhered to the current convention of regarding them as associated with induced hemolysis alone.

precipitates of denatured hemoglobin are characteristically seen in red cells by supravital staining, and sometimes, along with other marked morphological abnormalities, even in ordinary fixed stained films (Bezzi *et al.*, 1982). Considering these findings on red cells that are still circulating, one is led to surmise that in those that have been destroyed GSH reserves had been completely exhausted and massive Hb denaturation had taken place.

A different, complementary approach is to observe what changes occur *in vitro* upon exposure of red cells to potentially hemolytic agents. Numerous such experiments have been carried out, and the literature has been critically reviewed by Arese (1982). Classically, a major role in cell lysis was attributed to lipid peroxidation, but it now appears that this accompanies rather than causes hemolysis (see also Benatti *et al.*, 1981). An ideal test system would be one in which G6PD-deficient, but not G6PD-normal, red cells are lysed in the presence of a substance (or a metabolite or precursor thereof) that is known to cause hemolysis *in vivo*. Search for such a system has not been successful thus far, but it has been shown, for instance, that G6PD(−) red cells treated *in vitro* with the fava bean aglycone divicine lose normal deformability and become highly susceptible to mechanical lysis (Arese *et al.*, 1982). It is quite possible that this experiment mimics the *in vivo* situation, inasmuch as metabolic changes induced by divicine [such as rapid loss of GSH (Arese *et al.*, 1981)] may not be sufficient to cause hemolysis by themselves, but may cause sufficient membrane damage [formation of spectrin aggregates (Arese *et al.*, 1982)] for the cells to lyse as they are forced through capillaries.

In summary, acute hemolysis triggered by exogenous agents in G6PD deficiency not associated with CNSHD may involve a novel mechanism. However, it is also possible that the very same chronic changes that are likely to be responsible for hemolysis in CNSHD, by taking place on an abruptly massive scale, give rise to the dramatic acute hemolysis of patients with favism and related conditions.

Coexistence of Other Genetic Disorders

In principle, when two pathological conditions are encountered in the same person it means either that one causes the other or that the two coexist by chance. If both conditions are genetically determined and independently assorting, the latter must be the case. Because G6PD deficiency is common in populations in which thalassemia and hemoglobin S are also highly prevalent, these have been the most frequently encountered associations (see Table XIX). Much attention has been devoted particularly to the coexistence of homozygous sickle cell anemia with G6PD deficiency, because of an early suggestion that the latter could affect beneficially the course of the former (Lewis *et al.*, 1966). However, this has been amply disproven (Naylor *et al.*, 1960; Bienzle *et al.*, 1975; Praharaj and Choudhury, 1977; Ozsoylu and Altinoz, 1977; Gibbs *et al.*, 1980). In fact, the danger of acute hemolysis related to G6PD deficiency superimposed on the chronic hemolysis of sickle cell anemia is quite obvious, and severe hyperbilirubinemia has been observed in this context (Seeler, 1978; Ozsoylu, 1978). It has also been claimed that the frequency of G6PD deficiency is higher in AS heterozygotes than in the general population. Earlier references are given by Bernstein *et al.* (1980c), who suggest that HbS in heterozygotes might have a protective effect on the adverse manifestations of G6PD deficiency. However, according to their figures, this would imply a very high selective mortality (of the order of 50%) of G6PD-deficient males who do not have hemoglobin S, and this is not supported by the finding that in fact the frequency of G6PD deficiency is about the same in newborns and in adults (Bienzle *et al.*, 1976). At any rate, in the two largest series from Africa the coexistence of the two genetic abnormalities was no greater than expected by chance (Luzzatto and Allan, 1968; Nhonoli *et al.*, 1978).

G6PD and G6PD Deficiency in Nonerythroid Cells

Because of the common occurrence in the same species of multiple forms of enzymes with similar specificity (isozymes*), it is not easy in principle to be sure that an activity found in other cells or tissues can be attributed to the same enzyme that has been already fully characterized in erythrocytes. However, in the case of G6PD, genetic evidence offers the required proof, since, for instance, similar electrophoretic variation is observed between the B and A types in red cells and fibroblasts, and G6PD deficiency of red cells is also often expressed in other cells.

Although we have emphasized the housekeeping role of G6PD, this

---

* This term is often used inappropriately for allelic variants of human G6PD.

Table XIX. Interaction of G6PD Deficiency with Other Genetic Abnormalities[a]

Other condition	Frequency	Effect of other condition on G6PD deficiency	Effect of G6PD deficiency on other condition	Reference
Sickle cell anemia	Relatively common	Increased G6PD levels	None or slight	Bienzle et al. (1975), Gibbs et al. (1980)
Thalassemia	Relatively common	Increased G6PD levels	Slightly increased MCV; otherwise additive	Piomelli and Siniscalco (1969), Sanna et al. (1980)
GPI deficiency	Very rare	None	None	
PK deficiency	Single case	None	None	Meloni and Gaetoni (personal communication, 1983)
Gilbert disease	Rare	None	Intermittent increase in bilirubin	Panich et al. (1972)
CDA type II	Single case	None	Increased expression	Ventura et al. (1983)

[a] An entry of "none" indicates that the phenotypic manifestations are additive, without apparent interactions. For instance, a patient with CNSHD due to PK deficiency, who is also G6PD deficient, may develop favism, but in the steady state the clinical picture will not differ from that of any other PK-deficient patient who is not G6PD-deficient.

does not mean that all cells have the same level of enzyme. Indeed, if we look at solid tissues, we find an approximately tenfold range of variation from the lowest activity in muscle to the highest activity in brain and the adrenal gland (Table XX), and the ranking order tends to be preserved in various mammals. When considering the enzyme activity found in complex organs, the distribution can be, of course, quite uneven in different component cells. For instance, in rat lens and in ox adrenal most of the activity is localized in the cortex, whereas it is very low in the nucleus and in the medulla, respectively (Glock and McLean, 1954; Dovrat and Gershon, 1981). In the liver most of the activity is found in Kupffer cells, whereas it is low in hepatocytes (Teutsch and Rieder, 1979). In medulla

Table XX. G6PD Levels in Mammalian Tissues[a]

Organ	Species				
	Rat[b]	Rabbit[b]	Mouse[b]	Ox[b]	Man[c]
Seminal vescicles	0.1	—	—	—	—
Skeletal muscle	0.1	—	0.01	—	0.1
Cardiac muscle	0.3	—	0.02	—	0.2
Thyroid gland	—	0.2	—	—	—
Duodenal mucosa	—	0.2	—	—	—
Liver	0.5	—	0.3[e]	—	0.3
Testis	0.3	—	—	—	—
Pituitary	—	—	—	0.3	—
Placenta	0.4	—	—	—	—
Pancreas	—	—	—	—	0.5
Kidney	0.7	0.4, 0.3[d]	0.1	—	0.5
Prostate	0.3	—	—	—	0.5
Thymus	1.0	—	—	—	0.6
Adrenal gland	1.6	7.7	—	7.3, 0.7[d]	0.8
Lymph nodes	0.8	—	—	—	—
Brain	0.3	—	0.1	—	0.9
Lung	0.9	—	0.1	—	—
Spleen	3.1	1.1–0.2	—	—	—
Fibroblasts	—	—	—	—	6.7
Mononuclear cells	—	—	—	—	7.9
Granulocytes	—	—	—	—	32.8

[a] We have tabulated data only for the few species in which values for several tissues are available. Data are from males only and, when necessary, they have been converted to IU/grams of wet weight at 20°C.
[b] Glock and McLean (1954).
[c] G. Battistuzzi and L. Luzzatto, unpublished.
[d] Cortex and medulla, respectively.
[e] Yagil et al. (1974).

oblongata of rat, rabbit, and man, Sakharova *et al.* (1979) have been able to identify a special group of neurons with characteristically very high G6PD activity. In mouse testis Sertoli cells have more activity than the seminiferous tubules (Jones and Andrews, 1978). Muscle has very low activity in mammals and also in fishes (Champion *et al.*, 1975); moreover, most of the activity appears to be located in the connective tissue. Accordingly, G6PD activity is higher in atrophic muscle (Garcia-Buñuel and Garcia-Buñuel, 1980), and it is under neural control via estrogen level modulation. After denervation the G6PD level increases by 72%, and it goes back to normal values after reinnervation (Schaerf *et al.,* 1982). A similarly low level of activity is also found in tenocytes and chondrocytes of rabbits (Landi *et al.,* 1980).

It is quite apparent that very high G6PD activity is usually associated with structures producing steroids (medulla oblongata, adrenals) or fatty acid (Kupffer cells, mammary gland, developing brain). The impressive lactation-related changes taking place in the mammary gland have already been mentioned. A high activity is also observed in tumors compared to benign hyperplasia (Zampella *et al.,* 1982).

We do not yet know whether this considerable intertissue variation merely reflects postsynthetic differences (for instance, in the rate of G6PD degradation), or whether they may be dependent in some measure on different rates of gene transcription, implying that a tissue-specific transcriptional regulation does exist (see addendum). What is striking as more and more varieties of erythrocyte G6PD deficiency are investigated is the paucity of manifestations in other tissues, which makes quite a constrast to other red cell enzymopathies, where hemolytic anemia is often accompanied by other clinical signs, especially in the neuromuscular system.* This must mean one or both of the following. (1) The reduction of G6PD activity in Gd^- individuals is much less severe in cells other than erythrocytes. (2) In erythrocytes G6PD fulfills some role unique or peculiarly important to these cells. It is clear from Table XXI that factor 1 is generally true. Therefore, we may not need to postulate that factor 2 is also the case, although it seems not unlikely that the red cell, having a less structured cytoplasm and an autocannibalized metabolic machinery, is both less capable of detoxifying and more susceptible to damage by hydrogen peroxide and oxygen radicals.

---

* It is noteworthy that G6PD activity is *normally* extremely low in muscle (see Table XX); perhaps for this reason this tissue is not particularly sensitive to genetically determined G6PD deficiency.

Table XXI. Expression of G6PD Deficiency in Selected Cells and Tissues (Normal Values = 100)

Cell type or tissue	Percent of normal G6PD activity with G6PD($-$) variant			Known clinical manifestations
	A$-$	Mediterranean	Canton	
Erythrocytes[a]	15	<10	8	AHA
Granulocytes	90	25[b]	25[c]	None
Lymphocytes	—	—[b]	—	None
Platelets	—	19[d]	28[c]	None[e]
Liver	Reduced[f]	15[g]	49[c]	NNJ?[h], other?[i]
Lens	Reduced[j]	0[k]	—	Increased incidence of cataract[kl]
Sperm	16[m]	—	—	None

[a] Values from Tables XVI and XVII.
[b] Morellini et al. (1983).
[c] Chan et al. (1965).
[d] Hofmann et al. (1981).
[e] Enhanced platelet aggregation in vitro in response to ADP has been observed (Hofmann et al., 1981).
[f] Oluboyede et al. (1979): percentage not given because all samples were pathological.
[g] Panizon (1960).
[h] See text.
[i] Hyperbilirubinemia that may not be only hemolytic in origin has been reported in lobar pneumonia (Tugwell, 1973) and in other situations (Sidi et al., 1980).
[j] Zinkham (1961).
[k] Orzalesi et al. (1981).
[l] This is not found with G6PD Mahidol (Panich and Na-Nakorn, 1980[b]).
[m] Sarkar et al. (1977).

However, there are a few exceptions to the rule that G6PD deficiency lacks significant phenotypic expression in nonerythroid cells. Apart from those summarized in Table XXI, the leukocytes deserve special mention, both because they normally have a G6PD activity an order of magnitude higher than solid tissues (Table XX), and because of their function.

Granulocytes

In well-conducted studies of hospitalized children in Thailand (Lampe et al., 1975) and of hospitalized adults in Iran (Clark and Root, 1979), the frequency of G6PD deficiency was somewhat higher than in control groups, but the difference was not statistically significant. At the moment, there is no conclusive evidence that the considerable reduction in G6PD activity observed in granulocytes in a number of common Gd⁻

mutants causes significant functional impairment in these cells (see, for instance, Schilirò et al., 1976). The same is true even with the great majority of rare variants causing CNSHD. However, there have been two well-characterized families and one isolated patient (see p. 295) in whom leukocyte G6PD activity was extremely low (probably less than 2% of normal) and clinically significant susceptibility to infection was observed. In one family (Gray et al., 1973) there were three affected male sibs, and impaired killing of non-hydrogen peroxide-producing bacteria, such as *Staphylococcus aureus*, was demonstrated *in vitro*. In a 34-year-old man investigated by Vives Corrons et al. (1982) the findings were quite similar, and the patient's heterozygous mother also had mild hemolytic anemia. Interestingly, the functional abnormality of so severely G6PD-deficient granulocytes resembles that of granulocytes in another rare genetic disorder, chronic granulomatous disease (CGD) (Baehner, 1975). It is now clear that CGD is genetically heterogeneous. The more frequent form is X-linked and its basis is a deficiency of the granulocyte-specific cytochrome b_{-245} (Segal et al., 1982) (less frequent cases are autosomally inherited and in these the molecular basis is unknown). It seems likely that the phenotypic resemblance between CGD and severe granulocyte G6PD deficiency is based on an NADPH-linked pathway required for killing ingested bacteria, and which is also involved in the conventional nitroblue tetrazolium test. In X-linked CGD, NADPH cannot be utilized because of cytochrome b_{-245} deficiency. In severe G6PD deficiency affecting granulocytes NADPH is simply not produced in sufficient amounts. In addition, low levels of leukocyte G6PD have been reported in both the X-linked (Erickson et al., 1972) and the autosomal form of CGD (Corberand et al., 1978). However, this is a secondary abnormality, which may be artifactual (see Table XXII), and it has not been proven to contribute to the severity of expression of CGD.

Lymphocytes

Considerable differences in enzyme activity level have been observed in human B lymphocytes, T lymphocytes, and monocytes from venous blood, whether the values are expressed per protein content or per cell (Morellini et al., 1983; L. Luzzatto and G. Battistuzzi, unpublished results). The G6PD level of B lymphocytes is not significantly different from that of RBC, and approximately threefold, sixfold, and ten-

Table XXII. G6PD and Granulocyte Function

Condition	G6PD activity in granulocytes	NBT test[a]	Susceptibility to infection
Common G6PD deficiency	20–90%	Normal	Normal[b]
Chronic granulomatous disease	Normal but labile[c] or decreased[d]	Abnormal	Increased
G6PD deficiency with CNSHA (most cases)	Often markedly reduced	Normal	Normal
Very rare G6PD deficiency[e]	<5%	Abnormal	Increased (*Klebsiella pneumoniae, Eschenchia coli, Staphylococcus aureus*)

[a] Baehner and Nathan (1968).
[b] Although there is no evidence that G6PD-deficient subjects are prone to infection, it is not impossible that, once they have an acute infection, this may run a more severe course (Luzzatto, 1975).
[c] Erickson *et al.* (1972).
[d] Corberand *et al.* (1978).
[e] Cooper *et al.* (1972), Gray *et al.* (1973), Vives Corrons *et al.* (1982).

fold lower than that shown by T lymphocytes, monocytes, and granulocytes, respectively. The variation observed is not G6PD-specific, since it applies also to other enzymes involved in G6P metabolism.

Acquired Changes

Post-Translational Modifications

Further processing of a completed polypeptide chain is, to some extent, an obligatory stage in the biosynthesis of any protein. For instance, the N-terminal methionine is generally removed, and oligomeric molecules assemble in their definitive quaternary structure. In the case of G6PD this involves the association of two or four identical chains, an event that probably takes place spontaneously through mutual recognition of complementary surfaces, and is probably final. Indeed, dissociation to monomers is achieved *in vitro* only by rather drastic treatment or after removal of NADP by extensive dialysis. Dissociated monomers reassociate within milliseconds when NADP is added (Cancedda *et al.*, 1973), and apparently there is always enough NADP in cells to prevent dissociation, once the oligomer is formed (Kahler and Kirkman, 1983), so as to make subunit association a practically irreversible process in the cell (Goldstein and Gartler, 1979).

We have already mentioned that G6PD may be regulated after the protein is synthesized, since measurable amounts of inactive enzyme molecules are found in certain conditions (see p. 234). Post-translational modifications of G6PD have also been reported to occur at fertilization in sea urchins (Barber *et al.*, 1982), during fasting–refeeding experiments or in hormone-treated rat liver (Hori *et al.*, 1975) [these data have been questioned by Chang *et al.* (1979), who find no modifications], and in cancer cells (Hilf *et al.*, 1975; Hunter, 1980). For a more detailed discussion on post-translational modifications see the review papers by Dreyfus *et al.* (1978) and Luzzatto and Testa (1978). However, very little is known of the mechanisms that generate post-translational modifications of G6PD, and some of them, for instance, those described in the house fly, *Musca domestica,* may be artifacts of the extraction procedure (Gasperi *et al.*, 1978). Differences in G6PD structure in different cells are almost certainly post-translational (Dreyfus *et al.*, 1978), and they may be affected in mutants. Morellini *et al.* (1983) have compared leukocytes and erythrocytes of normal and G6PD-deficient subjects. In normal subjects the red blood cell enzyme, which is thought to have undergone post-translational modification (but see addendum), has higher affinity toward G6P than that from white blood cells. In G6PD(−) subjects this difference is abolished, and since contamination by white blood cells of the red cell enzyme was rigorously excluded, this must mean either that the mutant molecule is unaffected by the post-translational modification, or that this occurs at a much higher rate, so that even in white cells G6PD is completely modified. In either case, this genetically determined difference in events that affect enzyme kinetics supports the notion that post-translational changes may serve a physiological role.

Aging

Early work on the physiology of G6PD was more directed toward events in development, but as time goes on interest in aging has tended to develop as well. Senescence is associated with a decline in G6PD activity in a number of systems, such as rat liver (Iritani *et al.*, 1981) rat ovary (Leathem and Appel, 1977), other rat organs (Dovrat and Gershon,

1981), and human fibroblasts (De Mars, 1964) and blood cells (Gartler *et al.*, 1981).

Holliday and Tarrant (1972) have shown that during the senescent phase of *in vitro* cultured human fetal lung fibroblasts, strain MRC-5, a heat-labile fraction of G6PD, appears. Moreover, the shorter *in vitro* life span of fibroblasts that is found from patients with Werner syndrome, progeria, Cockayne syndrome, Bloom syndrome, Fanconi anemia, and ataxia telangectasia appears to correlate with an earlier appearance of this heat-labile fraction of the enzyme. These authors suggest that the observed changes can be ascribed to errors in transcription and/or translation of G6PD, thus supporting Orgel's protein-error theory of aging (Orgel, 1963). Other authors have questioned this interpretation. Duncan *et al.* (1977) propose that the heat-labile fraction occurs as a consequence of changes in the oligomeric state of the enzyme. Kahn *et al.* (1977) have suggested that the G6PD molecule is modified after its synthesis in senescent cells by a soluble factor that *in vitro* can convert normal G6PD into a heat-labile form. Recently, however, Holliday and Thompson (1983) have brought further support to the error theory by showing that normal cells grown in media containing paromomycin, an agent that reduces the fidelity of translation, produce an enzyme form comparable to that seen in senescent cells.

Fine Regulation

We have already discussed a variety of factors that help to determine G6PD activity levels. These differ in their nature and in their time scale. First, modifications of the enzyme molecule, whether genetic or acquired, may be permanent. Second, changes in enzyme activity, such as those related to development or to dietary stimuli, require a certain amount of restructuring of intermediary metabolism, which often involves the coordinated tuning of several enzyme functions; these are characterized by a delayed response, because the metabolic machinery has a certain built-in inertia. This relative inertia has its advantages, since confirmation of the stimulus is required before a great amount of energy is invested in readjusting metabolism. However, there are circumstances in which metabolic inertia could be detrimental or even fatal to the cell. Oxidant stress is a good example. Thus, there seems to be a need for a third type of regulation, which we may call "fine tuning," whose characteristic must lie in the capacity to display very rapid responses. A number of different mechanisms have been described in various organisms, with a number of effectors (some examples are listed in Table XXIII). We refer readers to the general review by Levy (1979) and to that by Luzzatto and Testa (1978) specifically for human erythrocyte G6PD.

A striking feature of G6PD has emerged from the study of human erythrocytes, but it is probably common to other somatic cells as well: namely, this enzyme operates normally at a rate that is a small fraction of its V_{max} [in erythrocytes this fraction is about 1% (Gaetani et al., 1974)]. This means that normally, unlike other key enzymes in other metabolic pathways, G6PD is not rate-limiting for the HMP, and that there is a vast untapped reserve of activity. It also means that there must be some mechanism whereby the rate of operation of the enzyme is normally restrained. The biochemical basis for this is certainly manifold. First, the intracellular concentration of the substrate, G6P, is rather stable and about one-half of the enzyme's K_m. Second, a variety of intracellular phosphate compounds can inhibit G6PD. Third, and perhaps most important, very little of the coenzyme is in the NADP form (in red cells 2% or less), while nearly all is in the NADPH form. As a result, G6PD finds itself normally in a condition of very much limiting concentration of this substrate and very severe product inhibition. This situation, apparently wasteful at first sight, places the cell in an ideal position to respond to an oxidant stress. In general this will be in the form of peroxide, and the first effect will be to oxidize NADPH (via glutathione peroxidase and glutathione reductase) and generate NADP. Thus substrate concentration increases and product inhibition is relieved at the same time. Even if nothing else happens, G6PD activity will increase by perhaps an order of magnitude, and since nothing else is required, the response will be immediate. Thus, the main controller for fine tuning is undoubtedly the NADP/(NADP + NADPH) ratio. How effective this control mechanism can be is expressed visually by the sigmoid dependence of G6PD activity on this ratio, observed both in intact cells (Luzzatto and Afolayan, 1971) and in cell-free extracts (Galiano et al., 1982—see addendum). A sigmoid curve as a function of NADP concentration, suggesting cooperativity in substrate binding, has also been observed with purified G6PD (Luzzatto, 1967; Luzzatto and Testa, 1978), although it has not been confirmed by others under somewhat different experimental conditions (Kirkman et al., 1980). There is also evidence that the normal restraint in intracellular G6PD activity (Gaetani et al., 1974) is not

Table XXIII. Examples of Quick-Acting Regulation of G6PD Activity

Effector(s)	System	Organism	Likely physiological role	References
NADP/NADPH	Nearly all cells	—	Rapid tuning of HMP activity[a]	Many
Glucose 6-phosphate	Lactating mammary gland	Rat	Enables operation of G6PD even in high NADPH[b]	Shreve and Levy (1980)
Palmitoyl-CoA/polyamines	Fertilized egg, regenerating liver	Yeast, sea urchin, rat	Control of lipid synthesis in dividing cells[c]	Mita and Yasumasu (1980)
Phosphoenol pyruvate (PEP)	—	Bacteria	Control of glucose metabolism through HMP versus Entner-Duodoroff pathway[d]	Turnail and Schlegel (1972)
Ribulose 1,5-diphosphate	Chloroplasts	Spinach	Control of HMP versus Calvin cycle[e]	Lendzian and Bassham (1975)

[a] By concentration-dependent substrate activation and product inhibition.
[b] By (competitive) inhibition of NADPH binding.
[c] Palmitoyl-CoA blocks G6PD by binding to it. Polyamines synthesized at time of DNA synthesis relieve the block, thus allowing G6PD to operate and provide the NADPH required for synthesis of membrane lipids.
[d] PEP affects differentially the NAD-linked versus the NADP-linked G6PD activity.
[e] Ribulose 1,5-diphosphate, which increases in concentration in the light, inhibits G6PD at a time when NADPH is already amply supplied by photosynthesis.

entirely accounted for by the factors mentioned above (Kirkman *et al.*, 1980; Wilson *et al.*, 1980), and that specific, previously undescribed, NADP- and NADPH-binding proteins may be involved. One of them has now been shown to be catalase (Kirkman and Gaetani, 1984—see addendum). However, it seems clear that from the physiological point of view the two main important features are the vast reserve in G6PD activity and how promptly much of it can be recruited by the change in the NADP/NADPH ratio.

It is relevant to ask how "fine tuning" is affected by genetic changes. We have already pointed out which enzyme properties are most important in allowing a deficient variant not to cause too much harm and even to become polymorphic. In crude approximation, increased substrate affinities will decrease restraint and thus easily enable a deficient variant to operate at a normal rate in a steady state in which the NADP/NADPH is higher than normal. The price to be paid is a decreased reserve. Under oxidant stress there is less room for the coenzyme ratio to shift; the maximal rate of G6PD activity (being too near the steady state rate) will be quickly reached, but it may be inadequate to avoid irreversible damage to the cell membrane. Thus, we understand, at least in first approximation, why kinetic properties of variants are important in preventing chronic hemolysis, but relatively unimportant in the pathophysiology of acute hemolytic attacks triggered by exogenous causes. Once restraint is removed, the only thing that matters is the total G6PD activity. Accordingly, the pattern of acute hemolysis has been rather uniform with different variants, but the range of potential offenders is broader, for instance, in subjects with G6PD Mediterranean (high substrate affinities but activity less than 5% of normal) than in subjects with G6PD A($-$) (nearly normal substrate affinities but activity 10–15% of normal).

Somatic Mutation of G6PD?

Mutation rates of 10^{-6}–10^{-8} have been measured in nondiploid rodent cell lines *in vitro*, and mutational events in human somatic cells must not be infrequent, judging from the only too dramatic *in vivo* evidence supplied by malignant tumors. In addition, somatic mutation within the immunoglobulin genes is regarded as a normal event in the special process of generation of antibody diversity. However, formal proof for a protein variant arising *in vivo* by somatic mutation in any other individual structural gene is lacking. We must also consider that if such an event occurred in an autosomal gene it would mostly pass unnoticed because the mutation might be recessive with respect to the unmutated allele. On the other hand, a mutated X-linked gene may become manifest more easily because it is haploid in somatic cells in both males and females. Perhaps this was the case with G6PD Verona, a variant with increased activity observed in the blood cells of a woman with a myelodysplastic syndrome which terminated in acute leukemia (Perona *et al.,* 1983). This variant was not found in any of the patient's relatives (although the strength of the negative family evidence was limited by the fact that the proposita had no offspring). More important, the patient's fibroblasts had only normal G6PD. We wonder whether a similar situation existed in another patient, reported by Cooper *et al.* (1972). This woman had, from the clinical description, a myeloproliferative disorder and severe G6PD deficiency in red cells and white cells. In this case the fibroblasts were not studied, but four brothers, three sisters, and the only living son had normal G6PD, which makes an inherited variant somewhat unlikely. One wonders whether in each of these two patients a somatic mutation produced a G6PD variant, the detection of which was made easier by the expansion of the mutated clone into a neoplastic growth.

G6PD POLYMORPHISM AND MALARIA SELECTION

The wealth of data on human polymorphic genes has reached stunning proportions (Mourant *et al.,* 1976), and a new, exponentially rising wave is mounting with the accumulation of data on restriction fragment length polymorphisms (RFLP) (Skolnick and White, 1982) at the DNA level. Yet, there are few cases in which we have any idea as to *why* gene frequencies are what they are. The G6PD system is one of the few in which the paramount role of an environmental selective agent, *Plasmodium falciparum* malaria, has been established.

Summary of Evidence

We state this as a fact on the grounds of compelling evidence reviewed elsewhere (Luzzatto and Testa, 1978; Luzzatto, 1979). It seems redundant to repeat the full argument, for which not enough space can be allowed here. We hope the reader will be content with a list of the now classical lines of evidence, for which full original references are given in the papers quoted above.

1. There is no population in which G6PD deficiency is frequent that has not been abundantly exposed to malaria over extended periods of time (dozens to hundreds of generations).

2. Although drift effects have almost certainly played a role in the present-day distribution of Gd^- alleles (see p. 265ff), as of any other gene, the impressive number of different Gd^- alleles that have reached polymorphic frequencies clearly show a pattern of convergent evolution, in which a similar phenotype has been selected from a background of independently arisen mutations.

3. Within populations that are otherwise genetically relatively homogeneous, the variance of Gd^- frequency is generally higher than that of other genes and, when this is tested, it is found to correlate with the degree of exposure to malaria.

4. In the only major clinical field survey in which severity of malaria infection was quantitatively measured in Gd^+/Gd^- heterozygous girls, these were found to have significantly lower levels of parasitemia than appropriate male and female control groups.

In vitro Culture Work

Having stated these established facts, we wish now to analyze here in some detail the more recent evidence accruing from *in vitro* experiments. Some initial attempts had already indicated that G6PD-deficient red cells were invaded at approximately normal rate (Luzzatto, 1974), but systematic work became possible only after the establishment of continuous cultures of *P. falciparum* (Trager and Jensen, 1976). Friedman (1979) then reported that the parasite cycle *in vitro* was essentially normal in G6PD-deficient (A⁻) red cells under "standard" culture conditions, but growth was significantly impaired under "oxidative stress" imposed by a higher pO_2 or by the addition of menadione or riboflavin. When similar experiments were carried out on G6PD-deficient red cells with the Mediterranean variant, impaired growth was seen even under standard conditions (Luzzatto, 1981). These experiments also identified clearly that the stage at which the impairment takes place is not invasion by the parasite, but its subsequent intracellular development. Reduced growth in culture in red cells from both hemizygous deficient males and heterozygous Gd^+/Gd^- females was confirmed by Roth et al. (1983).

However, the paradox of why Gd^+/Gd^- heterozygous girls, rather than Gd^- boys are relatively protected against malaria in a natural environment was not explained by these data. Indeed, the latter should be *more* resistant than the former if parasite development simply could not take place in G6PD (⁻) red cells. A possible explanation is suggested by further *in vitro* culture experiments in which the growth pattern of *P. falciparum* in G6PD(+) and G6PD(−) red cells was quantitated in successive cycles (Luzzatto et al., 1983). It became clear that the inhibition of growth in G6PD(−) cells is "leaky": a fraction of the parasites pull through, and this fraction increases as more passages in deficient cells are carried out. Eventually, the infection of G6PD(−) cells by parasites emerging from G6PD(−) cells is just as successful as that in control cultures (Table XXIV). The mechanism of this adaptation process is not yet known. In one possible model the parasite's G6PD gene might be involved. For example, one might speculate that, if *P. falciparum* had a *Gd* gene, this may be inactive in most circumstances. However, the gene may be induced in a G6PD(−) host cell environment, and redepression may have a lag lasting one or more schizogonic cycles. By this model, in Gd^- boys the parasite would have ample room for adaptation and subsequent successful development, whereas in Gd^+/Gd^- its development would be frustrated every time a parasite emerging from a G6PD(+) cell happens to invade a G6PD(−) cell (on the average, one-half of the infective events). From this point of view, the existence or otherwise of a *Gd* gene in the parasite becomes of special interest. Most previous attempts

Table XXIV. Dependence of *Plasmodium falciparum* Growth *in Vitro* on G6PD Status of Donor and Recipient Erythrocytes[a]

Type of transfer	Efficiency of transfer		
	Rings/1000 red cells at 24 hr	Schizonts/1000 red cells at 50 hr	Total parasites/ 1000 red cells at 75 hr
G6PD(+) → G6PD(+)	24	8.9	85
G6PD(+) → G6PD(−)	26	4.5	53
G6PD(−) → G6PD(−)	25	9.8	87

[a] From Luzzatto et al. (1983), by permission.

to demonstrate G6PD activity in *Plasmodia* failed* (Tsukamoto, 1974; Theakston *et al.,* 1976; Momen, 1979), but Hemplemann and Wilson (1981) produced evidence for a parasite-specific G6PD, although the possibility that this was a modified host-cell enzyme has not been strictly ruled out. In fact, according to the model proposed, G6PD expression would not be expected in parasites grown on normal cells, and it may be more promising to test for it in parasites grown in G6PD-deficient cells. Alternatively, a search for the *Gd* gene itself could be attempted since a genomic library of *P. falciparum* is now available (Goman *et al.,* 1982).

In the face of so much direct evidence on the protective role of G6PD deficiency against *P. falciparum,* it is interesting to note that a number of papers still refer to this interaction as a "hypothesis" or simply express disbelief. To count their number and compare it with the number of papers supporting the malaria model [among the most recent, see, for instance, Tzoneva *et al.* (1980), Hitzeroth and Bender (1980), Shatskaya *et al.* (1980*a*), Guggenmoos-Holzmann *et al.* (1981)] would hardly be a scientific approach. On the other hand, to identify the nature of the objections may help to identify which tests may be of use in the future. There seem to be three types of objections.

Objections

The Geographic Correlation between Malaria Endemicity and G6PD Deficiency Is Not Universal

In fact, there is not a single example of a population in which G6PD deficiency has reached a polymorphic frequency in the absence of exposure to malaria. The single reverse "exception" is the indigenous American population, who do not have G6PD deficiency in spite of malaria endemicity. It should be only too obvious that this fact in no way contradicts the concept of malaria selection, since a *Gd⁻* allele can hardly be expected to become polymorphic in a populaton if it does not happen to get there, or to arise *in situ* by mutation. It appears that the (probably very few) people who reached America through Bering's Strait did not carry a *Gd⁻* gene with them, and whether they have the same or a lower

---

* G6PD has been purified from other parasitic protozoa, for example, *Trypanosoma cruzi* (Funayama *et al.,* 1977) and *Leishmania tropica* (Walter, 1979).

overall mutation frequency than other populations we do not know (interestingly, Amerindians do not have any polymorphic hemoglobin variant either).

Within Malarious Areas Where G6PD Deficiency Is Prevalent, Malaria Selection Alone Does Not Always Quantitatively Account for the Microgeographic Distribution of Gd^- Gene Frequencies

For instance, Brown (1981) has carried out a critical analysis of the widely quoted Sardinian data (Siniscalco et al., 1966), and he has produced some epidemiologic data suggesting that the assumed inverse correlation between altitude and rate of malaria transmission is not as perfect as had been assumed. He also ably reviews historical evidence for gene input into the island from Carthaginians and from Jews deported from Rome, and concludes by questioning that "natural selection by malaria is the sole explanation for the distribution of the abnormal gene trait." In fact, no geneticist would seriously propose that, once a gene is subject to selection, migration and drift effects cease to operate! Indeed, we have amply discussed in a previous section several likely examples of spread by migration of various Gd^- alleles. But this does not remove the fact that when gene frequencies in Sardinian villages are analyzed, the Wahlund variance for G6PD and a few other genes is higher than that for all other genes (Piazza et al., 1972; Terrenato, 1976). Moreover, there must be a balancing factor to maintain a polymorphism in which hemizygous and homozygous children are at serious risk of dying from neonatal jaundice or from an attack of favism.

"The Clinical Data Are Controversial"

This statement paraphrases in short the gist of discussion paragraphs found in a number of papers (for instance, Gloria-Bottini et al., 1980) and it is simply inaccurate. It would hardly seem necessary to point out that, with an X-linked trait, data on males and females cannot be pooled or interchanged, whether in pedigree analysis or in calculating gene frequencies. Obviously the same must apply to studies of susceptibility to malaria. Yet, inexplicably, data obtained in males are still being compared with data obtained in females. In fact, the clinical data are impressively concordant in showing little or no protection against *P. falciparum* in G6PD-deficient boys [see compilation of earlier data in Luzzatto (1972) and more recent data by Martin *et al.* (1979); comment by Luzzatto and Bienzle (1979)], and significant protection in G6PD-deficient heterozygous girls (Bienzle *et al.*, 1972, 1979, 1981) [see also Duflo *et al.* (1979, 1982), who published a large series of 1822 patients, but unfortunately did not report on males and females separately].

Conclusion

In summary, there is no doubt that G6PD polymorphism is "complex," and gene frequencies are not determined by malaria alone (Bernstein and Bowman, 1980; Calabrese, 1982). However, the challenge of biological research is to dissect complex situations by identifying its components. *Plasmodium falciparum* selection favoring Gd^+/Gd^- heterozygotes is one clearcut component of the system, identified by *in vivo* and *in vitro* studies. If additional evidence is to be useful, it will have to be gathered by field studies of *heterozygotes*, for instance, in areas, such as the Middle East or Southeast Asia, where G6PD($-$) variants other than A($-$) are prevalent and malaria is still endemic; or by pinpointing further the molecular basis for the already established impairment of parasite growth in mixtures of G6PD($+$) and G6PD($-$) red cells *in vitro* (see addendum).

CONCLUDING REMARKS

A review of this sort hardly lends itself to a summary, and we shall not attempt one here. G6PD is but one of the hundreds of enzymes involved in intermediary metabolism, and it does exhibit a number of features in human genetics that are highly specific. Examples include its extreme variability in many populations, the pathology associated with G6PD deficiency, and the host–parasite interactions when G6PD-deficient cells are infected by malarial *Plasmodia*. Some of these features are much better understood now than they were in 1971, when H. N. Kirkman elegantly reviewed the topic in this series. On the other hand, G6PD is by no means the only human polymorphic enzyme; it is not the only X-linked marker; it is not the only enzyme whose deficiency causes hemolytic anemia; and by now it is no longer the only, even if it has been the first, human enzyme for which we have specific nucleic acid probes.

Of course one always wishes that a particular genetic system, apart from the problem-solving exercise it contributes in itself, may tell us something that has a wider biological significance. Motivations for research vary a great deal. Hematologists have worked on hemoglobins and G6PD not because they chose these systems, but because they had to solve the pathogenesis of genetically determined hemolytic anemias. At the other extreme, a molecular biologist interested in gene structure and expression will choose the most convenient and potentially informative system, quite regardless of species and of clinical implications. Until fairly recently the two approaches rarely converged, but from the spectacular progress of the hemoglobin work we have learnt that understanding regulation of mammalian globin genes and understanding the pathophysiology of thalassemias are nearly one and the same thing. How far is it likely that G6PD, quite apart from its own special problems, may become itself a model system? We have tried to emphasize in this review that G6PD typifies well the product of a ubiquitously expressed housekeeping gene. We think it is likely that genes in this category may have regulatory features significantly different from those pertaining to genes, such as globins, whose expression is confined to a highly specialized cell lineage. Such regulatory features of housekeeping genes must ultimately be written in the DNA sequence, whether within or near the transcribed portion of the gene, and they must ensure that expression is never turned off, while still perhaps leaving room for variation in transcription rate from one tissue to another and in response to environmental changes. In this respect G6PD, having graduated from hematology and biochemistry to molecular biology, may well be a useful model system.

Interest in G6PD from the point of view of enzymology is also likely to continue, because as the three-dimensional structure of the molecule is elucidated, the wealth of available natural mutants will give a readymade key to understanding which residues are crucial for substrate binding, regulation by effectors, and *in vivo* stability of the protein. Because of the increasingly fine mapping of the X chromosome, and because of its close linkage to factor VIII, to adrenal leukodystrophy, and to a fragile site associated with mental retardation, G6PD will remain an important tool in formal genetic analysis and in clinical genetics, especially once DNA polymorphisms become available. In view of the current interest in X-chromosome inactivation and of the ease of detection of its variants,

G6PD is also likely to continue to be important in the understanding of this phenomenon and in somatic cell genetics in general.

Finally, we think evolution deserves special mention, because in a biological system it is akin to hysteresis in a physical system: it depends in a unique way on the previous history of the system. On a macroscale, we have seen that the metabolic role of G6PD has been largely preserved in the course of evolution, but that considerable functional adaptation has taken place. We should learn in due course how this is reflected in the structure of the gene in various organisms. In human populations, mutations and selection have affected *Gd* more than any other single known gene. Thus far our attempts at unraveling the role of drift, selection, and second mutations in explaining contemporary gene frequencies are entirely speculative. However, sequence information at the DNA level should enable us on the one hand to identify double mutants, and on the other hand to look separately at polymorphisms in introns and flanking regions, most of them presumably not subject to selection, and to polymorphisms within translated regions, all of them potentially subject to selection. Thus, G6PD may indeed be a good model for the study of human microevolution.

ACKNOWLEDGMENTS.   We are very grateful to Dr. M. D'Urso, M. G. Persico, D. Toniolo, and G. Martini for the work we have done together over several years. We thank them and Dr. G. F. Gaetani, Dr. B. Migeon, and Dr. S. Wolf for communicating unpublished results. We are extremely grateful to Ruth Frearson for her invaluable role in preparing the manuscript, and we thank the Library Staff at the Royal Postgraduate Medical School for their cooperation in the literature search. G. B. was a Research Fellow supported by EMBO, on leave of absence from the Department of Genetics, University of Naples, Naples, Italy. Work in the authors' laboratory was supported by a Programme Grant from the Medical Research Council of Great Britain.

REFERENCES

Abraham, I., and Lucchesi, J. C., 1974, Dosage compensation of genes on the left and right arms of the X chromosome of *Drosophila pseudoobscura* and *Drosophila willistoni, Genetics* 78:1119–1126.

Adamson, J. W., Failkow, P. J., Murphy, S., Prchal, J. F., and Steinmann, L., 1976, Polycythemia vera: Stem-cell and probable clonal origin of the disease, *N. Engl. J. Med.*
295:913–916.

Afolayan, A., 1979, The plasma membrane of human erythrocyte with different levels of
glucose-6-phosphate dehydrogenase, *Int. J. Biochem.* **10**:361–365.

Afolayan, A., and Luzzatto, L., 1971, Genetic variants of human erythrocyte glucose-6-
phosphate dehydrogenase. I. Regulation of activity by oxidized and reduced nicotinamide adenine dinucleotide phosphate, *Biochemistry* **10**:415–419.

Aksoy, M., Dinçol, G., and Erdem, S., 1980, Survey on haemoglobin variants, β-thalassae-
mia, glucose-6-phosphate dehydrogenase deficiency and haptoglobin types in Turkish
people living in Manavgat, Serik and Boztepe (Antalya), *Hum. Hered.* **30**:3–6.

Allendorf, F. W., Christiansen, F. B., Dobron, T., Eanes, W. F. and Frijdenberg, O., 1979,
Electrophoretic variation in large mammals. I. The polar bear, *Thalartos maritimus,*
Hereditas **91**:19–22.

Anderson, J. E., and Giblett, E. R., 1975, Intraspecific red cell enzyme variation in the pig-
tailed Macaque *(Macaca nemestrina), Biochem. Genet.* **13**:189–212.

Andersson, L., Ryman, N., Rosenberg, R., and Stahl, G., 1981, Genetic variability in Atlantic herring *(Clupea harengus harengus):* Description of protein loci and population
data, *Hereditas* **95**:69–78.

Arese, P., 1982, Favism—A natural model for the study of hemolytic mechanisms, *Rev.
Pure Appl. Pharmacol. Sci.* **3**:123–183.

Arese, P., Bosia, A., Naitana, A., Gaetani, S., D'Aquino, M., and Gaetani, G. F., 1981, Effect
of divicine and isouramil on red cell metabolism in normal and G6PD-deficient (Mediterranean variant) subjects. Possible role in the genesis of favism, in: *The Red Cell:
Fifth Ann Arbor Conference,* pp. 725–744, Alan R. Liss, New York.

Arese, P., Naitana, A., Mannuzzu, L., Turrini, F., Haest, C. W. M., Fischer, T. M., and
Deuticke, B., 1982, Biochemical and micro-rheological modifications in normal and
glucose-6-phosphate dehydrogenase-deficient red cells treated with divicine, in:
Advances in Red Cell Biology (D. J. Weatherall, G. Fiorelli, and S. Gorini, eds.), pp.
375–379, Raven Press, New York.

Arnold, H., Löhr, G. W., Hasslinger, K., and Ludwig, R., 1981, Combined erythrocyte glu-
cosephosphate isomerase (GPI) and glucose-6-phosphate dehydrogenase (G6PD) deficiency in an Italian family, *Hum. Genet.* **57**:226–229.

Avise, J. C., Smith, M. H., Selander, R. K., Lawlor, T. E., and Ramsey, P. R., 1974, Biochemical polymorphism and systematics in the genus *Peromiscus.* V. Insular and mainland species of the subgenus *Haplomylomys, Syst. Zool.* **23**:226–238.

Ayala, F. J., Valentine, J. W., Hedgecock, D., and Barr, L. G., 1975, Deep-sea asteroids:
High genetic variability in a stable environment, *Evolution* **29**:203–212.

Azevedo, E., Kirkman, H. N., Morrow, A. C., and Motulsky, A. G., 1968, Variants of red
cell G6PD among asiatic indians, *Ann. Hum. Genet.* **31**:373–379.

Azim, A. A., Kamel, K., Gaballah, M. F., Sabry, F. H., Ibrahim, W., Selim, O., and Moafy,
N., 1974, Genetic blood markers and anthropometry of the populations in Aswan gov-
ernorate, Egypt, *Hum. Hered.* **24**:12–23.

Babalola, A. O. G., Beetlestone, J. G., and Luzzatto, L., 1976, Genetic variants of human
erythrocyte glucose-6-phosphate dehydrogenase. Kinetic and thermodynamic parameters of variants A, B and A⁻ in relation to quaternary structure, *J. Biol. Chem.*
251:2992–3002.

Backstrom, S., 1959, Activation of glucose-6-phosphate dehydrogenase in sea urchin
embryos of different developmental trends, *Exp. Cell. Res.* **18**:347–356.

Baehner, R. I., 1975, The growth and development of an understanding of chronic granulomatous disease, in: *The Phagocytic Cell in Host Resistance*, pp. 173–175, Raven Press, New York.

Baehner, R. L., and Nathan, D. G., 1968, Quantitative nitro blue tetrazolium test in chronic granulomatous disease, *N. Engl. J. Med.* **278**:971–978.

Baer, A., Lie-Injo, L.-E., Welch, Q. B., and Lewis, A. N., 1976, Genetic factors and malaria in Temuan, *Am. J. Hum. Genet.* **28**:179–188.

Balinsky, D., and Jenkins, T., 1967, Electrophoretic variants of glucose-6-phosphate dehydrogenase and phosphoglucomutase in Bantu and Coloured subjects, *S. Afr. J. Med. Sci.* **32**:96.

Balogh, A., Borbély, G., Cséke, Cs., Udvardy, J., and Farkas, G. L., 1979, Virus infection affects the molecular properties and activity of glucose-6-P dehydrogenase in *Anacystic nidulans*, a cyanobacterium: Novel aspect of metabolic control in a phage-infected cell, *FEBS Lett.* **105**:158–162.

Banerjee, S., and Fraenkel, D. G., 1972, Glucose-6-phosphate dehydrogenase from *Escherichia coli* and from a "high level" mutant, *J. Bacteriol.* **110**:155–160.

Banerjee, B., Saha, N., Daoud, Z. F., Khalaf, F. H., and Qudah, H., 1981, A genetic study of the Jordanians, *Hum. Hered.* **31**:65–69.

Barber, M. L., Kolan, D. M., Yabuta, C., and Nielsen, B., 1982, Mechanisms of glucose-6-phosphate dehydrogenase isozyme pattern changes at fertilization, *J. Exp. Zool.* **219**:369–376.

Barker, J. S. F., and Mulley, J. C., 1976, Isozyme variation in natural populations of *Drosophila buzzatii*, *Evolution* **30**:213–233.

Battistuzzi, G., Esan, G. J. F., Fasuan, F. A., Modiano, G., and Luzzatto, L., 1977a, Comparison of *Gd* A and *Gd* B activities in Nigerians. A study of the G6PD activity, *Am. J. Hum. Genet.* **29**:31–36.

Battistuzzi, G., Esan, G. J. F., Fasuan, F. A., Modiano, G., and Luzzatto, L., 1977b, Response to Nance letter, *Am. J. Hum. Genet.* **29**:543–544.

Battistuzzi, G., Morellini, M., Meloni, T., Gandini, E., and Luzzatto, L., 1982, Genetic factors in favism, in: *Advances in Red Blood Cell Biology* (D. J. Weatherall, G. Fiorelli, and S. Gorini, eds.), pp. 339–346, Raven Press, New York.

Bayoumi, R. A., Omer, A., Samuel, A. P. W., Saha, N., Sebai, Z. A., and Sabaa, H. M. A., 1979, Haemoglobin and erythrocytic glucose-6-phosphate dehydrogenase variants among selected tribes in Western Saudi Arabia, *Trop. Geogr. Med.* **31**:245–252.

Belote, J. M., and Lucchesi, J. C., 1980, Control of X chromosome transcription by the maleless gene in *Drosophila*, *Nature* **285**:573–575.

Benabadji, M., Merad, F., Benmoussa, M., Trabuchet, G., Junien, C., Dreyfus, J. C., and Kaplan, J. C., 1978, Heterogeneity of glucose-6-phosphate dehydrogenase deficiency in Algeria. Study in Northern Algeria with description of five new variants, *Hum. Genet.* **40**:177–184.

Benatti, U., Morelli, A., Meloni, T., Sparatore, B., Salamino, G., Michetti, M., Melloni, E., Pontremoli, S., and De Flora, A., 1981, Comparative patterns of *"in vitro"* oxidative hemolysis of normal and glucose 6-phosphate dehydrogenase (G6PD)-deficient erythrocytes, *FEBS Lett.* **128**:225–229.

Ben-Bassat, A., and Goldberg, I., 1980, Purification and properties of glucose-6-phosphate dehydrogenase (NADP$^+$/NAD$^+$) and 6-phosphogluconate dehydrogenase (NADP$^+$/NAD$^+$) from methanol-grown *Pseudomonas C*, *Biochim. Biophys. Acta* **611**:1–10.

Berg, K., and Bearn, A. G., 1968, Human serum protein polymorphism. A selected review, *Annu. Rev. Genet.* **2**:341–362.

Bernstein, S. C., and Bowman, J. E., 1980, G6PD/malaria hypothesis: A balanced or transient polymorphism, *Lancet* i:485.

Bernstein, S. C., Throckmorton, L. H., and Hubby, J. L., 1973, Still more genetic variability in natural populations, *Proc. Natl. Acad. Sci. USA* 70:3928.

Bernstein, S. C., Bowman, J. E., and Kaptue Noche, L., 1980a, Population studies in Cameroon: Hemoglobin S, glucose-6-phosphate dehydrogenase deficiency and *falciparum* malaria, *Hum. Hered.* 30:251–258.

Bernstein, S. C., Bowman, J. E., and Kaptue Noche, L., 1980b, Genetic variation in Cameroon: Thermostability variants of hemoglobin and of glucose-6-phosphate dehydrogenase, *Biochem. Genet.* 18:21–37.

Bernstein, S. C., Bowman, J. E., and Kaptue Noche, L., 1980c, Interaction of sickle cell trait and glucose-6-phosphate dehydrogenase deficiency in Cameroon, *Hum. Hered.* 30:7–11.

Bertin, T., Harris, J. E., Ferrell, R. E., and Schull, W. J., 1978, The Nubians of Kom Ombo: Serum and red cell protein types, *Hum. Hered.* 28:66–71.

Betke, K., Brewer, G. J., Kirkman, H. N., Luzzatto, L., Motulsky, A. G., Ramot, B., and Siniscalco, M., 1967, Standardization of procedures for the study of glucose-6-phosphate dehydrogenase: Report of a WHO Scientific Group, World Health Organization Technical Report Series 366.

Beutler, E., 1971, Abnormalities of the hexose monophosphate shunt, *Semin. Hematol.* 8:311–347.

Beutler, E., 1983, Glucose-6-phosphate dehydrogenase deficiency, in: *The Metabolic Basis of Inherited Disease* (J. B. Stanbury, J. B. Wyngaarden, D. S. Fredrickson, J. L. Goldstein, and M. S. Brown, eds.), 5th ed., pp. 1629–1653, McGraw-Hill, New York.

Beutler, E., and West, C., 1978, Glucose-6-phosphate variants in chimpanzee, *Biochem. Med.* 20:364–370.

Beutler, E., and Yoshida, A., 1973, Human glucose-6-phosphate dehydrogenase variants: A supplementary tabulation, *Ann. Hum. Genet. Lond.* 37:151–152.

Beutler, E., Yeh, M., and Fairbanks, V. F., 1962, The normal human female as a mosaic of X-chromosome activity: Studies using the gene for G-6-PD deficiency as a marker, *Proc. Natl. Acad. Sci. USA* 48:9–16.

Bezzi, T. M., Castaldi, G., Bergamini, M., and Scorrano, M., 1982, Morphological abnormalities of the red cells during hemolytic episode in a patient with glucose 6-phosphate dehydrogenase deficiency, *Haematologica (Pavia)* 67:147–148.

Bienzle, U., 1981, Glucose-6-phosphate dehydrogenase deficiency, Part 1: Tropical Africa, *Clin. Haematol.* 10:785–799.

Bienzle, U., Ayeni, O., Lucas, A. O., and Luzzatto, L., 1972, Glucose-6-phosphate dehydrogenase and malaria. Greater resistance of females heterozygous for enzyme deficiency and of males with nondeficient variant, *Lancet* i:107–110.

Bienzle, U., Sodeinde, O., Effiong, C. E., and Luzzatto, L., 1975, Glucose 6-phosphate dehydrogenase deficiency and sickle cell anemia: Frequency and features of the association in an African community, *Blood* 46:591–597.

Bienzle, U., Guggenmoos-Holzmann, I., and Luzzatto, L., 1979, Malaria and erythrocyte glucose-6-phosphate dehydrogenase variants in West Africa, *Am. J. Trop. Med. Hyg.* 28:619–621.

Bienzle, U., Guggenmoos-Holzmann, I., and Luzzatto, L., 1981, *Plasmodium falciparum* malaria and human red cells. 1. A genetic and clinical study in children, *Int. J. Epidemiol.* 10:9–15.

Bijlsma, R., 1978, Polymorphism at the G6PD and 6PGD loci in *Drosophila melanogaster*. II. Evidence for interaction in fitness, *Genet. Res.* **31**:227–237.

Bijlsma, R., and Van Delden, W., 1977, Polymorphism at the G6PD and 6PGD loci in *Drosophila melanogaster*. I. Evidence for selection in experimental population, *Genet. Res.* **30**:221–236.

Bijlsma, R., and Van der Meulen-Bruijns, C., 1979, Polymorphism at the G6PD and 6PGD loci in *Drosophila melanogaster*. III. Developmental and biochemical aspects, *Biochem. Genet.* **17**:1131–1143.

Bittner, R., Böhme, H.-J., Didt, L., Goltzsch, W., Hofmann, E., Levin, M. J., and Sparmann, G., 1978, Developmental changes in the levels of hepatic enzymes and their relation to metabolic functions, *Ad. Enzyme Reg.* **17**:37–57.

Blasi, F., and Toniolo, D., 1983, DNA methylation and X-chromosome inactivation, *Mol. Biol. Med.* **1**:271–274.

Bonnell, M. L., and Selander, R. K., 1974, Elephant seals: Genetic variation and near extinction, *Science* **184**:908–909.

Booth, P. B., Tills, D., Warlow, A., Kopeć, A. C., Mourant, A. E., Teesdale, P., and Hornabrook, R. W., 1982, Red cell antigen, serum protein and red cell enzyme polymorphisms in Karkar Islanders and inhabitants of the adjacent north coast of New Guinea, *Hum. Hered.* **32**:385–403.

Bouloux, C., Gomila, J., and Langaney, A., 1972, Hemotypology of the Bedik, *Hum. Biol.* **44**:289–302.

Bowman, J. T., and Simmons, J. R., 1973, Gene modulation in *Drosophila:* Dosage compensation of *PgD+* and *Zw+* genes, *Biochem. Genet.* **10**:319–331.

Bowman, J. E., Brubaker, R. R., Frischer, H., and Carson, P. E., 1967, Characterization of enterobacteria by starch-gel electrophoresis of glucose-6-phosphate dehydrogenase and phosphogluconate dehydrogenase, *J. Bacteriol.* **94**:544–551.

Boyer, S. H., and Graham, J. B., 1965, Linkage between the X chromosome loci for glucose-6-phosphate dehydrogenase electrophoretic variation and hemophilia A, *Am. J. Hum. Genet.* **17**:320–324.

Breguet, G., Ney, R., Kirk, R. L., and Blake, N. M., 1982, Genetic survey of an isolated community in Bali, Indonesia. II. Haemoglobin types and red cell isozymes, *Hum. Hered.* **32**:308–317.

Brewer, G. J., Gall, J. C., Honeyman, M., Gershowitz, H., Schreffler, D. C., Dern, R. J., and Hames, C., 1967, Inheritance of quantitative expression of erythrocyte glucose-6-phosphate dehydrogenase activity in the Negro—A twin study, *Biochem. Genet.* **1**:41–53.

Brinster, R. L., 1966, Glucose-6-phosphate dehydrogenase activity in preimplantation embryo, *Biochem. J.* **101**:161–163.

Brinster, R. L., 1970, Glucose-6-phosphate dehydrogenase activity in the early rabbit and mouse embryo, *Biochem. Genet.* **4**:669–676.

Brittnacher, J. G., Sims, S. R., and Ayala, F. J., 1978, Genetic differentiation between species of the genus *Speyeria (Lepidoptera nymphalidae), Evolution* **32**:199–210.

Brown, P. J., 1981, New considerations on the distribution of malaria, thalassemia, and glucose-6-phosphate dehydrogenase deficiency in Sardinia, *Hum. Biol.* **53**:367–382.

Bruce, E. J., and Ayala, F. J., 1978, Phylogenetic relationships between man and apes: Electrophoretic evidence, *Evolution* **33**:1040–1056.

Bryant, E. H., Van Dijk, H., and Van Delden, W., 1981, Genetic variability of the fare fly, *Musca autumnalis* de Geer, in relation to a population bottleneck, *Evolution* **35**:872–881.

Buettner-Janusch, J., Dame, L., Mason, G. A., and Sade, D. S., 1974, Primate red cell enzyme: Glucose-6-phosphate dehydrogenase and 6-phosphogluconate dehydrogenase, *Am. J. Phys. Anthropol.* **41**:7–14.

Burt, A. M., 1965, Glucose-6-phosphate dehydrogenase and chick neurogenesis. I. G6PD activity in embryonic brachial spinal cord, *Dev. Biol.* **12**:213–232.

Cabrera, V. M., Gonzales, A. M., and Gullon, A., 1980, Enzymatic polymorphism in *Drosophila subobscura* populations from the Canary Islands, *Evolution* **34**:875–887.

Cacciapuoti, A. F., and Lessie, T. G., 1977, Characterization of the fatty acid-sensitive glucose 6-phosphate dehydrogenase from *Pseudomonas cepacia, J. Bacteriol.* **132**:555–563.

Calabrese, E. J., 1982, Evolutionary loss of ascorbic acid synthesis: How it may have enhanced the survival interests of man, *Med. Hypotheses* **8**:173–175.

Cameron, D. G., and Vyse, E. R., 1978, Heterozygosity in Yellowstone Park elk, *Cervus canadensis, Biochem. Genet.* **16**:651–653.

Cancedda, R., Ogunmola, G. B., and Luzzatto, L., 1973, Genetic variants of human erythrocyte glucose-6-phosphate dehydrogenase, *Eur. J. Biochem.* **34**:199–204.

Carroll, A. J., Prchal, J. T., Crist, W. M., and Prchal, J. F., 1980, Cellular expression of Wiskott–Aldrich allele, *Lancet* **i**:601–602.

Carson, P. E., Flanagan, C. L., Ickes, C. E., and Alving, A., 1956, Enzymatic deficiency in primaquine-sensitive erythrocytes, *Science* **124**:484–485.

Carter, R., 1973, Enzyme variation in *Plasmodium berghei* and *Plasmodium vinchei, Parasitology* **66**:297–307.

Cavalli-Sforza, L. L., and Bodmer, W. F., 1971, *The Genetics of Human Populations,* W. H. Freeman, San Francisco.

Cavener, D. R., and Clegg, M. T., 1981, Evidence for biochemical and physiological differences between enzyme genotypes in *Drosophila melanogaster, Proc. Natl. Acad. Sci. USA* **78**:4444–4447.

Champion, M. J., Shaklee, J. B., and Witt, G. S., 1975, Developmental genetics of teleost isozymes, in: *Isozymes. III. Developmental Biology* (C. L. Markert, ed.), pp. 417–437, Academic Press, New York.

Chan, T. K., and Todd, D., 1972, Characteristics and distribution of glucose-6-phosphate dehydrogenase deficient variants in South China, *Am. J. Hum. Genet.* **24**:475–484.

Chan, T. K., Todd, D., and Wong, C. C., 1965, Tissue enzyme levels in erythrocyte glucose-6-phosphate dehydrogenase deficiency, *J. Lab. Clin. Med.* **66**:937–942.

Chan, T. K., Todd, D., and Lai, M. S. C., 1972, Glucose-6-phosphate dehydrogenase: Identity of erythrocyte and leukocyte enzyme with report of a new varient in Chinese, *Biochem. Genet.* **6**:119–130.

Chang, H.-L., Holten, D., and Karin, R., 1979, Distribution of the multiple molecular forms of glucose-6-phosphate dehydrogenase in different pathological states, *Can. J. Biochem.* **57**:396–401.

Chapman, V. M., and Shaws, T. B., 1976, Somatic cell genetics evidence for X chromosome linkage of three enzymes in the mouse, *Nature* **259**:665–667.

Cheun, H. L., 1966, Glucose-6-phosphate dehydrogenase activity in erythrocytes of experimental animals, *J. Clin. Pathol.* **19**:614–618.

Chockkalingam, K., and Board, P. G., 1980, Further evidence for heterogeneity of glucose-6-phosphate dehydrogenase deficiency in Papua New Guinea, *Hum. Genet.* **56**:209–212.

Chockkalingam, K., Board, P. G., and Breguet, G., 1982*a*, Glucose 6-phosphate dehydrogenase variants of Bali Island (Indonesia), *Hum. Genet.* **60**:60–62.

Chockkalingam, K., Board, P. G., and Nurse, G. T., 1982*b*, Glucose-6-phosphate dehydrogenase deficiency in Papua New Guinea: The description of 13 new variants, *Hum. Genet.* **60**:189–192.

Clark, M., and Root, R. K., 1979, Glucose-6-phosphate dehydrogenase deficiency and infection: A study of hospitalised patients in Iran, *Yale J. Biol. Med.* **52**:169–179.

Cooper, M. R., DeChatelet, L. R., McCall, C. E., LaVia, M. F., Spurr, C. L., and Baehner, R. L., 1972, Complete deficiency of leukocyte glucose-6-phosphate dehydrogenase with defective bactericidal activity, *J. Clin. Invest.* **51:**769–778.

Cooper, D. W., Johnston, P. G., Mutach, C. E., Sharman, C. B., Vanderberg, J. L., and Poole, W. E., 1975, Sex linked isozymes and sex chromosome evolution and inactivation in kangaroos, in: *Isozymes. III. Developmental Biology* (C. L. Markert, ed.), pp. 559–573, Academic Press, New York.

Corberand, J., De Larrard, B., Vergnes, H., and Corrière, J. P., 1978, Chronic granulomatous disease with leukocytic glucose-6-phosphate deficiency in a 28-month-old girl, *Am. J. Clin. Pathol.* **70:**296–300.

Corbo, R. M., Spennati, G. F., Scacchi, R., Palmarino, R., Della Penna, M. R., and Lucarelli, P., 1981, A survey of serum protein and enzyme polymorphisms in the district of L'Aquila (Italy), *Hum. Hered.* **31:**167–171.

Daneshbod, G., 1975, Erythrocyte glucose-6-phosphate dehydrogenase in Tehran, *Acta Haematol.* **53:**152–157.

Dao, M. L., Watson, J. J., Delaney, R., and Johnson, B. C., 1979, Purification of a high activity form of glucose-6-phosphate dehydrogenase from rat liver and effect of enzyme inactivation on its immunochemical reactivity, *J. Biol. Chem.* **254:**9441–9447.

Dao, M. L., Connor Johnson, B., and Hartman, P. E., 1982, Preparation of a monoclonal antibody to rat liver glucose-6-phosphate dehydrogenase and the study of its immunoreactivity with native and inactivated enzyme, *Proc. Natl. Acad. Sci. USA* **79:**2860–2864.

Davidson, R. G., Nitowsky, H. M., and Childs, B., 1963, Demonstration of two populations of cells in the human female heterozygous for glucose-6-phosphate variants, *Proc. Natl. Acad. Sci. USA* **50:**481–484.

Davidson, R. G., Childs, B., and Siniscalco, M., 1964, Genetic variations in the quantitative control of erythrocyte G6PD activity, *Am. J. Hum. Genet.* **28:**61–70.

De Flora, A., 1981, Present and future approaches to the correction of erythrocyte glucose-6-phosphate dehydrogenase deficiency, *Haematologica* **66:**691–701.

Dobzhansky, T. H., 1930, Genetical and environmental factors influencing the type of intersexes in *Drosophila melanogaster, Am. Nat.* **64:**261–271.

Donohue, T. M., Jr., and Barker, K. L., 1983, Glucose-6-phosphate dehydrogenase: Translational regulation of synthesis and regulation of processing of the enzyme in the uterus by estradiol, *Biochim. Biophys. Acta* **739:**148–157.

Dovrat, A., and Gershon, D., 1981, Rat lens superoxide dismutase and glucose-6-phosphate dehydrogenase: Studies on the catalytic activity and the fat of enzyme antigen as a function of age, *Exp. Eye Res.* **33:**651–661.

Dreyfus, J.-C., Kahn, A., and Schapira, F., 1978, Posttranslational modifications of enzymes, in: *Current Topics in Cellular Regulation,* Vol. 14 (B. L. Horecker, and E. R. Stadtman, eds.), pp. 243–275, Academic Press, New York.

Duflo, B., Diallo, A., Toure, K., and Soula, G., 1979, Le déficit en glucose-6-phosphate déshydrogénase au Mali: Épidémiologie et rôle pathologique, *Bull. Soc. Pathol. Exotique* **72:**258–264.

Duflo, B., Ranque, P., Quilici, M., Balique, H., Dembele, O., Diallo, D., Diallo, A.-N., Haidara, S., and Maiga, I., 1982, Déficit en glucose-6-phosphate-déshydrogénase et paludisme au Mali, *Nouv. Presse Méd.* **11:**2713.

Duncan, M. R., Dell'Orco, R. T., and Guthrie, P. L., 1977, Relationship of heat labile glucose-6-phosphate dehydrogenase and multiple molecular forms of the enzyme in senescent human fibroblasts, *J. Cell. Physiol.* **93:**49–56.

D'Urso, M., Battistuzzi, G., and Luzzatto, L., 1980, Genetic variants of human erythrocyte glucose-6-phosphate dehydrogenase: Automated procedure for characterization by column chromatography, *Anal. Biochem.* **108**:146–150.

D'Urso, M., Mareni, C., Toniolo, D., Piscopo, M., Schlessinger, D., and Luzzatto, L., 1983, Regulation of glucose-6-phosphate dehydrogenase expression in CHO–human fibroblast somatic cell hybrids, *Somat. Cell Genet.* **9**:429–443.

Elizondo, J., Sáenz, G. F., Páez, C. A., Ramón, M., García, M., Gutiérrez, A., and Estrada, M., 1982, G6PD-Puerto Limón: A new deficient variant of glucose-6-phosphate dehydrogenase associated with congenital nonspherocytoc hemolytic anemia, *Hum. Genet.* **62**:110–112.

Erickson, R. P., and Harper, K., 1980, A major autosomal gene effect on activity of glucose 6-phosphate dehydrogenase segregating between recombinant inbred lines of mice, *Genet. Res. Camb.* **36**:91–97.

Erickson, R. P., Stites, D. P., Fudenberg, H. H., and Epstein, C. J., 1972, Altered levels of glucose-6-phosphate dehydrogenase stabilizing factors in X-linked chronic granulomatous disease, *J. Lab. Clin. Med.* **80**:644–653.

Erikson, K., Halkka, O., Lokki, J., and Saura, A., 1976, Enzyme polymorphism in feral, outbred and inbred rats *(Rattus norvegicus), Heredity* **37**:341–349.

Everett, W. D., Yoshida, A., and Pearlman, E., 1977, Hemoglobin E and glucose-6-phosphate deficiency in the Khmer Air Force (Cambodia), *Am. J. Trop. Med. Hyg.* **26**:597–601.

Fenu, M. P., Finazzi, G., Manoussakis, C., Palomba, V., and Fiorelli, G., 1982, Glucose-6-phosphate dehydrogenase deficiency: Genetic heterogeneity in Sardinia, *Ann. Hum. Genet.* **46**:105–114.

Fernandez, M. N., and Fairbanks, V. F., 1968, Glucose-6-phosphate dehydrogenase in the Philippines: Report of a new variant G6PD Panay, *Mayo Clin. Proc.* **43**:645–660.

Ferraris, A. M., Giuntini, P., Galiano, S., and Gaetani, G. F., 1981, 2-Deoxy-glucose-6-phosphate utilization in the study of glucose-6-phosphate dehydrogenase mosaicism, *Am. J. Hum. Genet.* **33**:307–313.

Ferraris, A. M., Canepa, L., Mareni, C., Baule, G., Meloni, T., Salvidio, E., Forteleoni, G., and Gaetani, G. F., 1983, Reexpression of normal stem cells in erythroleukemia during remission, *Blood* **62**:177–179.

Ferrell, R. E., Bertin, T., Young, R., Barton, S. A., Murillo, F., and Schull, W. J., 1978, The Aymara of Western Bolivia. IV. Gene frequencies for eight blood groups and 19 protein and erythrocyte enzyme systems, *Am. J. Hum. Genet.* **30**:539–549.

Ferrell, R. E., Bertin, T., Barton, S. A., Rothhammer, F., and Schull, W. J., 1980, The Multinational Andean Genetic and Health Program. IX. Gene frequencies and rare variants of 20 serum proteins and erythrocyte enzymes in the Aymara of Chile, *Am. J. Hum. Genet.* **39**:92–102.

Fialkow, P. J., 1979, Clonal origin of human tumors, *Ann. Rev. Med.* **30**:135–143.

Fialkow, P. J., Gartler, S. M., and Yoshida, A., 1967, Clonal origin of chronic myelocytic leukemia in man, *Proc. Natl. Acad. Sci. USA* **58**:1468–1471.

Fialkow, P. J., Klein, E., Klein, G., Clifford, P., and Singh, S., 1973, Immunoglobulin and G-6-PD as markers of cellular origin in Burkitt lymphoma, *J. Exp. Med.* **138**:89–102.

Fialkow, P. J., Jacobson, R. J., and Papayannopoulou, T., 1977, Chronic myelocytic leukemia: Clonal origin in a stem cell common to the granulocyte, erythrocyte, platelet and monocyte/macrophage, *Am. J. Med.* **63**:125–130.

Fialkow, P. J., Denman, A. M., Jacobson, R. J., and Lowenthal, M. N., 1978, Chronic myelocytic leukemia: Origin of some lymphocytes from leukemic stem cells, *J. Clin. Invest.* **62**:815–823.

Filippi, G., Rinaldi, A., Archidiancono, N., Rocchi, M., Balaza, I., and Siniscalco, M., 1983, Linkage between G6PD and fragile-X syndrome, *Am. J. Med. Genet.* **15**:113–119.

Fincham, J. R. S., Day P. R., and Radford, A., 1979, *Fungal Genetics*, 3rd ed., Blackwell Scientific Publications, Oxford.

Fiorelli, G., Finazzi, G., Manoussakis, C., Palomba, V., and Fenu, M. P., 1982, G6PD deficiency in Sardinia: Genetic heterogeneity and clinical implications, in: *Advances in Red Cell Biology* (D. J. Weatherall, ed.), pp. 399–408, Raven Press, New York.

Fisher, R. A., Putt, W., and Hackel, E., 1976, An investigation of the products of 53 gene loci in three species of wild Canidae: *Canis lupus, Canis latrans,* and *Canis familiaris, Biochem. Genet.* **14**:963–974.

Flynn, T. P., Johnson, G. J., and Allen, D. W., 1981, Mechanisms of decreased erythrocyte deformability and survival in glucose-6-phosphate dehydrogenase mutants, *Prog. Clin. Biol. Res.* **56**:231–245.

Fraenkel, D. G., 1968, Selection of *Escherichia coli* mutants lacking glucose-6-phosphate dehydrogenase or gluconate-6-phosphate dehydrogenase, *J. Bacteriol.* **95**:1267–1271.

Friedman, M. J., 1979, Oxidant damage mediates variant red cell resistance to malaria, *Nature* **280**:245–247.

Fujii, H., Miwa, S., Tani, K., Takegawa, S., Fujinami, N., Takahashi, K., Nakayama, S., Konno, M., and Sato, T., 1981, Glucose 6-phosphate dehydrogenase variants: A unique variant (G6PD Kobe) showed an extremely increased affinity for galactose 6-phosphate and a new variant (G6PD Sapporo) resembling G6PD Pea Ridge, *Hum. Genet.* **58**:405–407.

Funayama, S., Funayama, S., Ito, I. Y., and Veiga, L. A., 1977, *Trypanosoma cruzi:* Kinetic properties of glucose 6-phosphate dehydrogenase, *Exp. Parasitol.* **43**:376–381.

Gaetani, G. F., Parker, J. C., and Kirkman, N. H., 1974, Intracellular restraint: A new basis for the limitation in response to oxidative stress in human erythrocytes containing low-activity variants of glucose-6-phosphate dehydrogenase, *Proc. Natl. Acad. Sci. USA* **71**:3584–3587.

Gaetani, G. F., Mareni, C., Salvidio, E., Gatiano, S., Meloni, T., and Arese, P., 1979, Favism: Erythrocyte metabolism during haemolysis and reticulocytosis, *Br. J. Haematol.* **43**:39–48.

Gaetani, G. F., Ferraris, A. M., Galiano, S., Giuntini, P., Canepa, L., and D'Urso, M., 1982, Primary thrombocythemia: Clonal origin of platelets, erythrocytes and granulocytes in a Gd^B/Gd^Mediterranean subject, *Blood* **59**:76–79.

Garcia-Bunuel, L., and Garcia-Bunuel, V. M., 1980, Connective tissue metabolism in normal and atrophic skeletal muscle, *J. Neurosci.* **47**:69–77.

Gartler, S. M., and Andina, R. J., 1976, Mammalian X-chromosome inactivation, in: *Advances in Human Genetics,* Vol. 7 (H. Harris and K. Hirschhorn, eds.), pp. 99–140, Plenum Press, New York.

Gartler, S. M., and Cole, R. E., 1981, Recent developments in the study of mammalian X-chromosome inactivation, in: *Mechanisms of Sex Differentiation in Animals and Man* (C. R. Austin and R. G. Edwards, eds.), pp. 113–143, Academic Press, New York.

Gartler, S. M., Hornung, S. K., and Motulsky, A. G., 1981, Effect of chronologic age on induction of cystathione synthase, uroporphyrinogen. I. Synthase, and glucose 6-phosphate dehydrogenase activities in lymphocytes, *Proc. Natl. Acad. Sci. USA* **78**:1916–1919.

Gartside, D. F., Dessauer, H. C., and Joanen, T., 1977, Genic homozygosity in an ancient reptile *(Alligator mississippiensis), Biochem. Genet.* **15**:655–854.

Gasperi, G., Malacrida, A., Cima, L., Sacchi, L., and Grigolo, A., 1978, The *in vitro* conversion of a specific molecular form of glucose-6-phosphate dehydrogenase from *Musca domestica* L., *J. Histochem. Cytochem.* **26**:850–854.

Gealy, W. J., Dwyer, J. M., and Harley, J. B., 1980, Allelic exclusion of glucose-6-phosphate dehydrogenase in platelets and T lymphocytes from a Wiskott–Aldrich syndrome carrier, *Lancet* **i**:63–65.

Geer, B. W., Bowman, J. T., and Simmons, J. R., 1974, The pentose phosphate shunt in the wild type and glucose-6-phosphate deficient *Drosophila melanogaster*, *J. Exp. Zool.* **187**:77–86.

Geer, B. W., Kamiak, S. N., Kidd, K. R., Nishimura, R. A., and Yemm, S. J., 1976, Regulation of the oxidative NADP-enzyme tissue levels in *Drosophila melanogaster*. I. Modulation by dietary carbohydrate and lipid, *J. Exp. Zool.* **195**:15–32.

Geer, B. W., Woodward, C. G., and Marshall, S. D., 1978, Regulation of the oxidative NADP-enzyme tissue levels in *Drosophila melanogaster*. II. The biochemical basis of dietary carbohydrate and D-glycerate modulation, *J. Exp. Zool.* **203**:391–402.

Geer, B. W., Lindel, D. L., and Lindel, D. M., 1979, Relationships of oxidative pentose phosphate pathway to lipid synthesis in *Drosophila melanogaster*, *Biochem. Genet.* **17**:881–895.

Gelpi, A. P., and King, M. C., 1977, New data on glucose-6-phosphate dehydrogenase deficiency in Saudi Arabia: G6PD variants, and the association between enzyme deficiency and hemoglobin S, *Hum. Hered.* **27**:285–291.

Gherardi, M., Bierme, R., Corrand, J., Pris, J., and Vergnes, H., 1976, Distribution of G6PD types in the population of Southwest France: Common variants and new variants, *Hum. Hered.* **26**:279–289.

Gibbs, W. N., Gray, R., and Lowry, M., 1979, Glucose-6-phosphate dehydrogenase deficiency and neonatal jaundice in Jamaica, *Br. J. Haematol.* **43**:263–274.

Gibbs, W. N., Wardle, J., and Sergeant, G. R., 1980, Glucose-6-phosphate dehydrogenase deficiency and homozygous sickle cell disease in Jamaica, *Br. J. Haematol.* **45**:73–80.

Gill, P., 1981, Enzyme variation in the grasshopper *Chorthippus brunneus* (Thunberg), *Biol. J. Linn. Soc.* **15**:247–258.

Glock, G. E., and McLean, P., 1953, Further studies on the properties and assay of glucose-6-phosphate dehydrogenase of rat liver, *Biochem. J.* **55**:400–408.

Glock, G. E., and McLean, P., 1954, Levels of enzymes of the direct oxidative pathway of carbohydrate metabolism in mammalian tissues and tumours, *Biochem. J.* **56**:171–175.

Gloria-Bottini, F., Falsi, A. M., Mortera, J., and Bottini, E., 1980, The relations between G-6-PD deficiency, thalassemia and malaria. Further analysis of data from Sardinia and the Po Valley, *Experientia* **36**:541–543.

Goldstein, L., and Gartler, S. M., 1979, The irreversibility of subunit associations in glucose-6-phosphate dehydrogenase and a suggestion regarding an early step in cellular morphogenesis, *Exp. Cell Res.* **122**:185–190.

Goman, M., Langley, G., Hyde, J. E., Yankovsky, N. K., Zolg, J. W., and Scaife, J. G., 1982, The establishment of genomic DNA libraries for the human malaria parasite *Plasmodium falciparum;* identification of individual clones by hybridisation, *Mol. Biochem. Parasitol.* **5**:391–400.

Goubern, M., and Portet, R., 1981, Modulation of malic enzyme and glucose-6-phosphate dehydrogenase activities in some tissues of cold acclimated rats, *Comp. Biochem. Physiol.* **69B**:237–241.

Graves, J. E., and Somero, G. N., 1982, Electrophoretic and functional isozymic evolution in four species of Eastern Pacific barracudas from different thermal environments, *Evolution* **36**:97–106.

Gray, G. R., Klebanoff, S. J., Stamatoyannopoulos, G., Austin, T., Naiman, S. C., Yoshida, A., Kliman, M. R., and Robinson, G. C. F., 1973, Neutrophil dysfunction, chronic granulomatous disease, and non-spherocytic haemolytic anaemia caused by complete deficiency of glucose-6-phosphate dehydrogenase, *Lancet* ii:530–534.

Grech, J. L., and Vicatou, M., 1973, Glucose-6-phosphate dehydrogenase deficiency in Maltese newborn infants, *Br. J. Haematol.* 25:261–269.

Green, C. D., Skarda, J., and Barry, J. M., 1971, Regulation of glucose 6-phosphate dehydrogenase formation in mammary organ culture, *Biochim. Biophys. Acta* 244:377–387.

Greenbaum, I. F., and Baker, R. J., 1976, Evolutionary relationships in macrotus *(Mammalia chiroptera):* Biochemical variation and karyology, *Syst. Zool.* 25:15–25.

Guggenmoos-Holzmann, I., Bienzle, U., and Luzzatto, L., 1981, *Plasmodium falciparum* malaria and human red cells. II. Red cell genetic traits and resistance against malaria, *Int. J. Epidemiol.* 10:16–22.

Guries, R. P., and Ledig, T. F. 1982, Genetic diversity and population structure in pitch pine *(Pinus rigida* mill.), *Evolution* 36:387–402.

Gvozdev, V. A., Gerasimova, T. I., Kogan, G. L., and Braslavskaya, O. Y., 1976, Role of the pentose phosphate pathway in metabolism of *Drosophila melanogaster* elucidated by mutations affecting glucose-6-phosphate and 6-phosphogluconate dehydrogenases, *FEBS Lett.* 64:85–88.

Gvozdev, V. A., Gerasimova, T. I., Kogan, G. L., and Rosovsky, J. M., 1977, Investigations on the organization of genetic loci in *Drosophila melanogaster:* Lethal mutations affecting 6-phosphogluconate dehydrogenase and their suppression, *Mol. Gen. Genet.* 153:191–198.

Haghighi, B., and Levy, H. R., 1982a, Glucose-6-phosphate dehydrogenase from *Leuconostoc mesenteroides.* Conformational transitions induced by nicotinamide adenine dinucleotide, nicotinamide adenine dinucleotide phosphate, and glucose 6-phosphate monitored by fluorescent probes, *Biochemistry* 21:5421–6428.

Haghighi, B., and Levy, H. R., 1982b, Glucose-6-phosphate dehydrogenase from *Leuconostoc mesenteroides.* Kinetics of reassociation and reactivation from inactive subunits, *Biochemistry* 21:6429–6434.

Halliday, R. B., 1981, Heterogeneity and genetic distance in sibling species of meat ants *(Iridomyrmex purpureus* group), *Evolution* 35:234–242.

Hedayat, Sh., Farhud, D. D., Montazami, K., and Ghadirian, P., 1981, The pattern of bean consumption, laboratory findings in patients with favism, G6PD deficient, and a control group, *J. Trop. Pediatr.* 27:110–113.

Hemplemann, E., and Wilson, R. J. M., 1981, Detection of glucose-6-phosphate dehydrogenase in malarial parasites, *Mol. Biochem. Parasitol.* 2:197–2004.

Hiernaux, J., 1976, Blood polymorphism frequencies in the Sara Majingay of Chad, *Ann. Hum. Biol.* 3:127–140.

Hilf, R., Ichowica, R., Bartley, J. C., and Abraham, S., 1975, Multiple molecular form of glucose-6-phosphate dehydrogenase in normal, preneoplastic and neoplastic tissues in mice, *Cancer Res.* 35:2109–2116.

Hitzeroth, H.. W., and Bender, K., 1980, Erythrocyte glucose 6 phosphate dehydrogenase and 6 phosphogluconate dehydrogenase genetic polymorphisms in South African Negroes, with a note on G-6-PD and the malaria hypothesis, *Hum. Genet.* 54:233–242.

Hitzeroth, H. W., and Bender, K., 1981, Age-dependency of somatic selection in South African Negro G-6-PD heterozygotes, *Hum. Genet.* 58:338–343.

Hizi, A., and Yagil, G., 1974a, On the mechanism of glucose-6-phosphate dehydrogenase regulation in mouse liver. 2. Purification and properties of the mouse liver enzyme, *Eur. J. Biochem.* 45:201–209.

Hizi, A., and Yagil, G., 1974b, On the mechanism of glucose-6-phosphate dehydrogenase regulation in mouse liver. 3. The rate of enzyme synthesis and degradation, *Eur. J. Biochem.* **45**:211–221.

Hofmann, J., Bosia, A., Arese, P., Losche, W., Pescarmona, G. P., Tazartos, O., and Till, U., 1981, Glucose-6-phosphate dehydrogenase deficiency in human platelets and its effect on platelet aggregation, *Acta Biol. Med. Germ.* **40**:1707–1714.

Holliday, R., and Tarrant, G. M., 1972, Altered enzymes in aging human fibroblasts, *Nature* **238**:26–30.

Holliday, R., and Thompson, K. V. A., 1983, Genetic effects on the longevity of cultured human fibroblasts. III. Correlations with altered glucose-6-phosphate dehydrogenase, *Gerontology* **29**:89–96.

Hori, S. H., and Matsui, M., 1967, Effects of hormones on hepatic glucose-6-phosphate dehydrogenase of rat, *J. Hystochem. Cytochem.* **15**:530–534.

Hori, S. H., and Tanda, S., 1980, Purification and properties of wild type and mutant glucose 6 phosphate dehydrogenase and 6-phosphogluconate dehydrogenase from *Drosophila melanogaster, Jpn. J. Genet.* **55**:211–223.

Hori, S. H., Yonezawa, S., Mochizuki, Y., Sado, Y., and Kamada, T., 1975, Evolutionary aspects of animal glucose 6-phosphate dehydrogenase isozymes, in: *Isozymes. IV. Genetics and Evolution* (C. L. Markert, ed.), pp. 839–852, Academic Press, New York.

Hughes, B. M., and Lucchesi, J. C., 1977, Genetic rescue of a lethal "null" activity allele for 6-phosphogluconate dehydrogenase in *Drosophila melanogaster, Science* **196**:1114–1115.

Hunter, L., 1980, Glucose-6-phosphate dehydrogenase isoenzymes in cultured human cell lines: Separation by isoelectric focusing, *Anal. Biochem.* **101**:78–87.

Iritani, N., Fukuda, H., and Fukuda, E., 1981, Age-dependent modifications of lipogenic enzymes, *Biochim. Biophys. Acta* **665**:636–639.

Jansson, S.-E., Hekali, R., Gripenberg, J., Härkönen, M., and Vuopio, P., 1980, Membrane characteristics and metabolic properties of glucose-6-phosphate dehydrogenase deficient red cells, *Br. J. Haematol.* **46**:79–87.

Jenkins, T., Harpending, H. C., Gordon, H., Keraan, M. M., and Johnston, S., 1971, Red-cell-enzyme polymorphisms in the Khoisan peoples of Southern Africa, *Am. J. Hum. Genet.* **23**:513–532.

Jenkins, T., Lane, A. B., Nurse, G. T., and Tanaka, J., 1975, Sero-genetic studies on the G/wi and G//ana San of Botswana, *Hum. Hered.* **25**:318–328.

Johnson, B. C., and Sassoon, H. F., 1967, Studies on the induction of liver glucose-6-phosphate dehydrogenase in the rat, in: *Advances in Enzyme Regulation,* Vol. 5 (G. Weber, ed.), pp. 93–106, Pergamon Press, Oxford.

Johnson, G. J., Allen, D. W., Cadman, S., Fairbanks, V. F., White, J. G., Lampkin, B. C., and Kaplan, M. E., 1979, Red-cell-membrane polypeptide aggregates in glucose-6-phosphate dehydrogenase mutants with chronic hemolytic disease. A clue to the mechanism of hemolysis, *N. Engl. J. Med.* **301**:522–527.

Johnson, M. S., and Michevich, M. F., 1977, Variability and evolutionary rates of characters, *Evolution* **31**:642–648.

Johnson, M. S., Clarke, B., and Murray, J., 1977, Genetic variation and reproductive isolation in *Partula, Evolution* **31**:115–126.

Jones, J. T., and Andrews, S. J., 1978, Glucose 6 phosphate dehydrogenase activity in somatic and germinal cells of mouse testis, *J. Reprod. Fertil.* **54**:357–362.

Kahan, B., and De Mars, R., 1975, Localized depression on the human inactive X chromosome in mouse–human cell hybrids, *Proc. Natl. Acad. Sci. USA* **72**:1510–1514.

Kahler, S. G., and Kirkman, H. N., 1983, Intracellular glucose-6-phosphate dehydrogenase does not monomerize in human erythrocytes, *J. Biol. Chem.* **258**:717–718.

Kahn, S., 1978, G6PD variants, *Hum. Genet. (Suppl. 1)* **1978**:37–44.

Kahn, A., Boivin, P., and Lagneau, J., 1973, Phénotypes de la glucose-6-phosphate déshydrogénase érythrocytaire dans la race noire. Étude de 301 noirs vivant en France et description de 9 variantes différentes. Fréquence élevée d'une enzyme déficitaire de migration "B," *Humangenetik* **18**:261–270.

Kahn, A., Guillonzo, A., Liebovitch, M. P., Cottreau, D., Bouvel, M., and Dreyfus, J.-C., 1977, Heat lability of G6PD in some senescent human cultured cells. Evidence for its post-synthetic nature, *Biochem. Biophys. Res. Commun.* **77**:760–766.

Kamel, K., 'Umar, M., Ibrahim, W., Mansour, A., Gaballah, F., Selim, O., Azim, A., Hamza, S., Sabry, F., Moafy, N., El-Naggar, A., and Hoerman, K., 1975, Anthropological studies among Lybians. Erythrocyte genetic factors, serum haptoglobins phenotypes and anthropometry, *Am. J. Phys. Anthropol.* **43**:103–111.

Karayalcin, G., Acs, H., and Lanzkowsky, P., 1979, G-6-PD deficiency and hyperbilirubinemia: In black American full-term infants, *N.Y. State J. Med.* **1979**(January):22–24.

Kato, N., Sahm, H., Schütte, H., and Wagner, F., 1979, Purification and properties of glucose-6-phosphate dehydrogenase and 6-phosphogluconate dehydrogenase from a methanol-utilizing yeast, *Candida boidinii, Biochim. Biophys. Acta* **566**:1–11.

Kazazian, H. H. J. R., Young, W. J., and Childs, B., 1965, X linked 6-phosphogluconate dehydrogenase in *Drosophila:* Subunit associations, *Science* **150**:1601.

Keats, B., 1983, Genetic mapping: X chromosome, *Hum. Genet.* **64**:28–32.

Kelley, D. S., Watson, J. J., Mack, D. O., and Johnson, B. C., 1975, Glucose-6-phosphate dehydrogenase is not induced in mammalian liver by dietary carbohydrate, *Nutr. Rep. Int.* **12**:121–135.

Kirkman, H.N., 1971, Glucose-6-phosphate dehydrogenase, in: *Advances in Human Genetics,* Vol. 2 (H. Harris and K. Hirschhorn, eds.), pp. 1–60, Plenum Press, New York.

Kirkman, H. N., and Lie-Injo, L. E., 1969, Variants of G6PD in Indonesia, *Nature* **221**:959.

Kirkman, H. N., Doxiadis, S. A., Valaes, T., Tassopoulos, N., and Brinson, A. G., 1965, Diverse characteristics of glucose-6-phosphate dehydrogenase from Greek children, *J. Lab. Clin. Med.* **65**:212–221.

Kirkman, H. N., Wilson, W. G., and Clemons, E. H., 1980, Regulation of glucose-6-phosphate dehydrogenase. I. Intact red cells, *J. Lab. Clin. Med.* **95**:877–887.

Komma, D. J., 1966, Effect of sex transformation genes on glucose-6-phosphate dehydrogenase activity in *Drosophila melanogaster, Genetics* **54**:497–503.

Komma, D. J., 1968*a*, Glucose-6-phosphate dehydrogenase in *Drosophila:* A sex-influenced electrophoretic variant, *Biochem. Genet.* **1**:229–237.

Komma, D. J., 1968*b*, Glucose-6-phosphate dehydrogenase in *Drosophila:* Sexual effect on structure, *Biochem. Genet.* **1**:337–346.

Krahl, M. E., Keltch, A. K., Walters, C. P., and Clowes, G. H. A., 1955, Glucose-6-phosphate and 6-phosphogluconate dehydrogenases from egg of the sea urchin, *Arbacia punctulata, J. Gen. Physiol.* **38**:431–439.

Kukulansky, T., and Yagil, G., 1979, On the effect of insulin on glucose-6-phosphate dehydrogenase and fatty acid synthetase activity in mouse liver, *Horm. Metab. Res.* **11**:14–19.

Kurtz, J. W., and Wells, W. W., 1981, Induction of glucose-6-phosphate dehydrogenase in primary cultures of adult rat hepatocytes. Requirement for insulin and dexamethasone, *J. Biol. Chem.* **256**:10870–10875.

Lampe, R. M., Kirdpon, S., and Mansuwan, P., 1975, G6PD deficiency in Thai children with typhoid, *J. Pediatr.* **87**:576–585.

Landi, A. P., Altman, F. P., Pringle, J., and Landi, A., 1980, Oxidative enzyme metabolism in rabbit intrasynovial flexor tendons. I. Changes in enzyme activity of tenocytes with age, *J. Surg. Res.* **29**:276–280.

Larson, A., 1980, Paedomorphosis in relation to rates of morphological and molecular evolution in the salamander *Aneides flavipunctatus (Amphibia Plethodontidae), Evolution* **34**:1–17.

Laudenslager, E. J., 1978, Variation in the genetic structure of *Peromyscus* populations. I. Genetic heterozygosity—its relationship to adaptive divergence, *Biochem. Genet.* **16**:1165.

Lawrie Ahlberg, C. C., Maroni, G., Bewley, G. C., Lucchesi, J. C., and Weir, B. S., 1980, Quantitative genetic variation of enzyme activities in natural populations of *Drosophila melanogaster, Proc. Natl. Acad. Sci. USA* **77**:1073–1077.

Lawrie-Ahlberg, C. C., Williamson, J. H., Cochrane, B. J., Wilton, A. N., and Chasalow, F. I., 1981, Autosomal factors with correlated effects on the activities of glucose-6-phosphate and 6-phosphogluconate dehydrogenases in *Drosophila melanogaster, Genetics* **99**:127–150.

Leathem, J. H., and Appel, N. M., 1977, Adrenal and gonadal glucose-6-phosphate dehydrogenase activity in aging rats, *J. Endocrinol.* **75**:433–434.

Ledig, F. T., and Conkle, M. T., 1983, Gene diversity and genetic structure in a narrow endemic species, Torrey pine (*Pinus torreyana* Parry ex Carr) *Evolution* **37**:79–85.

Lee, C.-Y., Langley, C. H., and Burkhart, J., 1978, Purification and molecular weight determination of glucose-6-phosphate dehydrogenase and malic enzyme from mouse and *Drosophila, Anal. Biochem.* **86**:697–706.

Lee, C.-Y., Yuan, J. H., Moser, D., and Kramer, J. M., 1979, Purification and characterization of mouse glucose-6-phosphate dehydrogenase, *Mol. Cell. Biochem.* **24**:67–73.

Lefèvre-Witier, P., and Vergnes, H., 1977, Enzyme polymorphisms of Ideles populations (Ahaggar, Algeria) and the Iwellemeden Kel Kummer Twaregs (Menaka, Mali), *Hum. Hered.* **27**:454–469.

Le Gall, J. Y., le Gall, M., Godin, Y., and Serre, J. L., 1982, A study of genetic markers of the blood in four Central African population groups, *Hum. Hered.* **32**:418–427.

Lendzian, K., and Bassham, J. A., 1975, Regulation of G6PD in spinach chloroplasts by ribulose 1,5 diphosphate and NADPH/NADP$^+$ ratios, *Biochim. Biophys. Acta* **396**:260–275.

Lenzerini, L., Khan, P. M., Filippi, G., Rattazzi, M. C., Ray, A. K., and Siniscalco, M., 1969, Characterization of glucose-6-phosphate dehydrogenase variants. I. Occurrence of a G6PD Seattle-like variant in Sardinia and its interaction with the G6PD Mediterranean variant, *Am. J. Hum. Genet.* **21**:142–153.

Lester, L. J., and Selander, R. K., 1979, Population genetics of haplodiploid insects, *Genetics* **92**:1329–1345.

Lester, S. C., Korn, N. J., and DeMars, R., 1982, Derepression of genes on the human inactive X chromosome: Evidence for differences in locus-specific rates of derepression and rates of transfer of active and inactive genes after DNA-mediated transformation, *Somat. Cell Genet.* **8**:265–284.

Levin, D. A., 1977, The organization of genetic variability in *Phlox drummondii, Evolution* **31**:477–494.

Levin, D. A., 1978, Genetic variation in annual *Phlox:* Self-compatible versus self-incompatible species, *Evolution* **32**:245–263.

Levy, H. R., 1979, Glucose-6-phosphate dehydrogenases, in: *Advances in Enzymology,* Vol. 48 (A. Meister, ed.), pp. 97–192, Wiley, New York.

Lewis, R. A., Kay, R. W., and Hathorn, M., 1966, Sickle cell disease and glucose-6-phosphate dehydrogenase, *Acta Haematol.* **35**:399–410.

Lie-Injo,L. E., 1969, Distribution of genetic red cell defects in South-East Asia, *Trans. R. Soc. Trop. Med. Hyg.* **63**:664–674.

Linder, D., and Gartler, S. M., 1965, Glucose-6-phosphate dehydrogenase mosaicism. Utilization of a cell marker in the study of leiomyomas, *Science* **150**:67–69.

Listay, R. M., and Evans, R. J., 1980, Inactive X chromosome DNA does not function in DNA-mediated cell transformation for hypoxanthine phosphoribosyltransferase gene, *Proc. Natl. Acad. Sci. USA* **77**:4895–4898.

Livingstone, F. B., 1967, *Abnormal Hemoglobins in Human Populations,* Aldine, Chicago.

Livingstone, D. R., 1981, Induction of enzymes as a mechanism for the seasonal control of metabolism in marine invertebrates: G6PD from the mantle and hepatopancreas of the common mussel *Mytilus edulis L, Comp. Biochem. Physiol.* **69B**:147–156.

Lobo, Z., and Maitra, P. K., 1982, Pentose phosphate pathway mutants of yeast, *Mol. Gen. Genet.* **185**:367–368.

Lucchesi, J. C., and Rawls, J. M., Jr., 1973, Regulation of gene function: A comparison of enzyme activity levels in relation to gene dosage in diploids and triploids of *Drosophila melanogaster, Biochem. Genet.* **9**:41–51.

Lucchesi, J. C., Rawls, J. M., and Maroni, G., 1974, Gene dosage compensation in metafemales (3X:2A) of *Drosophila, Nature* **248**:564–567.

Lucchesi, J. C., Belote, J. M., and Maroni, G., 1977, X linked gene activity in metamales (XY:3A) of *Drosophila, Chromosoma* **65**:1–7.

Lucotte, G., 1979, Génétique des populations, spéciation et taxonomie chez les babouins: II. Similitudes génétiques comparées entre différentes espéces: *Papio papio, P. anubis, P. cynocephalus,* et *P. hamadryas* basées sur les données du polymorphisme des enzymes erythrocytaires, *Biochem. Syst. Ecol.* **7**:245–251.

Lucotte, G., 1980, Polymorphisme électrophorétique des protéines et enzymes sériques et érythrocytaires chez le Chimpanzé *(Pan troglodytes), Hum. Genet.* **54**:97–102.

Lucotte, G., and Ruffié, J., 1982, Variation électrophorétique et spéciation chez les différentes espèces de singes anthropoides, *Hum. Genet.* **61**:310–317.

Luzzatto, L., 1967, Regulation of the activity of glucose 6 phosphate dehydrogenase by NADP$^+$ and NADPH, *Biochem. Biophys. Acta* **146**:18–25.

Luzzatto, L., 1972, Genetics and biochemistry of glucose 6-phosphate dehydrogenase variants in Nigeria, in: *VI. Internationales Symposium über Struktur und Funktion der Erythrocyten, Berlin, 1970, pp. 267–272, Akademie-Verlag, Berlin.*

Luzzatto, L., 1973a, Studies of polymorphic traits for the characterization of populations: African populations South of the Sahara, *Is. J. Med. Sci.* **9**:1181–1194.

Luzzatto, L., 1973b, New developments in G6PD deficiency, *Is. J. Med. Sci.* **9**:1484–1498.

Luzzatto, L., 1974, Genetic factors in malaria, *Bull. WHO* **50**:195–202.

Luzzatto, L., 1975, Inherited haemolytic states: Glucose 6-phosphate dehydrogenase deficiency, *Clin. Hematol.* **4**:83–108.

Luzzatto, L., 1979, Genetics of red cell and susceptibility to malaria, *Blood* **54**:961–976.

Luzzatto, L., 1980, Genetics of human red cells and susceptibility to malaria, in: *Modern Genetic Concepts and Techniques in the Study of Parasites* (F. Michal, ed.), Tropical Diseases Research Series No. 4, pp. 257–274, Schwabe & Co. Basel.

Luzzatto, L., and Afolayan, A., 1971, Genetic variants of human erythrocyte glucose 6-phosphate dehydrogenase. II. *In vitro* and *in vivo* function of the A⁻ variant, *Biochemistry* **10**:420–424.

Luzzatto, L., and Allan, N. C., 1965, Different properties of glucose 6-phosphate dehydrogenase from human erythrocytes with normal and abnormal enzyme levels, *Biochem. Biophys. Res. Commun.* **21**:547–554.

Luzzatto, L., and Bienzle, U., 1979, The malaria/G6PD hypothesis, *Lancet* **i**:1183–1184.

Luzzatto, L., and Gartler, S. M., 1983, Switching off blocks of genes, *Nature* **301**:375.

Luzzatto, L., and Lewis, E. A., 1972, Acute erythraemic myelosis in Ibadan, *Dokita (J. Univ. Ibadan Med. Students Assoc.)* **1972**(June).

Luzzatto, L., and Testa, U., 1978, Human erythrocyte glucose 6-phosphate dehydrogenase: Structure and function in normal and mutant subjects, *Curr. Top. Hematol.* **1**:1–70.

Luzzatto, L., Usanga, E. A., Bienzle, U., Esan, G. F. J., and Fasuan, F. A., 1979a, Imbalance in X-chromosome expression: Evidence for a human X-linked gene affecting growth of hemopoietic cells, *Science* **205**:1418–1420.

Luzzatto, L., Familusi, J. B., Williams, C. K. O., Junaid, T. A., Rotoli, B., and Alfinito, F., 1979b, The PNH abnormality in myeloproliferative disorders: Association of PNH and acute erythremic myelosis in two children, *Haematologica* **64**:13–30.

Luzzatto, L., Sodeinde, O., and Martini, G., 1983, Genetic variation in the hose and adaptive phenomena in *Plasmodium falciparum* infection, in: *Malaria and the Red Cell*, Ciba Foundation Symposium, pp. 159–173, Pitman, London.

Lyon, M. F., 1961, Gene action in the X chromosome of the mouse, *Nature* **190**:372–373.

Madvig, P., and Abraham, S., 1980, Enzyme activities during development of some organs of the rat, *J. Nutr.* **110**:100–104.

Maroni, G., and Plaut, W., 1973, Dosage compensation in *Drosophila melanogaster* triploids. II. Glucose 6 phosphate dehydrogenase activity, *Genetics* **74**:331–342.

Martin, G. R., 1982, X-chromosome inactivation in mammals, *Cell* **29**:721–724.

Martin, S. K., Miller, L. H., Alling, D., Okoye, V. C., Esan, G. J. F., Osunkoya, B. O., and Deane, M., 1979, Severe malaria and glucose-6-phosphate dehydrogenase: A reappraisal of the malaria/G6PD hypothesis, *Lancet* **i**:524–526.

Martin-DeLeon, P. A., Wolf, S. F., Persico, M. G., Toniolo, D., and Migeon, B. R., 1984, Localization of the G6PD locus in mouse and man by *in situ* hybridization: further evidence for an inverted order of homologous X-linked genes, *Somatic Cell Genet.*, in press.

Mashburn, S. J., Sharitz, R. R., and Smith, M. H., 1978, Genetic variation among *Typha* populations of the Southeastern United States, *Evolution* **32**:681–685.

Mathai, C. K., Ohno, S., and Beuter, E., 1966, Sex linkage of the glucose 6 phosphate dehydrogenase gene in *Equidae, Nature* **210**:115–116.

Matsuoka, N., and Hori, S. H., 1980, Immunological relatedness of hexose 6-phosphate dehydrogenase and glucose 6-phosphate dehydrogenase in echinoderms, *Comp. Biochem. Physiol.* **65B**:191–198.

Max, S. R., and Knudsen, J. F., 1980, Effect of sex hormones on glucose-6-phosphate dehydrogenase in rat levator ani muscle, *Mol. Cell. Endocrinol.* **17**:111–118.

McCracken, G. F., and Brussard, P., 1980, The population biology of the white-lipped land snail *Triodopsis albolabris:* Genetic variability, *Evolution* **34**:92–104.

McCurdy, P. R., and Mahmood, L., 1970, Red cell glucose-6-phosphate dehydrogenase deficiency in Pakistan, *J. Lab. Clin. Med.* **76**:943–948.

McCurdy, P. R., Kirkman, H. N., Naiman, J. L., Jim, R. T. S., and Pickard, B. M., 1966, A Chinese variant of G6PD, *J. Lab. Clin. Med.* **67**:374.

McCurdy, P. R., Blackwell, R. Q., Todd, D., Tso, S. C., and Tuchinda, S., 1970, Further studies on glucose-6-phosphate dehydrogenase deficiency in Chinese subjects, *J. Lab. Clin. Med.* **75**:788–797.

McCurdy, P. R., Schneer, J. H., and Hansen, I. M., 1972, Red cell glucose-6-phosphate dehydrogenase variants in Rumania, *Rev. Eur. Études Clin. Biol.* **17**:66–69.

McCurdy, P. R., Maldonado, N., Dillon, D. E., and Conrad, M. E., 1973, Variants of glucose

6 phosphae dehydrogenase (G6PD) associated with G6PD deficiency in Puerto Ricans, *J. Lab. Clin. Med.* **82**:432–437.

McCurdy, P. R., Kamel, K., and Selim, O., 1974, Heterogeneity of red cell glucose-6-phosphate dehydrogenase (G-6-PD) deficiency in Egypt, *J. Lab. Clin. Med.* **84**:673–680.

McKusick, V. A., 1978, *Mendelian Inheritance in Man. Catalogue of Autosomal Dominant, Autosomal Recessive and X Linked Phenotypes,* 5th ed., Johns Hopkins University Press, Baltimore.

McLoughlin, K., Blake, N. M., Korarome, J., and Alpers, W., 1982, Blood group, red cell enzyme and serum protein types in an Asaro village, Eastern Highlands, Papua New Guinea, *Hum. Hered.* **32**:160–165.

Meloni, T., Cagnazzo, G., Dore, A., and Cutillo, S., 1973, Phenobarbital for prevention of hyperbilirubinaemia in glucose-6-phosphate dehydrogenase-deficient newborn infants, *J. Pediatr.* **82**:1048–1051.

Metcalf, R. A., Marlin, J. C., and Whitt, G. S., 1975, Low level of genetic heterozygosity in hymenoptera, *Nature* **257**:792–794.

Migeon, B. R., Norum, R. A., and Corsaro, C. M., 1974, Isolation and analysis of somatic hybrids derived from two human diploid cells, *Proc. Nat. Acad. Sci. USA* **71**:937–941.

Migeon, B. R., Sprenkle, J. A., and Do, T. T., 1979, Stability of the "two active X" phenotype in triploid somatic cells, *Cell* **18**:637–641.

Migeon, B. R., Wolf, S. F., Mareni, C., and Axelman, J., 1982*a*, Depression with decreased expression of the *G6PD* locus on the inactive X chromosome in normal human cells, *Cell* **29**:595–600.

Migeon, B. R., Moser, H. W., Moser, A. B., Axelman, J. A., Sillence, D., and Norum, R. A., 1982*b*, Linkage between loci for adrenoleukodystrophy (ALD) and G6PD, Human Gene Mapping 6: Oslo Conference (1981) (Abstract), *Cytogenet. Cell Genet.* **32**:298–299.

Milkman, R., 1975, Allozyme variation in *E. coli* of diverse natural origins, in: *Isozymes. IV. Genetics and Evolution* (C. L. Markert, ed.), pp. 274–285, Academic Press, New York.

Mita, M., and Yasumasu, I., 1980, Inhibition of glucose-6-phosphate dehydrogenase and 6-phosphogluconate dehydrogenase in sea urchin eggs by palmitoyl-coenzyme A and reversal by polyamines, *Arch. Biochem. Biophys.* **201**:322–329.

Miwa, S., 1980, Glucose 6-phosphate dehydrogenase variants in Japan, *Hemoglobin* **4**:781–787.

Miwa, S., 1981, Pyruvate kinase deficiency and other enzymopathies of the Embden-Meyerhof pathway, *Clin. Haematol.* **10**:57–80.

Modiano, G., 1976, Genetically determined quantitative protein variations in man, excluding immunoglobulins, *Mem. Acc. Naz. Lincei Ser. 8* **13**:55–437.

Modiano, G., Battistuzzi, G., Esan, G. J. F., Testa, U., and Luzzatto, L., 1979, Genetic heterogeneity of "normal" human erythrocyte glucose-6-phosphate dehydrogenase: An isoelectrophoretic polymorphism, *Proc. Natl. Acad. Sci. USA* **76**:852–856.

Mohandas, T., Sparkes, R. S., Hellkuhl, B., Grzeschik, K. H., and Shapiro, L. J., 1980, Expression of an X-linked gene from an inactive human X chromosome in mouse–human hybrid cells: Further evidence for the noninactivation of the steroid sulfatase locus in man, *Proc. Natl. Acad. Sci. USA* **77**:6759–6763.

Mohandas, T., Sparkes, R. S., and Shapiro, L. J., 1981, Reactivation of an inactive human X chromosome: Evidence for X inactivation by DNA methylation, *Science* **211**:393–396.

Momen, H., 1979, Biochemistry of intraerythrocytic parasites. II. Comparative studies in carbohydrate metabolism, *Ann. Trop. Med. Parasitol.* **73**:117–121.

Momen, H., and Salles, C. A., 1981, An electrophoretic analysis of variation in the glucose-

6-phosphate dehydrogenase and malate dehydrogenase of *Vibrio colerae, Vibrio para-haemolyticus* and *Vibrio fluvialis, J. Appl. Bacteriol.* **51**:425–432.

Morelli, A., Benatti, U., Lenzerini, L., Sparatore, B., Salamino, F., Melloni, E., Michetti, M., Pontremoli, S., and De Flora, A., The interference of leukocytes and platelets with measurement of glucose-6-phosphate dehydrogenase activity of erythrocytes with low activity variants of the enzyme, *Blood* **58**:642–644.

Morellini, M., Colonna-Romano, S., Meloni, T., Battistuzzi, G., and Gandini, E., 1983, Glucose-6-phosphate dehydrogenase of leukocyte subpopulations in normal and enzyme deficient individuals, *Clin. Lab. Haematol.,* in press.

Mortlock, R., 1962, Gluconate metabolism of *Pasteurella pestis, J. Bacteriol.* **84**:53–59.

Mourant, A. E., Kopeć, A. C., and Domaniewska-Sobczak, K., 1976, *The Distribution of the Human Blood Groups and Other Polymorphisms,* 2nd ed., Oxford University Press, London.

Mourant, A. E., Tills, D., Kopeć, A. C., Warlow, A., Teesdale, P., Booth, P. B., and Hornabrook, R. W., 1981, Red cell antigen, serum protein, and red cell enzyme polymorphsms in inhabitants of the Jimi Valley, Western Highlands, New Guinea, *Hum. Genet.* **59**:77–80.

Mourant, A. E., Tills, D., Kopeć, A. C., Warlow, A., Teesdale, P., Booth, P. B., and Hornabrook, R. W., 1982, Red cell antigen, serum protein and red cell enzyme polymorphisms in Eastern Highlanders of New Guinea, *Hum. Hered.* **32**:374–384.

Muller, H. J., League, B. B., and Offerman, C. A., 1931, Effects of dosage changes of sex-linked genes and the compensatory effect of other gene differences between male and female, *Anat. Rec. Suppl.* **51**:110.

Nakamura, T., Yoshimoto, K., Aoyama, K., and Ichihara, A., 1982, Hormonal regulations of glucose-6-phosphate dehydrogenase and lipogenesis in primary cultures of rat hepatocytes, *J. Biochem.* **91**:681–693.

Nakatsuji, T., and Miwa, S., 1979, Incidence and characteristics of glucose-6-phosphate dehydrogenase variants in Japan, *Hum. Genet.* **51**:297–305.

Nance, W. E., 1967, Quantitative studies of G6PD in a Nigerian population, *Clin. Res.* **16**:66.

Nance, W. E., 1977, Quantitative studies of glucose 6-phosphate dehydrogenase, *Am. J. Hum. Genet.* **29**:537–543.

Naylor, J., Rosenthal, I., Grossman, A., Schulman, I., and Yi-Yung Hsia, D., 1960, Activity of glucose-6-phosphate dehydrogenase in erythrocytes of patients with abnormal hemoglobins, *Pediatrics* **26**:285–292.

Naylor, H. B., Fukin, G. M., and McDuff, C. R., 1961, Effect of temperature on growth and virulence of *Pasteurella pestis, J. Bacteriol.* **81**:649–655.

Nevo, E., 1978, Genetic variation in natural populations: Patterns and theory, *Theor. Popul. Biol.* **13**:121–177.

Nhonoli, A. M., Kujwalile, J. M., Kigoni, E. P., and Masawe, A. E. J., 1978, Correlation of glucose-6-phosphate dehydrogenase (G-6-PD) deficiency and sickle cell trait (Hb-AS), *Trop. Geogr. Med.* **30**:99–101.

Nobrega, F. G., Maia, J. C. C., Colli, W., and Saldanha, P. H., 1970, Heterogeneity of erythrocyte G6PD activity and electrophoretic patterns among representatives of different classes of vertebrates, *Comp. Bichem. Physiol.* **33**:191–199.

Nozawa, K., Takayashi, S., and Okura, Y., 1975, Blood protein polymorphisms and population structure of the Japanese Macaque, *Macaca fuscata fuscata,* in: *Isozymes. IV. Genetics and Evolution* (C. L. Markert, ed.), pp. 225–241, Academic Press, New York.

Nurse, G. T., and Jenkins, T., 1975, The Griqua of Campbell, Cape Province, South Africa, *Am. J. Anthropol.* **43**:71–78.

Nurse, G. T., Botha, M. C., and Jenkins, T., 1977, Sero-genetic studies on the San of South West Africa, *Hum. Hered.* **27**:81–98.

Nyhan, W. L., Bakay, B., Connor, J. D., Marks, J. F., and Keele, D. K., 1970, Hemizygous expression of glucose-6-phosphate dehydrogenase in erythrocytes of heterozygotes for Lesch–Nyhan syndrome, *Proc. Natl. Acad. Sci. USA* **65**:214–218.

Oakeshott, J. G., Chamber, G. K., Gibson, J. B., Eanes, W. F., and Willcocks, D. A., 1983, Geographic variation in G6PD and PGD allele frequencies in *Drosophila melanogaster, Heredity* **50**:67–72.

Ohnishi, K.-I., and Hori, S. H., 1977, A comparative study of invertebrate glucose 6-phosphate dehydrogenases, *Jpn. J. Genet.* **52**:95–106.

Ohno, S., Poole, J., and Gustavson, I., 1965, Sex linkage of erythrocyte G6PD in two species of wild hares, *Science* **150**:1737–1738.

Ohno, S., Payne, H. W., Morrison, M., and Beutler, E., 1966, Hexose-6-phosphate dehydrogenase found in human liver, *Science* **153**:1015–1016.

Oka, K.-I., Takahashi, T., and Hori, S. H., 1981, Differential effect of NADPH/NADP⁺ ratio on the activities of hexose-6-phosphate dehydrogenase and glucose-6-phosphate dehydrogenase, *Biochem. Biophys. Acta* **662**:318–325.

Oluboyede, O. A., Esan, G. J. F., Francis, T. I., and Luzzatto, L., 1979, Genetically determined deficiency of glucose-6-phosphate dehydrogenase (type A⁻) is expressed in the liver, *J. Lab. Clin. Med.* **93**:783–789.

Oni, S. B., Osunkoya, B. O., and Luzzatto, L., 1970, Paroxysmal nocturnal hemoglobinuria: Evidence for monoclonal origin of abnormal cells, *Blood* **36**:145–152.

Orgel, L. E., 1963, The maintenance of accuracy of protein synthesis and its relevance to aging, *Proc. Natl. Acad. Sci. USA* **49**:517–521.

Orzalesi, N., Sorcinelli, R., and Guiso, G., 1981, Increased incidence of cataracts in male subjects deficient in glucose-6-phosphate dehydrogenase, *Arch. Ophthalmol.* **99**:69–70.

Owusu, S. K., and Opare-Manta, A., 1972, Electrophoretic characterisation of glucose-6-phosphate dehydrogenase in Ghana, *Lancet* **ii**:44.

Ozsoylu, S., 1978, Sickle cell disease, G-6-PD deficiency, and jaundice, *J. Pediatr.* **93**:898.

Ozsoylu, S., and Altinoz, N., 1977, Sickle cell anaemia in Turkey, *Scand. J. Haematol.* **19**:85–92.

Pai, G. S., Sprenkle, J. A., Do, T. T., Mareni, C. E., and Migeon, B. R., 1980, Localization of loci for hypoxanthine phosphoriboxyltransferase and glucose-6-phosphate dehydrogenase and biochemical evidence of non-random X chromosome expression from studies of a human X-autosome translocation, *Proc. Natl. Acad. Sci. USA* **77**:2810–2813.

Palmour, R. M., Cronin, J. E., Childs, A., and Grunbaum, B. W., 1980, Studies of primate protein variation and evolution: Microelectrophoretic detection, *Biochem. Genet.* **18**:793–808.

Panich, V., 1973, The occurrence of G-6-PD Union in Thailand, *Humangenetik* **17**:169–171.

Panich, V., 1974, G-6-PD variants in Laotians, *Hum. Hered.* **24**:285–290.

Panich, V., 1980, Glucose-6-phosphate dehydrogenase in Thailand: The occurrence of three electrophoretic variants among 1157 nondeficient males, *Hum. Genet.* **53**:227–228.

Panich, V., 1981, Glucose-6-phosphate dehydrogenase deficiency, Part 2: Tropical Asia, *Clin. Haematol.* **10**:800–814.

Panich, V., 1982, Glucose-6-phosphate dehydrogenase deficiency: Genetic heterogeneity in Asia, in: *Advances in Red Cell Biology* (D. J. Weatherall, G. Fiorelli, and S. Gorino, eds.), pp. 329–338, Raven Press, New York.

Panich, V., and Na-Nakorn, S., 1980a, G-6-PD variants in Thailand, *J. Med. Assoc. Thailand* **63**:537–543.

Panich, V., and Na-Nakorn, S., 1980b, G6PD deficiency in senile cataracts, *Hum. Genet.* **55:**123–124.

Panich, V., and Sungnate, T., 1973, Characterization of glucose-6-phosphate dehydrogenase in Thailand. The occurrence of 6 variants among 50 G-6-PD deficient Thai, *Humangenetik* **18:**39–46.

Panich, V., Sungnate, T., and Pootrakul, P., 1972, Gilbert's syndrome associated with glucose 6-phosphate dehydrogenase deficiency, *J. Med. Assoc. Thailand* **55:**483–491.

Panich, V., Na-Nakorn, S., and Wasi, P. 1980a, G-6-PD variants in Chinese in Thailand, *Southeast Asian J. Trop. Med. Public Health* **11:**250–254.

Panich, V., Bumrungtrakul, P., Jitjai, C., Kamolmatayakul, S., Khoprasert, B., Klaisuvan, C., Kongmuang, U., Maneechai, P., Pornpatkul, M., Ruengrairatanoroje, P., Surapruk, P., and Viriyayudhakorn, S., 1980b, Glucose-6-phosphate dehydrogenase deficiency in South Vietnamese, *Hum. Hered.* **30:**361–364.

Panizon, F., 1960, Dimostrazione della anomalia enzimatica nel fegato di soggetti con difetto eritrocitario di glucoso-6-fosfato deidrogenasi, *Boll. Soc. Ital. Biol. Sper.* **36:**106–107.

Panizon, G., Zacchello, F., Sartori, A., and Addis, S., 1970, The ratio between normal and sensitive erythrocytes in heterozygous glucose-6-phosphate dehydrogenase deficient women, *Acta Haematol.* **43:**291–295.

Patton, J. L., Yong, S. Y., and Myers, P., 1975, Genetic and morphologic divergence among introduced rat populations *(Rattus rattus)* of the Galapagos Archipelago, Ecuador, *Syst. Zool.* **24:**296–310.

Perona, G., Guidi, G. C., Tummarello, D., Mareni, C., Battistuzzi, G., and Luzzatto, L., 1983, A new glucose 6-phosphate dehydrogenase variant (G-6-PD Verona) in a patient with myelodysplastic syndrome, *Scand. J. Haematol.* **30:**407–414.

Persico, M. G., Toniolo, D., Nobile, C., D'Urso, M., and Luzzatto, L., 1981, cDNA sequences of human glucose 6-phosphate dehydrogenase cloned in pBR322, *Nature* **294:**778–780.

Persico, M., Battistuzzi, G., Mareni, C., Nobile, C., D'Urso, M., Toniolo, D., and Luzzatto, L., 1982, Genetic variants of human glucose 6-phosphate dehydrogenase (G6PD): Studies of turnover and of G6PD-specific mRNA, in: *Advances in Red Cell Biology* (D. J. Weatherall, G. Fiorelli, and S. Gorini, eds.), pp. 309–318, Raven Press, New York.

Piazza, A., Belvedere, M. C., Bernoco, D., Conighi, C., Contu, L., Curtoni, E. S., Mattiuz, P. L., Mayer, W., Richiardi, P., Scudeller, G., and Ceppellini, R., 1972, HLA and other genetic polymorphisms in Sardinia in relation to malaria selection, in: *Histocompatibility Testing,* pp. 73–83, Munksgaard, Copenhagen.

Piomelli, S., and Siniscalco, M., 1969, The haematological effects of glucose-6-phosphate dehydrogenase deficiency and thalassaemia trait: Interaction between the two genes at the phenotype level, *Br. J. Haematol.* **16:**537–545.

Piomelli, S., Corash, L. M., Davenport, D. D., Miraglia, J., and Amorosi, E. L., 1968, *In vivo* lability of glucose-6-phosphate dehydrogenase in Gd^A and $Gd^{Mediterranean}$ deficiency, *J. Clin. Invest.* **47:**940–946.

Praharaj, K. C., and Choudhury, U., 1977, Sickle cell anemia and its association with G6-P-D deficiency in Orissa, *Ind. Pediatr.* **14:**279–284.

Prakash, S., 1977, Genetic divergence in closely related sibling species: *Drosophila pseudoobscura, Drosophila persimilis* and *Drosophila miranda, Evolution* **31:**14–23.

Prchal, J. T., Carroll, A. J., Prchal, J. F., Crist, W. M., Skalka, H. W., Gealy, W. J., Harley, J., and Malluh, A., 1980, Wiskott-Aldrich syndrome: Cellular impairments and their implication for carrier detection, *Blood* **56:**1048–1054.

Purrello, M., Nussbaum, R., Rinaldi, A., Filippi G., Traccis, S., Latte, B., and Siniscalco,

M., 1984, Old and new genetics help ordering loci at the telomere of the human X-chromosome long arm, *Hum. Genet.* **65**:295–299.

Race, R. R., and Sanger, R., 1975, *Blood Groups in Man,* 6th ed., Blackwell Scientific Publications, Oxford.

Ramot, B., Bauminger, S., Brok, F., Gafni, D., and Shwartz, J., 1964, Characterization of glucose-6-phosphate dehydrogenase in Jewish mutants, *J. Lab. Clin. Med.* **64**:895–904.

Rattazzi, M. C., Lenzerini, L., Khan, P. M., and Luzzatto, L., 1969, Characterization of glucose-6-phosphate dehydrogenase variants. II. G6PD Kephalonia, G6PD Attica, and G6PD "Seattle-like" found in Greece, *Am. J. Hum. Genet.* **21**:154–167.

Rattazzi, M. C., Corash, L. M., Van Zanen, G. E., Jaffe, E. R., and Piomelli, S., 1971, G6PD deficiency and chronic hemolysis: Four new mutants—relationships between clinical syndrome and enzyme kinetics, *Blood* **38**:205–218.

Rawls, J. M., and Lucchesi, J. C., 1974a, Regulation of enzyme activities in *Drosophila.* I. The detection of regulatory loci by gene dosage response, *Genet. Res.* **24**:59–72.

Rawls, J. M., and Lucchesi, J. C., 1974b, Regulation of enzyme activities in *Drosophila.* II. Characterization of enzyme responses in aneuploid flies, *Genet. Res.* **24**:73–80.

Reys, L., Manso, C., and Stamatoyannopoulos, G., 1970, Genetic studies on Southeastern Bantu of Mozambique. I. Variants of glucose-6-phosphate dehydrogenase, *Am. J. Hum. Genet.* **22**:203–215.

Rice-Evans, C., Rush, J., Omorphos, S. C., and Flynn, D. M., 1981, Erythrocyte membrane abnormalities in glucose-6-phosphate dehydrogenase deficiency of the Mediterranean and A-types, *FEBS Lett.* **136**:148–152.

Richardson, B. J., Czuppon, A. B., and Sharman, G. B. 1971, Inheritance of G6PD variation in kangaroos, *Nature New Biol.* **230**:154–155.

Riggs, A. D., 1975, X-inactivation, differentiation, and DNA methylation, *Cytogenet. Cell Genet.* **14**:9–25.

Rinaldi, A., Filippi, G., and Siniscalco, M., 1976, Variability of red cell phenotypes between and within individuals in an unbiased sample of 77 certain heterozygotes for G6PD deficiency in Sardinians, *Am. J. Hum. Genet.* **28**:496–505.

Ritte, U., and Pashtan, A., 1982, Extreme levels of genetic variability in two Red Sea *Cerithium* speciesl *(Gasteropoda cerithidae), Evolution* **36**:403–407.

Romeo, G., and Migeon, B. R., 1975, Stability of X chromosomal inactivation in human somatic cells transformed by SV-40, *Humangenetik* **29**:165–170.

Roose, M. L., and Gottlieb, L. D., 1976, Genetic and biochemical consequences of polyploidy in *Tragopogon, Evolution* **30**:818–830.

Rosenstraus, M., and Chasin, L. A., 1975, Isolation of mammalian cell mutants deficient in glucose-6-phosphate dehydrogenase activity: Linkage to hypoxanthine phosphoribosyl transferase, *Proc. Natl. Acad. Sci. USA* **72**:493–497.

Roth, E. F., Jr, Raventos-Suarez, C., Rinaldi, A., and Nagel, R. L., 1983, Glucose-6-phosphate dehydrogenase deficiency inhibits *in vitro* growth of *Plasmodium falciparum, Proc. Natl. Acad. Sci. USA* **80**:298–299.

Roux, P., Karabus, C. D., and Hartley, P. S., 1982, The effect of glucose-6-phosphate dehydrogenase deficiency on the severity of neonatal jaundice in Cape Town, *S. Afr. Med. J.* **1982**(22 May):781–782.

Rudack Garcia, D., and Holten, D., 1974, Inhibition of rat liver glucose-6-phosphate dehydrogenase synthesis by glucagon, *J. Biol. Chem.* **250**:3960–3965.

Ryman, N., Beckman, G., Bruun Petersen, G., and Reuterwall, C., 1977, Variability of red cell enzymes and genetic implications of management policies in Scandinavian moose *(Alces alces), Hereditas* **85**:157–162.

Saha, N., Elamin, F. M., and Samuel, A. P. W., 1983a, Electrophoretic and quantitative studies of red cell G6PD in the one-humped camel *(Camelus dromedarius)* in the Sudan, *Comp. Biochem. Physiol.* **75B**:189–194.

Saha, N., Samuel, A. P. W., Omer, A., and Hoffbrand, A. V., 1983*b*, The inter- and intra-tribal distribution of red cell G6PD phenotypes in Sudan, *Hum. Hered.* **33**:39–43.

Sakharova, A. V., Salimova, N. B., and Sakharov, D. A., 1979, Peculiar cells notable for very high activity of glucose-6-phosphate dehydrogenase in the mammalian medulla oblongata, a histochemical and electron microscopic study, *Neuroscience* **4**:1173–1177.

Saldanha, P. H., Lebensztajn, B., and Itskan, S. B., 1976, Activity of G6PD among Indians living in a malarial region of Mato Grosso and its implication to the Indian-Mixed populations in Brazil, *Hum. Hered.* **26**:241–251.

Samuel, A. P. W., Saha, A., Omer,A., and Hoffbrand, A. V., 1981, Quantitative expression of G6PD activity of different phenotypes of G6PD and haemoglobin in a Sudanese population, *Hum. Hered.* **31**:110–115.

Sanna, G., Frau, F., Melis, M. A., Galanello, R., De Virgiliis, S. and Cao, A., 1980, Inter-action between the glucose-6-phosphate dehydrogenase deficiency and thalassaemia genes at phenotype level, *Br. J. Haematol.* **44**:555–561.

Sansone, G., Perroni, L., Testa, U., Mareni, C., and Luzzatto, L., 1981, New genetic variants of glucose 6-phosphate dehydrogenase (G6PD) in Italy, *Ann. Hum. Genet.* **45**:97–104.

Sarkar, S., Nelson, A. J., and Jones, O. W., 1977, Glucose-6-phosphate dehydrogenase (G6PD) activity of human sperm, *J. Med. Genet.* **14**:250–255.

Savant, S., Parikh, N., and Chhatpar, H. S., 1982, Phosphate mediated regulation of some of the enzymes of carbohydrate metabolism in *Neurospora crassa, Experientia* **38**:310–312.

Schaerf, F. W., Patz, T., and Max, S. R., 1982, Estrogen modulates neural control of muscle glucose-6-phosphate dehydrogenase, *J. Neurochem.* **38**:1765–1767.

Schilirò, G., Russo, A., Mauro, L., Pizzarelli, G., and Marino, S., 1976, Leukocyte function and characterization of leukocyte glucose-6-phosphate dehydrogenase in Sicilian mutants, *Pediatr. Res.* **10**:739–742.

Schilirò, G., Russo, A., Curreri, R., Marino, S., Sciotto, A., and Russo, G., 1979, Glucose-6-phosphate dehydrogenase deficiency in Sicily. Incidence, biochemical characteristics and clinical implications, *Clin. Genet.* **15**:183–188.

Schmitt, L. H., 1978, Genetic variation in isolated populations of the Australian bush rat, *Rattus fuscipes, Evolution* **32**:1–14.

Scott, W. A., and Mahoney, E., 1976, Defects of glucose-6-phosphate and 6-phosphogluco-nate dehydrogenases in *Neurospora* and their pleiotropic effects, in: *Current Topics in Cellular Regulation,* Vol. 10 (B. L. Horecker and E. R. Stadtman, eds.), pp. 205–236, Academic Press, New York.

Scozzari, R., Trippa, G., Santachiara-Benerecetti, S. A., Terrenato, L., Iodice, C., and Benincasa, A., 1981, Further genetic heterogeneity of human red cell phosphoglucomutase-1: A non-electrophoretic polymorphism, *Ann. Hum. Genet.* **45**:313–322.

Seecof, R. L., Kaplan, W. D., and Fuch, D. G., 1969, Dosage compensation for enzyme activities in *Drosophila melanogaster, Proc. Natl. Acad. Sci. USA* **62**:528–535.

Segal, A. W., Cross, A. R., Garcia, R. C., Borregaard, N., Valerius, N. H., Soothill, J. F., and Jones, O. T. G., 1982, Absence of cytochrome b_{-248} in chronic granulomatous disease: A multicentre European evaluation of its incidence and relevance, *N. Engl. J. Med.* **308**:245–251.

Serov, O. L., Zakijan, S. M., Khlebodarova, T. M., and Korochkin, L. I., 1976, Allelic expression in intergeneric fox hybrids *(Alopex lagopus × Vulpes vulpes).* I. Comparative electrophoretic studies on blood enzymes and proteins in Arctic and silver foxes, *Biochem. Genet.* **14**:1091.

Serov, O. L., Zakijan, S. M., and Kulichkov, V. A., 1978a, Allelic expression in intergeneric fox hybrids *(Alopex lagopus* × *Vulpes vulpes).* III. Regulation of the expression of the parental alleles at the *Gpd* locus linked to the X chromosome, *Biochem. Genet.* **16:**145–157.

Serov, O. L., Zakijan, S. M., and Kulichkov, V. A., 1978b, Analysis of mechanisms regulating the expression of parental alleles at the *GPD* locus in mule erythrocytes, *Biochem. Genet.* **16:**379–386.

Shaklee, J. B., and Tamaru, C. S., 1981, Biochemical and morphological evolution of Hawaian bonefishes *(Albula), Syst. Zool.* **30:**125–146.

Shatskaya, T. L., Krasnopolskaya, K. D., Tzoneva, M., Mavrudieva, M., and Toncheva, D., 1980a, Variants of erythrocyte glucose-6-phosphate dehydrogenase (G6PD) in Bulgarian populations, *Hum. Genet.* **54:**115–117.

Shatskaya, T. L., Krasnopolskaya, K. D., and Zakharova, T. V., 1980b, Regularities of distribution of *Gd⁻* alleles in Azerbaijan. III. Identification of G6PD mutant forms, *Genetica* **16:**2217–2225.

Shaw, C. R., 1966, Glucose-6-phosphate dehydrogenase: Homologous molecules in deer mouse and man, *Science* **153:**1013–1015.

Shaw, C. R., and Barto, E., 1965, Autosomally determined polymorphism of glucose-6-phosphate dehydrogenase in *Peromyscus, Science* **148:**1099–1100.

Shreve, D. S., and Levy, H. R., 1980, Kinetic mechanism of glucose-6-phosphate dehydrogenase from the lactating rat mammary gland, *J. Biol. Chem.* **255:**2670–2677.

Sicard, D., Kaplan, J.-C., and Labie, D., 1978, Haemoglobinopathies and G.-6-P.D. deficiency in Laos, *Lancet* **ii:**571–572.

Sidell, B. D., Otto, R. G., and Powers, D. A., 1978, A biochemical method for distinction of striped bass and white perch larvae, *Copeia* **1978:**340–343.

Sidi, Y., Aderka, D., Brok-Simoni, G., Benjamin, D., Ramot, B., and Pinkhas, J., 1980, Viral hepatitis with extreme hyperbilirubinemia, massive hemolysis and encephalopathy in a patient with a new G6PD variant, *Isr. J. Med. Sci.* **16:**130–133.

Silagi, S., Darlington, G., and Bruce, S. A., 1969, Hybridization of two biochemically marked human cell lines, *Proc. Natl. Acad. Sci. USA* **62:**1085–1092.

Silva-Pando, M., Carrion-Angosto, A., and Ruiz-Amil, Y. M., 1978, G6PDH of hepatopancreas of Mejillon, *Rev. Espan, Fisiol. (Barcelona)* **34:**1–8.

Simonsen, V., 1982, Electrophoretic variation in large mammals. II. The red fox, *Vulpes vulpes,* the stoat, *Mustela erminea,* the weasel, *M. nivalis,* the pole cat, *M. putorius,* the pine marten, *Martes martes,* the beech marten, *Martes martes,* the beech marten, *M. foina,* and the badger, *Meles meles, Hereditas* **96:**299–305.

Simonsen, V., Allendorf, F. W., Eanes, W. F., and Kapel, F. O., 1982a, Electrophoretic variation in large mammals. III. The ringed seal, *Pusa hispida,* the harp seal, *Pagophilus groenlandicus,* and the hooded seal, *Cystophora cristata, Heriditas* **97:**87–90.

Simonsen, V., Born, E. W., and Kristensen, T., 1982b, Electrophoretic variation in large mammals. IV. The Atlantic walrus, *Obodenus rosmarus rosmarus (L), Hereditas* **97:**91–94.

Siniscalco, M., Filippi, G., and Latte, B., 1964, Recombination between protan and deutan genes; data on their relative positions in respect to the G6PD locus, *Nature* **204:**1062–1064.

Siniscalco, M., Bernini, L., Filippi, G., Latte, B., Khan, P. M., Piomelli, S., and Rattazzi, M., 1966, Population genetics of haemoglobin variants, thalassaemia and glucose-6-phosphate dehydrogenase deficiency, with particular reference to the malaria hypothesis, *Bull. WHO* **34:**379–393.

Siniscalco, M., Klinger, H. P., Eagle, H., Koprowski, H., Fujimoto, W. Y., and Seegmiller,

J. E., 1969, Evidence for intergenic complementation in hybrid cells derived from two human diploid strains each carrying an X-linked mutation, *Proc. Natl. Acad. Sci. USA* **62**:793–799.

Sites, J. W., and Greenbaum, I. F., 1983, Chromosome evolution in the iguanid lizard *Sceloporus grammicus*. II. Allozyme variation, *Evolution* **37**:54–65.

Skolnick, M. H., and White, R., 1982, Strategies for detecting and characterizing restriction fragment length polymorphisms (RFLP's), *Cytogenet. Cell Genet.* **32**:58–67.

Smith, J. E., Ryer, K., and Wallace, L., 1976, Glucose-6-phosphate dehydrogenase deficiency in a dog, *Enzyme* **21**:379–383.

Snyder, T. P., 1974, Lack of allozymic variability in three bee species, *Evolution* **28**:687–689.

Solanki, D. L., McCurdy, P. R., and MacDermott, R. P., 1982, Chronic lymphocytic leukemia: A monoclonal disease, *Am. J. Hematol.* **13**:159–162.

Stamato, T. D., MacKenzie, L., Pagani, J. M., and Weinstein, R., 1982, Mutagen treatment of single Chinese hamster ovary cells produces colonies mosaic for glucose-6-phosphate dehydrogenase activity, *Somat. Cell Genet.* **8**:643–651.

Stamatoyannopoulos, G., Voigtlander, V., Kotsakis, P., and Akrivakis, A., 1971, Genetic diversity of the "Mediterranean" glucose-6-phosphate dehydrogenase deficiency phenotype, *J. Clin. Invest.* **50**:1253–1261.

Stanbury, J. B., Wyngaarden, J. B., Fredrickson, D. S., Goldstein, J. L., and Brown, M. S., eds., 1983, *The Metabolic Basis of Inherited Disease*, 5th ed., McGraw-Hill, New York.

Steele, M. W., 1976, On the evolution of X-chromosome inactivation in mammals and the clinical consequences to man: A hypothesis, *Med. Hypotheses* **2**:195–199.

Steele, M. W., and Migeon, B. R., 1973, Sex difference in activity of glucose-6-phosphate dehydrogenase in fetal lung cells, *Biochem. Genet.* **9**:163–168.

Steele, M. W., Young, W. J., and Childs, B., 1968, Glucose-6-phosphate dehydrogenase in *Drosophila melanogaster:* Starch gel electrophoretic variation due to molecular instability, *Biochem. Genet.* **2**:159–175.

Steele, M. W., Young, W. J., and Childs, B., 1969, Genetic regulation of glucose-6-phosphate dehydrogenase activity in *Drosophila melanogaster, Biochem. Genet.* **3**:359–370.

Steiman, I., Kaufman, S., Zaidman, J. L., and Leiba, H., 1978, Combined glucose phosphate isomerase and glucose-6-phosphate dehydrogenase deficiency of erythrocytes, *Isr. J. Med. Sci.* **14**:1186–1190.

Steinbach, R. A., Sahm, H., and Schütte, H., 1978, Purification and regulation of glucose-6-phosphate dehydrogenase from obligate methanol-utilizing bacterium *Methylomonas M15, Eur. J. Biochem.* **87**:409–415.

Stewart, B. R., and Merriam, J. R., 1974, Segmental aneuploidy and enzyme activity as a method for cytogenetic localization in *Drosophila* melanogaster, *Genetics* **76**:301–309.

Stewart, B. R., and Merriam, J. R., 1975, Regulation of gene activity by dosage compensation at the chromosomal level in *Drosophila, Genetics* **79**:635–647.

Stewart, B. R., and Merriam, J. R., 1980, Dosage compensation, in: *The Genetics and Biology in Drosophila* (M. Ashburner and T. R. F. Wright, eds.), Vol. 2, pp. 107–140, Academic Press, New York.

Swanson, L. V., and Barker, K. L., 1983, Antagonistic effects of progesterone on estradiol-induced synthesis and degradation of uterine glucose-6-phosphate dehydrogenase, *Endocrinology* **112**:459–465.

Taggart, J., Ferguson, A., and Mason, F. M., 1981, Genetic variation in Irish populations of brown trout *(Salmo trutta L.):* Electrophoretic anaysis of allozymes, *Comp. Biochem. Physiol.* **69B**:393–412.

Takahashi, K., Fujii, H., Takegawa, S., Tani, K., Hirono, A., Takizawa, T., Kawakatsu, T., and Miwa, S., 1982, A new glucose-6-phosphate dehydrogenase variant (G6PD Nagano) associated with congenital hemolytic anemia, *Hum. Genet.* **62**:368–370.

Tantravahi, U., Kirschner, D. A., Beauregard, L., Page, L., Kunkel, L., and Latt, S., 1983, Cytologic and molecular analysis of 46,XXq- cells to identify a DNA segment that might serve as a probe for a putative human X chromosome inactivation center, *Hum. Genet.* **64**:33–38.

Tashian, R. E., Brewer, G. J., Lehmann, H., Davies, D. A., and Rucknagel, D. L., 1967, Further studies on Xavante indians. V. Genetic variability in some serum and erythrocyte enzyme, hemoglobin, and the urinary excretion of β-aminoisobutyric acid, *Am. J. Hum. Genet.* **19**:524–531.

Tepperman, H. M., and Tepperman, J., 1963, On the response of hepatic G6PD activity to changes in diet composition and food intake pattern, in: *Advances in Enzyme Regulation,* Vol. 1 (G. Weber, ed.), pp. 121–136, Pergamon Press, New York.

Tepperman, H. M., and Tepperman, J., 1965, Effect of saturated fat diets on rat liver NADP-linked enzymes, *Am. J. Physiol.* **209**:773–780.

Terrenato, L., 1976, Variabilita genetica in Sardegna, in: *Genetica di Popolazioni,* Atti Convegni Lincei, Rome, Vol. 14, pp. 187–214.

Terzi, M., Piras, A., and Simi, S., 1978, Generation of variability of glucose-6-phosphate dehydrogenase after explanation *in vitro* of somatic cells, in: *Symposium on Genetics of Somatic Cells,* 14th International Congress of Genetics, Moscow.

Testa, U., Meloni, T., Lania, A., Battistuzzi, G., Cutillo, S., and Luzzatto, L., 1980, Genetic heterogeneity of glucose 6-phosphate dehydrogenase deficiency in Sardinia, *Hum. Genet.* **56**:99–105.

Teutsch, H. F., and Rieder, H., 1979, NADP-dependent dehydrogenases in rat liver parenchima. II. Comparison of qualitative and quantitative glucose-6-phosphate dehydrogenase distribution patterns with particular reference to sex differences, *Histochemistry* **60**:43–52.

Theakston, R. D. G., Fletcher, K. A., and Moore, G. A., 1976, Glucose-6-phosphate and 6-phosphogluconate dehydrogenase activities in human erythrocytes infected with *Plasmodium falciparum, Ann. Trop. Med. Parasitol.* **70**:125–127.

Toncheva, D., Evrev, T., and Tzoneva, M., 1982, G6PD in immature and mature human brain. Electrophoretic and enzyme kinetic studies, *Hum. Hered.* **32**:193–196.

Toniolo, D., Persico, M. G., Battistuzzi, G., and Luzzatto, L., 1984a, Partial purification and characterization of the mRNA for human glucose-6-phosphate dehydrogenase, *Mol. Biol. Med.,* in press.

Toniolo, D., D'Urso, M., Martini, G., Persico, M., Tufano, V., Battistuzzi, G., and Luzzatto, L., 1984, Specific methylation pattern at the 3′ end of the human housekeeping gene, glucose 6-phosphate dehydrogenase, *EMBO Journal,* **3**:1987–1995.

Trager, W., and Jensen, J. B., 1976, Human malaria parasites in continuous culture, *Science* **193**:673–675.

Trujillo, J. M., Walden, B., O'Neil, P., and Anstall, H. B., 1965, Sex linkage of G6PD in the horse and donkey, *Science* **148**:1603–1604.

Tsukamoto, M., 1974, Differential detection of soluble enzymes specific to a rodent malaria parasite, *Plasmodium berghei,* by electrophoresis on polyacrylamide gels, *Trop. Med.* **16**:55–69.

Tugwell, P., 1973, Glucose-6-phosphate dehydrogenase deficiency in Nigerians with jaundice associated with lobar pneumonia, *Lancet* **i**:968–970.

Tunail, N., and Schlegel, H. G., 1972, Phosphoenolpyruvate, a new inhibitor of glucose 6-phosphate dehydrogenase, *Biochem. Biophys. Res. Commun.* **49**:1554–1560.

Turner, T. R., 1981, Blood protein variation in a population of Ethiopian Vervet monkeys *(Cercopithecus aethiops aethiops), Am. J. Phys. Anthropol.* **55**:225–232.

Tzoneva, M., Boshnakova, E., Mavrudieva, M., Proynova, M., 1975, Widespreading of G6PD deficiency among the populations in some regions of Bulgaria, *Acta Med. Bulg.* **3**:38–43.

Tzoneva, M., Bulanov, A. G., Mavrudieva, M., Lalchev, S., Toncheva, D., and Tanev, D., 1980, Frequency of glucose-6-phosphate dehydrogenase deficiency in relation to altitude: A malaria hypothesis, *Bull WHO* **58**:659–662.

Usanga, E. A., Bienzle, U., Cancedda, R., Fasuan, F. A., Ajayi, O., and Luzzatto, L., 1977, Genetic variants of human erythrocyte glucose 6-phosphate dehydrogenase: New variants in West Africa characterized by column chromatography, *Ann. Hum. Genet. Lond.* **40**:279–286.

Varvio Aho, S., and Pamilo, P., 1979, Genetic differentiation of *Gerris lacustris* populations, *Hereditas* **90**:237–249.

Venolia, L., and Gartler, S. M., 1983, Comparison of transformation efficiency of human active and inactive X-chromosomal DNA, *Nature* **302**:82–83.

Ventura, A., Panizon, G.,Soranzo, M. R., Veneziano, G., Sansone, G., Testa, U., and Luzzatto, L., 1983, Congenital dyserythropoietic anaemia type II associated with a new type of G6PD deficiency (G6PD Gabrovizza), *Acta Haematol.* **71**:227–234.

Vergnes, H., and Cabannes, R., 1976, Polymorphism of erythrocyte and serum enzyme systems in the Gagu of the Ivory Coast, *Ann. Hum. Biol.* **3**:423–429.

Vergnes, H., Puget, A., and Gouarderas, C., 1974, Comparative study of red cell enzyme polymorphism in the pika and rabbit, *Anim. Blood Groups Biochem. Genet.* **5**:181–188.

Vergnes, H., Gherardi, M., and Bouloux, G., 1975, Erythrocyte glucose-6-phosphate dehydrogenase in the Niokolonko (Malinke of the Niokolo) of Eastern Senegal. Identification of a slow variant with normal activity (Tacoma-like), *Hum. Hered.* **25**:80–87.

Vergnes, H., Sevin, A., Sevin, J., and Jaeger, G., 1979a, Population genetic studies of the Aka Pygmies (Central Africa). A survey of red cell and serum enzymes, *Hum. Genet.* **48**:343–355.

Vergnes, H., Gherardi, M., Lefevre-Witier, P., Jaeger, G., and Benabadji, M., 1979b, Genetic variants of human glucose-6-phosphate dehydrogenase in a Saharian and Pygmy family, *Hum. Hered.* **29**:50–56.

Vergnes, H., Sevin, A., and Brun, H., 1982, Kinetic characteristics of different glucose-6-phosphate dehydrogenase variants and their hemolytic incidence in man, *Enzyme* **27**:204–214.

Vives Corrons, J. L., and Pujades, A., 1982, Heterogeneity of "Mediterranean Type" glucose-6-phosphate dehydrogenase (G6PD) deficiency in Spain and description of two new variants associated with favism, *Hum. Genet.* **60**:216–221.

Vives Corrons, J. L., Feliu, E., Pujades, M. A., Cardellach, F., Rozman, C., Carreras, A., Jou, J. M., Vallespí, M. T., and Zuazu, F. J., 1982, Severe glucose-6-phosphate dehydrogenase (G6PD) deficiency associated with chronic hemolytic anemia, granulocyte dysfunction, and increased susceptibility to infections: Description of a new molecular variant (G6PD Barcelona), *Blood* **59**:428–433.

Wagner, A. E. and Briscoe, D. A., 1983, An absence of enzyme variability within two species of *Trigona (Hymenoptera), Heredity* **50**:97–103.

Wallace, R. A., 1961, Enzymatic patterns in the developing frog embryo, *Dev. Biol.* **3**:486–515.

Walter, R. D., 1979, Purification and properties of glucose-6-phosphate dehydrogenase from *Leishmania tropica* promastigotes, *Tropenmed. Parasit.* **30**:3–8.

Ward, P. S., 1980, Genetic variation and population differentiation in the *Rhytidoponera impressa* group, a species complex of ponerine ants *(Hymenoptera formicidae), Evolution* **34**:1060–1076.

Welch, S. G., Aidley, D. J., Barry, J. V., Carter, N. D., Culliford, B. J., Huntsman, R. G., Jenkins, G. C., Powell, R. B., and Parr, C. W., 1975, Blood group, serum protein and red cell enzyme polymorphisms in a population from the Seychelle Islands, *Hum. Hered.* **25**:346–353.

Welch, S. G., McGregor, I. A., and Williams, K., 1978a, A new variant of human erythrocyte G6PD occurring at a high frequency amongst the population of two villages in the Gambia, West Africa, *Hum. Genet.* **40**:305–309.

Welch, S. G., Lee, J., McGregor, I. A., and Williams, K., 1978b, Red cell glucose 6 phosphate dehydrogenase genotypes of the population of two West African villages, *Hum. Genet.* **43**:315–320.

Werth, G., and Müller, G., 1967, Vererbarer glucose-6-phosphatdehydrogenasemangel, *Klin. Wochenschr.* **45**:265–269.

Wild, D., and Hellkuhl, B., 1976, Isolation of mammalian cell mutants deficient in glucose 6-phosphate dehydrogenase by means of a replicating technique, *Hum. Genet.* **32**:315–322.

Willcox, M. C., and Beckman, L., 1981, Haemoglobin variants, β-thalassaemia and G-6-PD types in Liberia, *Hum. Hered.* **31**:339–347.

Williams, C. K. O., Ogunmola, G. B., Abugo, O., Ukaejiofo, E. O., and Esan, G. J. F., 1983, Polycythaemia rubra vera associated with unbalanced expression of the X chromosome and monoclonalith of T lymphocytes, *Acta Haematol.* **70**:229–235.

Williams, C. K. O., Esan, G. J. F., Luzzatto, L., Town, M. -M., and Ogunmola, G. B., 1984, X-linked somatic-cell selection and polycythemia rubra vera, *New Engl. J. Med.* **310**:1265.

Wilson, W. G., Kirkman, H. N., and Clemons, E. H., 1980, Regulation of glucose-6-phosphate dehydrogenase. II. Resealed red cell ghosts, *J. Lab. Clin. Med.* **95**:888–896.

Winans, G. A., 1980, Geographic variation in the milkfish *Chanos chanos.* I. Biochemical evidence, *Evolution* **34**:558–574.

Winberry, L., and Holten, D., 1977, Rat liver G6PD. Dietary induction of the rate of synthesis, *J. Biol. Chem.* **252**:7796–7801.

Wolf, R. E., Jr., Prather, D. M., and Shea, F. M., 1979, Growth rate dependent alteration of 6 phosphogluconate and glucose-6-phosphate dehydrogenase levels in *Escherichia coli* K 12, *J. Bacteriol.* **139**:1093–1096.

Wright, D. A., 1975, Expression of enzyme phenotypes in hybrid embryos, in: *Isozymes. IV. Genetics and Evolution* (C. L. Markert, ed.), pp. 649–664, Academic Press, New York.

Wright, D. A., and Shaw, C. R., 1970, Time of expression of genes controlling specific enzymes in *Drosophila* embryos, *Biochem. Genet.* **4**:385–394.

Wright, D. A., Richards, C. M., and Nace, G. W., 1980, Inheritance of enzymes and blood proteins in the leopard frog, *Rana pipiens:* The linkage groups established, *Biochem. Genet.* **18**:591–616.

Wurdeman, R., Berdanier, C. D., and Tobin, R. B., 1978, Enzyme overshoot in starved-refed rats: Role of the adrenal glucocorticoid, *J. Nutr.* **108**:1457–1461.

Yagil, G., Shimron, F., and Hizi, A., 1974, On the mechanism of glucose-6-phosphate dehydrogenase regulation in mouse liver. 1. Characterization of the system, *Eur. J. Biochem.* **45**:189–200.

Yamauchi, T., and Goldberg, E., 1974, Asynchronous expression of glucose-6-phosphate dehydrogenase in splake trout embryos, *Dev. Biol.* **39**:63–68.

Yamauchi, T., Stegeman, J. J., and Goldberg, E., 1975, The effects of starvation and temperature acclimation on pentose phosphate pathway dehydrogenases in brook trout liver, *Arch. Biochem. Biophys.* **167**:13–20.

Yoshida, A., 1967, Human G6PD: Purification and characterization of Negro type variant (A+) and comparison with normal enzyme (B+), *Biochem. Genet.* **1**:81–88.

Yoshida, A., 1970, Amino acid substitution (histidine to tyrosine) in a glucose 6-phosphate dehydrogenase variant (G6PD Hektoen) associated with overproduction, *J. Mol. Biol.* **52**:483–490.

Yoshida, A., 1973, Hemolytic anemia and G-6-PD deficiency, *Science* **179**:532–537.

Yoshida, A., 1975, Evolution of glucose 6-phosphate dehydrogenase and hexose 6-phosphate dehydrogenase, in: *Isozymes. IV. Genetics and Evolution* (C. L. Markert, ed.), pp. 853–866, Academic Press, New York.

Yoshida, A., and Beutler, E., 1978, Human glucose-6-phosphate dehydrogenase variants: A supplementary tabulation, *Ann. Hum. Genet. Lond.* **41**:347–355.

Yoshida, A., and Beutler, E., 1983, G-6-PD variants: Another up-date, *Ann. Hum. Genet.* **47**:25–38.

Yoshida, A., Baur, E. W., and Motulsky, A. G., 1970, A Philippino glucose-6-phosphate dehydrogenase variant (G6PD Union) with enzyme deficiency and altered substrate specificity, *Blood* **35**:506–513.

Yoshida, A., Beutler, E., and Motulsky, A. G., 1971, Human glucose-6-phosphate dehydrogenase variants, *Bull. WHO* **45**:243–253.

Yoshida, A., Giblett, E. R., and Malcom, L. A., 1973, Heterogeneous distribution of glucose 6 phosphate dehydrogenase variants with enzyme deficiency in the Markham Valley area of New Guinea, *Ann. Hum. Genet.* **37**:145–150.

Young, W. J., 1966, X linked electrophoretic variation in 6-phosphogluconate dehydrogenase in *Drosophila melanogaster, J. Hered.* **57**:58.

Young, W. J., Porter, J. E., and Childs, B., 1964, G6PD in *Drosophila:* X linked electrophoretic variants, *Science* **143**:140–141.

Zampella, E. J., Bradley, E. L., and Pretlow, T. G., 1982, Glucose-6-phosphate dehydrogenase: A possible indicator for prostatic carcinoma, *Cancer* **49**:384–387.

Zavala, C., Herner, G., and Fialkow, P. J., 1978, Evidence for selection in cultured diploid fibroblast strains, *Exp. Cell Res.* **117**:137–144.

Zera, A. J., 1981, Genetic structure of two species of waterstriders *(Gerridae hemiptera)* with differing degree of winglessness, *Evolution* **35**:218–225.

Zinkham, W., 1961, A deficiency of glucose-6-phosphate dehydrogenase activity in lens from individuals with primaquine-sensitive erythrocytes, *Bull. Johns Hopkins Hosp.* **109**:206–210.

Chapter 5

Steroid Sulfatase Deficiency and the Genetics of the Short Arm of the Human X Chromosome

Larry J. Shapiro

Departments of Pediatrics and Biological Chemistry
School of Medicine
University of California at Los Angeles
Los Angeles, California

INTRODUCTION

It is considered axiomatic in human genetics that the study of relatively rare disorders may yield far more in dividends than might be anticipated based on the incidence of the condition in question. This has clearly been demonstrated in studies of human steroid sulfatase deficiency and the steroid sulfatase system during the past few years. Investigations of this infrequent human variation have led to expanded studies of sulfated steroid metabolism, the physiological control of epidermal keratinization, estrogen biosynthesis in pregnancy, testosterone biosynthesis, and the molecular mechanism of X-chromosome inactivation and the escape of inactivation of certain portions of the human X. In addition, the availability of a readily scoreable marker for the distal human short arm provides the potential basis for a number of observations regarding X/Y interchange involving this portion of the X and has raised a number of evolutionary issues as well. Further studies may help clarify several of these questions and substantially add to our understanding of a variety of human X-chromosome disorders, such as X aneuploid states, XX males, and true hermaphrodites.

SULFATED STEROIDS AND THEIR METABOLISM

Sulfated steroids are relatively ubiquitous compounds found in a variety of body fluids and tissues in quantitatively significant amounts. Until relatively recently, there has been surprisingly little interest in studying the biochemistry or metabolism of these substances, as they were thought to represent metabolic end products that had been conjugated with sulfuric acids soley to render them more water soluble so that they might be excreted. In the 1930s the existence of acid-labile conjugates of steroids and glucuronic acid or sulfuric acid were identified in urine, which explained the previous observations that acid hydrolysis of urine greatly increased the yield of steroids that could be extracted into organic solvents (Schachter and Marrian, 1938). Munson *et al.* (1944) identified sulfated dehydroisoandrosterone (DHEA) in human urine, and in the 1950s and 1960s sulfoconjugates of a number of other 3-β-hydroxy-Δ^5-steroids were identified. With the development of sensitive chemical methods of measurement, radioimmunoassay, and chromatographic methods of separation it became possible to accurately isolate and quantitate these compounds and to begin to unravel their physiological implications. This work became relevant if for no other reason than that DHEAS represents the most abundant steroid present in plasma except for cholesterol and its sulfate. For a complete background, an excellent review of the biochemistry of sulfated steroids by Roberts and Lieberman (1970) can be consulted.

3-β-Hydroxy-steroid sulfates are formed enzymatically by sulfotransferase-mediated reactions in a variety of tissues utilizing a number of substrates, all presumably using 3'-phosphoadenosyl-5'-phosphosulfate (PAPS) as the sulfate donor (Roy *et al.*, 1970). This pathway has been demonstrated in the adrenal gland, liver, skin, testis, and placenta. Whether or not all of these sulfotransferase activities correspond to a single gene product or are derived from multiple loci is not yet clear. The physiological effectors that modulate the degree of sulfation of free steroids is also not known. As will be discussed in considerable detail, a neutral pH optimum microsomal steroid sulfatase capable of hydrolyzing many of these steroid sulfate esters is distributed ubiquitously in mammalian tissues. Thus, the interconversion of free steroids and steroid sulfates occurs readily in many anatomic locations.

While several of the sulfated steroids, such as DHEAS and estrone

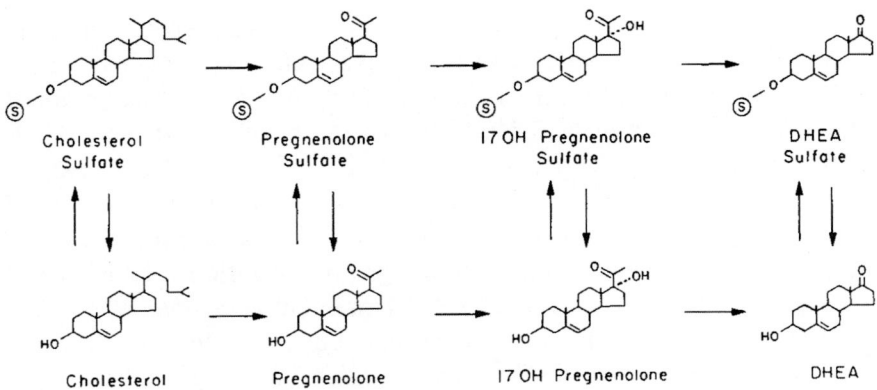

Fig. 1. Interconversion of free 3β-hydroxysteroids and their sulfates. The pathway of metabolism from cholesterol sulfate to DHEAS and from cholesterol to DHEA is shown. It is presumed but not proven that the same enzymes catalyze analogous reactions with either free steroids or steroid sulfates as substrates. At any point, free steroids may be esterified with PAPS as the sulfate donor, and sulfated steroids can be hydrolyzed by STS.

sulfate, are not capable of binding to relevant receptor proteins, these sulfated compounds clearly play an important role in the intermediary metabolism and general economy of steroid hormones. This was elegantly demonstrated by administration of sulfated cholesterol or pregnenolone labeled with both ³H and ³⁵S to human subjects (Calvin et al., 1963; Roberts et al., 1964). After isolating DHEAS from the urine of these individuals, it was shown that the ³⁵S/³H ratio was the same in this steroid as in the sulfated conjugate originally injected. This implies that a number of metabolic reactions took place without prior desulfation of the molecule. Presumably these interconversions were mediated by the same enzyme systems that would normally metabolize the free steroids (Fig. 1). At any rate, it now seems clear that sulfated steroids may be important intermediaries in steroid hormone synthesis.

Cholesterol Sulfate

Cholesterol sulfate (CS) is found in a variety of tissues and fluids, including the adrenal gland, brain, liver, kidney, plasma, urine, feces, bile, aortic plaques, gallstones, red cell membranes, and seminal fluid (Dreyer and Lieberman 1965, 1967; Moser et al., 1966). Normal plasma levels of this steroid are approximately 150–300 μ/dl (Bergner and Shapiro, 1981). Much of the plasma CS is apparently associated with low-density lipoportein (LDL) (Epstein *et al.*, 1981*a*). The excessive amount of CS contained within the LDL isolated from patients with steroid sulfatase deficiency probably contributes to an abnormal electronegative charge of the lipoprotein in these patients. The normal physiological role of cholesterol sulfate is uncertain. Red cell membranes and presumably other cell membranes as well contain high concentrations of cholesterol sulfate (Elias, 1981; Bleau *et al.*, 1974, 1975; Lalumiere *et al.*, 1975). This amphipathic molecule is avidly taken up from incubation media when red cells are suspended in cholesterol sulfate-containing solutions. The addition of cholesterol sulfate to red cell membrane appears to promote osmotic stability both *in vivo* and *in vitro*. Another area to which significant interest has been directed is the association of cholesterol sulfate with sperm membranes (Bleau and Van den Heuvel, 1974; Lalumiere *et al.*, 1976; Langlais *et al.*, 1981; Legault *et al.*, 1979). Human spermatozoa actively absorb labeled cholesterol sulfate, which is concentrated in the region of the acrosome. It has been speculated that, as in the red cell, cholesterol sulfate stabilizes acrosomal membranes and must be removed in the process of sperm capacitation. There is a very potent steroid sulfatase in human female reproductive tract extracts, which theoretically could carry out this reaction. It is of note, however, that secretion of steroid sulfatase enzyme into any extracellular environment has not been demonstrated.

The other principal site where cholesterol sulfate has been studied is as a constituent of the stratum corneum of the epidermis. This aspect has received attention primarily following the elucidation of the role of steroid sulfatase deficiency in X-linked ichthyosis. It has been pointed out that solvent extraction of lipids from stratum corneum allows dissolution of this layer into individual cells and that reconstitution with lipid causes these cells to reaggregate (Smith *et al.*, 1980). In addition, it has been noted that 80% of all lipids in the stratum corneum are found in cell membranes and in intercellular spaces (Epstein *et al.*, 1981*b*). The observation that a variety of disorders of lipid metabolism appear to interfere with stratum corneum adhesion has added credence to these models. Several theories have been put forth suggesting a specific role for cholesterol sulfate in promoting epidermal cohesion either through ionic properties or through changes in thermal transition properties of stratum corneum lips. Numerous examples of ichthyosis in association with administration of cholesterol synthesis inhibitors have been described (Anderson and Martt, 1965; Ruiter and Meyler, 1960; Simpson *et al.*, 1964; Winkelmann *et al.*, 1963), and the ratio of cholesterol sulfate to other stratum corneum lipids may prove to be of critical importance (Borgaonkar *et al.*, 1974). Further work needs to be carried out in all of these areas to definitively establish the role of cholesterol sulfate in these biologic membranes.

DHEA Sulfate

In contrast to some of the other steroid sulfates, there has been great interest in the physiology of DHEAS (De Peretti and Forest, 1978; Korth-Schutz *et al.*, 1976; Reiter *et al.*, 1977). DHEAS is present in appreciable amounts in cord blood rapidly diminishes in concentration during the first months of life. Levels remain low until 5–7 years of age, when they begin a gradual rise to adult values. On the average, this rise begins 1–2 years earlier in females than in males and heralds the onset of adrenarche. Most of the DHEAS in blood probably arises from adrenal secretion. Production rates of DHEAS for adults are on the order of 6–10 mg/day (Reiter *et al.*, 1977). The normal human testis is probably not responsible for very much secretion of DHEAS. The levels of DHEAS in surgically adrenalectomized or exogenously suppressed patients confirm that the adrenal is the principal site of origin for circulating DHEAS.

DHEAS is an important precursor of estriol production during human pregnancy (Shapiro, 1982). While this relationship is well established, the potential role of DHEAS as a substrate for testosterone and androgen production is unclear (Chapdelaine *et al.*, 1965; Horton and Tait, 1967; McDonald *et al.*, 1965). The transfer factors observed for DHEAS → DHEA suggest that this interconversion is quantitatively important in normal individuals (Rosenfield *et al.*, 1982). One group has noted that much of the plasma-free DHEA seems to arise from peripheral desulfation of DHEAS rather than direct secretion of DHEA by the adrenal glands. Since it has been well established that DHEA can be further metabolized by a number of endocrine and peripheral tissues to androstenedione and testosterone, some consideration has recently been given to the possibility that DHEAS may be a physiologically significant precursor of plasma testosterone. The accumulated data make it seem clear that plasma DHEAS is not a major precursor of testosterone production, being responsible for no more than 15% of the testosterone made in nor-

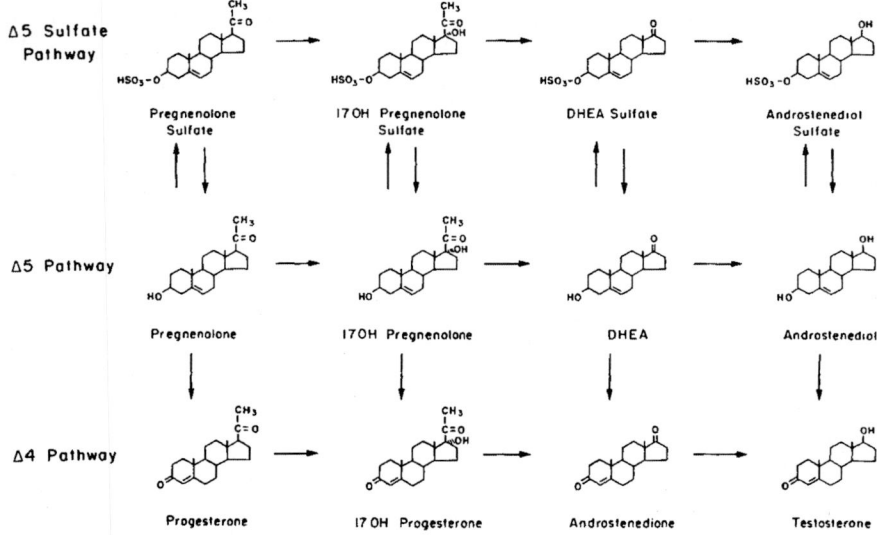

Fig. 2. Potential pathways for testicular testosterone production from cholesterol. The relative flux of intermediates down the Δ^4, Δ^5, or sulfated steroid pathways is not known with certainty for all human developmental stages or situations of varying hormonal stimulation.

mal females, and probably no more than 1% of the testosterone production in adult males (Horton and Tait, 1967). Within the testes per se, however, it is difficult to get precise information about the contribution of steroid sulfates as precursors for testosterone hormonogenesis (Dominguez *et al.,* 1975; Huhtaniemi, 1977; Notation, 1975; Payne, 1980; Siiteri and Wilson, 1974; Vihko and Ruokonen, 1974, 1975). Recent data suggest that older concepts about the relative importance of the Δ^5 versus Δ^4 pathways of steroid biosynthesis in human testes may be incorrect (Fig. 2). The Δ^5 intermediates are present in the greatest quantities, and the largest fraction of these 3-β-hydroxy-Δ^5-steroids in testicular extracts are present as sulfate conjugates. Testicular extracts can make use of labeled sulfated steroids for testosterone production, and the level of testicular steroid sulfatase activity is responsive to exogenous HCG stimulation. If sulfated steroids are important precursors of testosterone within the Leydig cell, steroid sulfatase deficiency could impact on the ability of the Leydig cell to respond to HCG and to make testosterone. In addition, a number of other potential roles for DHEAS in the regulation of caloric expenditure and as a contributor to longevity have received recent interest in both the scientific and lay press.

Another potential role for steroid sulfatase in endocrine physiology is that the peripheral response to sulfated steroids could well be regulated by local tissue activity of this enzyme. It has been speculated that the fetal sheep hypothalamus has its exposure to active estrogen controlled by the amount of steroid sulfatase activity, which acts locally to desulfate estrone sulfate, the principal circulating estrogen in sheep (Lakshima and Balasubramanian, 1981; Siiteri and Wilson, 1974). Similarly, it has been argued that the seminiferous tubules are particularly rich in steroid sulfatase activity and that this enzyme may regulate the physiological exposure of the seminiferous tubules to the effects of active metabolites of steroid monosulfates (Notation, 1975). Clearly, much further work will need to be undertaken regarding the potential role of steroid sulfates as intermediates in hormone biosynthesis. It must be remembered, however, that many of these reactions take place in anatomical compartments that are difficult to sample and that plasma steady state levels of hormones and the metabolism of labeled tracers placed in the bloodstream may not reflect what is taking place at a tissue level. Furthermore, species differences and alterations in metabolic pathways with development will surely be appreciated.

DHEAS and Estrogen Production

A major and the best established role for sulfated steroids as precursors of more active hormones comes through studies of human pregnancies. DHEAS secreted either by the maternal adrenal glands early in pregnancy or the fetal adrenal glands later in pregnancy appears to be the major precursor for the very large amounts of estrogen produced during a normal pregnancy (Siiteri and MacDonald, 1963, 1966; Warren and Timberlake, 1964). When substrate supply is interrupted, as occurs in fetuses with hypoplastic adrenal glands, estrogen production is markedly reduced. When pregnant women are given ACTH, stimulation of estrogen production is seen, and when the maternal adrenals are suppressed with dexamethasone, estrogen production diminishes. Furthermore, administration of DHEAS loads to pregnant women results in augmentation of estrogen production rates, and perfused placentas are capable of converting DHEAS into estrogens. Thus, the role of DHEAS and 16-hydroxy-DHEAS as precursors of estrogens in normal human pregnancies seems well established. Evidence derived from the study of patients with genetic defects in steroid sulfatase activity have even further sub-stantiated this precursor–product relationship.

STEROID SULFATASE (STS)

Many mammalian tissues and a few nonmammalian sources as well contain an enzymatic activity or activities capable of hydrolyzing a broad range of 3-β-hydroxy-steroid sulfates and structurally related synthetic sulfate ester (Rose, 1982; Roy, 1970). In early studies employing synthetic sulfates as substrates, a variety of genetically distinct sulfatases became grouped together operationally as the arylsulfatases. Such tissue arylsul-fatase activity was originally separated into type 1 and type 2 enzymes (Table I). Type 1 arylsulfatases are relatively insensitive to inhibition by sulfate or phosphate ion, but are strongly inhibited by cyanide. Type 2 enzymes are quite sensitive to sulfate and phosphate inhibition, but are partially activated by exposure to chloride ions. Subsequently, at least three arylsulfatase activities were separated by chromatographic and elec-trophoretic procedures and were termed arylsulfatases A, B, and C. The first two represent type 2 enzymes and the latter represents the type 1 enzyme. In addition, it is now clear that arylsulfatases A and B are lyso-somal in their location and have acid pH optima. The natural substrate for arylsulfatase A is galactocerebroside-3-sulfate and a gene specifying this enzyme activity is located on human chromosome 22 (De Luca *et al.*, 1979; Kolodny and Moser, 1983). Deficiency of arylsulfatase A activ-ity results in the well-known disorder of metachromatic leukodystrophy, which probably exists in a variety of allelic forms. The natural substrate for arylsulfatase B is galactosamine-4-sulfate residues in dermatan sulfate (McKusick and Neufeld, 1983). This exohydrolase recognizes terminal *N*-acetylgalactosamine-4-sulfate residues and desulfates them. This activity seems to be encoded on human chromosome 5 and a deficiency of enzyme activity results in mucopolysaccharidosis Type VI or the Maro-teaux–Lamy syndrome. The remaining arylsulfatase activity is particu-late (sediments with the 100,000 $\times$ g fraction of cell extracts), and has a neutral to slightly alkaline pH optimum. The natural substrates for this enzyme activity are thought to be 3-β-hydroxysteroid sulfates. Arylsul-fatases A and B hydrolyze nitrocatechol sulfate quite effectively, while

Table I. Properties of Arylsulfatases

	Type 1 enzyme: Arylsulfatase C	Type 2 enzymes	
		Arylsulfatase A	Arylsulfatase B
Natural substrate	Cholesterol sulfate DHEA sulfate 16-OH DHEA sulfate Estrone sulfate Estriolsulfate Pregnenolone sulfate 17-OH pregnenolone sulfate Others?	Galactosyl sulfatide Lactosyl sulfatide Psychosine sulfate Ascorbic acid sulfate	N-Acetyl galactosamine-4-sulfate (in dermatan sulfate) UDP-N-Acetyl galactosamine-4-sulfate Chondroitin-4-sulfate
Artificial substrate	4-Methylumbelliferyl sulfate P-Nitrophenylsulfate Others	Nitrocatechol sulfate 4-Methylumbelliferyl sulfate Others	Nitrocatechol sulfate 4-Methylumbelliferyl sulfate Others
pH Optimum	7.7–8.2	4.6–5.1	6.0
Activator	±SDS	Chloride	Chloride
Inhibitor	CN^-	SO_4^{2-}, PO_4^{2-}, Ba^{2+}	SO_4, PO_4^{3-}, P_2O_7
Glycoprotein	+	+	+
Subunit MW	57–60 kd	50 kd	50 kd
Subcellular location	"Microsomal"	Lysosomal	Lysosomal
Chromosomal assignment	$Xp22.3 \rightarrow Xpter$	22q13.31–22qter	5
Genetic deficiency	Placental sulfatase deficiency X-Linked ichthyosis Multiple sulfatase deficiency	Metachromatic leukodystrophy Multiple sulfatase deficiency	Mucopolysaccharidosis VI Maroteaux–Lamy syndrome Multiple sulfatase deficiency

arylsulfatase C does not. In contrast, p-nitrophenyl sulfate is more avidly recognized by arylsulfatase C. All three classes of sulfatases appear to act quite efficiently on the fluorogenic substrate 4-methylumbelliferyl sulfate. As will be discussed below (p. 340), it is still open to some debate as to whether or not arylsulfatase C corresponds exactly to steroid sulfatase.

The question of the number of discrete steroid sulfatases that might exist in human or mammalian tissues has been the subject of much controversy (Bleau *et al.*, 1971; French and Warren, 1967; Hameister *et al.*, 1979; Iwamori *et al.*, 1976; Zuckerman and Hagerman, 1966). Utilizing kinetic data, it has been observed that many of the sulfated steroids inhibit the hydrolysis of one another, but do so in a noncompetitive fashion when analyzed by Lineweaver–Burk plots. Furthermore, during several attempts at purification of steroid sulfatases, it has been observed that the relative specific activities toward various steroid sulfate substrates increase to a differing extent (Iwamori *et al.*, 1976; Zuckerman and Hagerman, 1966). Finally, some properties, such as pH optima for the various substrates and thermal stability of enzyme activity when assayed with different substrates, suggest the existence of separable isozymes for these various activities. Several facts should be borne in mind when interpreting these results, however. First, most of these studies have been carried out with crude microsomal preparations or solubilized partially purified enzyme. Therefore, a variety of additional factors could influence the kinetic results obtained with these impure enzyme preparations. There is ample precedent for alteration of pH optimum and other parameters in such crude preparations, and many multisubstrate enzymes show slightly differing properties toward various potential substrates. Most preparations of steroid sulfatase do not show classical Michaelis–Menten kinetics with natural steroidal substrates (Gauthier *et al.*, 1978) and therefore determination of competitive versus noncompetitive inhibition is difficult. Finally, some of the enzyme substrates utilized in these assays have only limited solubility and may in fact exist in micelles rather than in solution. Considerable evidence cogently argues in favor of there being only a single genetically determined steroid sulfatase in most mammalian tissues. First, with two possible exceptions (Erickson *et al.*, 1983; Mathew and Balasubramanian, 1982), no physical separation of any of the sulfatases appears to have occurred even during rather substantial purification. Second, antibodies (including monoclonal antibodies) against steroid sulfatase precipitate all enzyme activities (Erickson *et al.*, 1983; L. J. Shapiro, unpublished results). Third, all of these activities appear to map to the same region of the short arm of the human X chromosome in human–rodent somatic cell hybrids (Mohandas *et al.*, 1979; Muller *et al.*, 1980c). Finally, all activities appear to be lost coordinately in patients with steroid sulfatase deficiency (all of whom seem to belong to a single complementation group by cell fusion studies) (Shapiro and Mohandas, 1980).

The enzyme can be solubilized with the use of a variety of detergents. Some degree of purification of rat liver steroid sulfatase and human placental sulfatase has been achieved by several groups (Gauthier *et al.*, 1978; Iwamori *et al.*, 1976; McNaught and France, 1980; Noel *et al.*, 1983; Epstein and Bonifus, 1984). The results of these analyses are somewhat discrepant, however. Molecular weights ranging from 23,000 to over one million have been reported. This probably reflects incompletely solubilized enzyme in some of these preparations, which is either aggregated due to hydrophobic domains, or to which small pieces of microsomal membranes have remained attached as well as attendant adsorbed phospholipid. Three laboratories seem to agree that the placental enzyme has a subunit of molecular weight of between 57,000 and 62,000. Some microheterogeneity in subunit size may exist for a variety of reasons. The enzyme appears to be a glycoprotein, as is manifested by its binding to and elution from concanavalin A (Noel et al., 1983b). Substantial hydrophobic domains also probably exist, which result in rapid reaggregation of the enzyme. A dimeric form of the enzyme appears to be active, but the actual state of the ezyme in microsomal membranes is not clear. Neutron inactivation analysis suggests a functional in situ molecular weight of up to 533,000 (Noel et al., 1983a). Work ongoing in several laboratories should help to elucidate a number of these structural details in the near future. Steroid sulfatase can be inhibited by a number of physiological and synthetic steroids. This has led to suggestions that pharmacological modification of steroid sulfatase activity in pregnancy might be an effective means of controlling estrogen production and perhaps even be a useful adjunct in the prevention of prematurity. Steroid sulfatase appears to have no cofactor requirements and seems to be unaffected by divalent cation concentration, reducing agents, etc. Once solubilized, detergent needs to be present during all manipulations to prevent spontaneous reaggregation. The enzyme is remarkably stable to heat, pH alterations, exposure to urea, and a variety of other procedures.

In light of recent observations regarding the biosynthesis and processing of another microsomal enzyme, 3-hydroxy-3-methyl glutaryl CoA reductase (HMG CoA reductase) (Liscom et al., 1983), it is interesting to speculate that steroid sulfatase may share some features in common. HMG CoA reductase is also a glycoprotein and apparently has a significant hydrophobic region, which contains the carbohydrate and is embedded in the microsomal membrane. HMG CoA reductase can be released from the microsomal membrane by treatment with a calcium-dependent protease, giving rise to a much smaller protein that retains antigenic and enzymatic activity but has lost its carbohydrate. Similar analyses have not yet been carried out for steroid sulfatase, and future experiments will hopefully shed light on the biosynthesis, degradation, and posttranslational processing that occur during the life cycle of this enzyme. Such studies could be important for understanding the biogenesis of organelles and could prove relevant to such human genetic defects as steroid sulfatase deficiency and multiple sulfatase deficiency.

STEROID SULFATASE DEFICIENCY

France and Liggins (1969) investigated two pregnancies in a New Zealand woman that were associated with strikingly low estriol excretion (France, 1979). They were able to show that the placentas from these pregnancies had markedly reduced activities of 3-β-hydroxy-steroid sulfatase, with preservation of the other enzymes necessary for aromatization of precursors to estrogens (France and Liggins, 1969; France et al., 1973). In subsequent work, they showed that women carrying an affected fetus responded normally to a load of free DHEA with an increase in estrogen excretion, but that DHEAS could not be used as a precursor in vivo. During the ensuing years, many additional cases of steroid sulfatase deficiency have been detected during pregnancy by this means (diminished estriol levels) [reviewed in Crawford, (1982) and France (1979]. In all instances, the fetus in question was a male and no physiological abnormalities other than the low estrogen levels were noted. However, many of these pregnancies were characterized by lack of cervical dilatation at the onset of labor, with some degree of prolongation of gestation due to failure to initiate parturition (Table II). Similar findings have been observed in a number of other clinical situations in which estrogen production is impaired.

Prenatal metabolic consequences of steroid sulfatase deficiency have been extensively studied. The maternal urinary excretion of a variety of sulfated steroids is abnormal (Taylor, 1982; Taylor and Shackleton, 1979). The maternal urinary 16-hydroxy-DHEAS levels are elevated more than 20-fold above normal (Beastall et al., 1976; France et al., 1973; Oakey et al., 1974; Taylor and Shackleton, 1979). Similarly, DHEAS levels in amniotic fluid of affected pregnancies are increased (Braunstein et al., 1976; Oakey et al., 1974; Osathanondh et al., 1976). Cord blood DHEAS and 16-hydroxy-DHEAS are usually normal, although in one instance, an apparent DHEAS elevation was described (France et al., 1973; Osathanondh et al., 1976; Tabei and Heinrichs, 1976; Taylor and Shackleton, 1979). Early on, there was some confusion about the bio-

Table II. Clinical Features of Steroid Sulfatase Deficiency[a]

Normal karyotype
  X-Linked inheritance
  Diminished maternal estriol excretion and levels
  Delayed parturition*
  Ichthyosis
  Elevated cholesterol sulfate levels
  Normal DHEAS, testosterone, FSH, LH
  Elevated DHEAS, 16-OH DHEAS prenatally
  Abnormal lipoprotein electrophoretic mobility
  Corneal opacities
  Cryptorchidism*
  Testicular tumors*

Abnormal karyotype
  Mental retardation
  Short stature
  Stippled epiphyses
  Nasal hypoplasia
  Other abnormalities as above
  Loss of STS locus and other genes in Xp22.3 → Xpter as result of deletion or
    translocation

[a] Asterisk denotes variable feature.

chemical and genetic aspects of this condition. Employing different assay techniques, the New Zealand group reported very low levels of arylsulfatases A and B in the placenta of an affected child, but on subsequent evaluation of this subject in later life, peripheral leukocytes showed normal levels of arylsulfatases A and B (France *et al.*, 1976). They interpreted these findings to mean that the genetic lesion resulted in a diminution of all arylsulfatase activities in the placenta, but not in somatic tissues. These observations were subsequently refuted when consistent assay techniques using sulfated steroids were applied to affected placentas and to cultured fibroblasts (Shapiro *et al.*, 1977). Thus it has become clear that, with the exception of the disorder of multiple sulfatase deficiency, defects of arylsulfatases A, B, and C are genetically distinct, and patients with steroid sulfatase deficiency have no evidence of lysosomal accumulation of any substrates. Biochemically, absence of enzyme activity has been documented in placenta (France and Liggins, 1969), cultured skin fibroblasts (Shapiro *et al.*, 1977), cultured epidermal cells (Kubilus *et al.*, 1979), leukocytes (Epstein and Leventhal, 1981) hair roots (Dancis *et al.*, 1983; Meyer *et al.*, 1979), epidermis (DeGroot *et al.*, 1980; Epstein and

Leventhal, 1981; Jobsis *et al.*, 1980; Koppe *et al.*, 1978; Ruokonen and Oikarinen, 1981), stratum corneum (Baden *et al.*, 1980), and even fingernail clippings (Baden *et al.*, 1980) of affected subjects. During early investigations, the marked sex predilection of this disorder for males suggested X-linked inheritance. Confirmation of this suggestion did not come until application of fibroblast culture techniques in family studies was undertaken.

Clinical Features of Steroid Sulfatase Deficiency

Clincial manifestations of stored sulfatase deficiency can be grouped into three areas: impaired placental estrogen production, ichthyosis, and altered gonadal function. The latter finding is more recent and will require further verification. As indicated above, the prenatal manifestations of steroid sulfatase deficiency were the first to be appreciated. Since 1969, a large number of cases ascertained during pregnancy have been described. A recent review includes clinical details on 70 patients reported in the literature (Crawford, 1982). By definition, all affected pregnancies have been associated with markedly diminished estriol production and with striking deficiency of steroid sulfatase activity assayed with a variety of substrates. However, there is an obvious ascertainment bias in such compilations, since serum or urinary estriol determinations were in fact the mode of recognition of each of the patients. The majority of these affected pregnancies were delivered by Caesarian section or following pharmacological induction of labor, but a significant number were born following spontaneous vaginal delivery. It would be of considerable interest to study a series of pregnancies prospectively ascertained by the presence in the family of subjects with X-linked ichthyosis. In similar families, a retrospective assessment of the incidence of Caesarian section, stillbirth, etc., would remove the bias of having obstetrical observers who are primed to intervene in these pregnancies at the earliest sign of difficulty. A single pregnancy studied in which the fetus had steroid sulfatase deficiency due to a distinct autosomal mutation (multiple sulfatase deficiency) was associated with a similar degree of impaired estrogen production (Steinmann *et al.*, 1981). A variety of abnormalities of estrogen precursor levels has been reported both prenatally and postnatally. It seems prudent at this juncture to conclude that steroid sulfatase deficiency is always associated with decreased estrogen biosynthesis, but that variations in the duration of pregnancy and the frequency with which obstetrical intervention is required are far more variable (Crawford, 1982).

X-Linked Ichthyosis

Ichthyosis is a descriptive term used in relation to a number of genetic and acquired skin disorders characterized by hyperkeratosis leading to a scaly appearance. A variety of systemic illnesses as well as a number of drugs can produce this phenotype. Ichthyosis has been noted as a component of a number of complex syndromes. In addition, a group of well-defined and genetically discrete conditions have been described in which ichthyosis is the sole recognized component (Marks and DyFes, 1978). These include autosomal dominant ichthyosis vulgaris, autosomal recessive lamellar ichthyosis, and X-linked ichthyosis. It is likely that there is a significant degree of heterogeneity in at least the former two conditions. In 1863, Sedgwick described a family with ichthyosis that was clearly inherited in an X-linked fashion. A number of similar families were subsequently reported, enabling Cockayne (1933) to propose that sex-linked ichthyosis was a clearly definable entity. Although many pedigrees were subsequently written about in the medical literature, it was not until the meticulous work of Wells, Kerr, and colleagues in the 1960s that clear clinicial delineation of the various ichthyoses was achieved (Kerr and Wells, 1965; McNaught and France, 1980; Wells and Jennings, 1967; Wells and Kerr, 1965, 1966a,b). They studied a number of families in the UK and were able to establish an array of clinical and histological criteria for the classification of these disorders. Autosomal recessive lamellar ichthyosis is the most severe of these conditions. Manifestations are frequently obvious at birth and include ectropion and eclabion and a "collodoin membrane." Some recessively inherited cases are associated with striking erythroderma when the collodoin membrane is shed (Marks and DyFes, 1978). In later life, there are generalized large, coarse, scales and the palms and soles are noticeably thickened. Histologically, there is an increased epidermal mitotic index with moderate to marked hyperkeratosis and a normal granular layer.

Autosomal dominant ichthyosis vulgaris is probably the most common and the mildest of these entities. It is rarely present at birth, but usually appears during the first year of life. It is frequently associated with

Table III. The Common Genetic Ichthyoses

	X-Linked ichthyosis	Lamellar ichthyosis	Ichthyosis vulgaris
Inheritance	X-Linked	Autosomal recessive	Autosomal dominant
Age of onset	Four to six months, may be present at birth	Birth	Usually about 1 year
Severity	++	+++ to ++++	+
Erythroderma	−	Occasional	−
Atopy	−	−	+
Seasonal fluctuation	+	−	+
Size of scale	Moderate	Large	Small to moderate
Associated features	Steroid sulfatase deficiency; decreased fetal–maternal estriol production; delayed parturition; collodion membrane (rare); cryptorchidism; testicular tumors	Collodion membrane (occasional); ectropion; eclabion (occasional)	−
Thickening of palms and soles	−	+	±
Incidence	One in 6000 males	Rare	One in 1000
Response to retinoids	−	+	±
Histology	Normal granular layer; hyperkeratosis	Increased mitotic index; normal granular layer	Diminished granular layer

atopy and eczema. The forehead and cheeks may be mildly affected, but the flexor surfaces are spared. The palms and soles are often thickened, and there is a tendency for symptoms to improve with increasing age. Histologically a diminished or absent granular layer in the epidermis is said to be characteristic (Table III).

X-Linked ichthyosis affects about one in 6000 males. This incidence seems remarkably constant in a variety of racial and ethnic groups. In contrast to dominant ichthyosis vulgaris, which it resembles most closely, X-linked ichthyosis may be present at birth (although more typically at 3–6 months of age). It is usually somewhat more severe and particularly involves the neck and trunk more extensively than does the autosomal dominant variety. Palms and soles are spared, but flexor surfaces may be affected in X-linked patients. Histology of skin biopsies from X-linked patients is usually normal except for the thickened stratum corneum (Kerr and Wells, 1965; McNaught and France, 1980; Wells and Jennings, 1967; Wells and Kerr, 1965, 1966a,b). The scales themselves are often larger, thicker, and darker than in the vulgaris patients (Fig. 3). The ichthyosis in X-linked subjects may grow worse with age, while autosomal dominant varieties often improve. No consistent abnormalities are observed in female heterozygotes for the X-linked form. Sporadic reports of dry skin are difficult to interpret. Hemizygous males with X-linked ichthyosis usually have corneal opacities detectable by slit lamp examination. Heterozygotes are said to have similar opacities, although milder in degree. Careful inspection of the original report describing this finding in female carriers indicates that many normal control subjects were found to have opacities of a comparable extent (Sever *et al.*, 1968). Two women presumably affected by X-linked ichthyosis have been described in a single pedigree (Stern, 1973). This is apparently the result of consanguinity and so the affected sisters are presumably homozygotes. Both kinds of

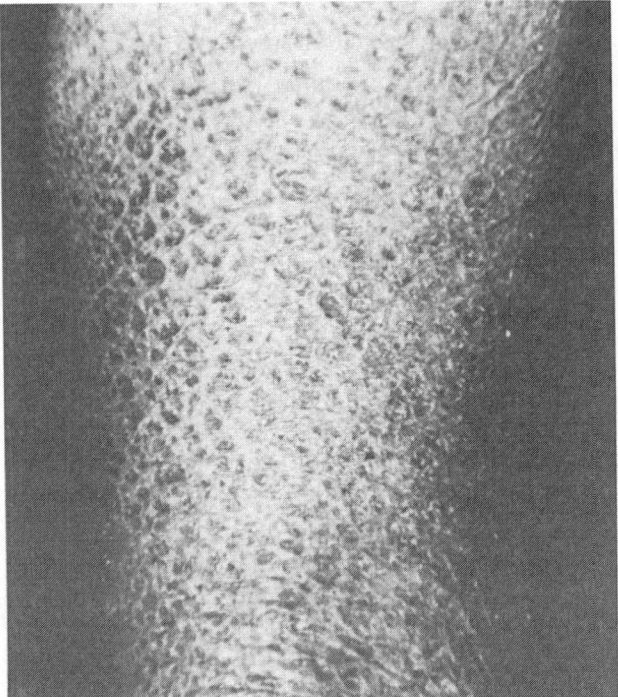

Fig. 3. The clinical appearance of X-linked ichthyosis. Note darkened scales, which become more pronounced with age, and are particularly marked on extremities, trunk, and flanks.

ichthyosis may show seasonal variations, with improvement being seen in warm or hot weather.

Treatment of all the ichthyoses is currently undergoing substantial reevaluation. Dominant ichthyosis vulgaris is often mild enough not to require treatment, and when it does, it often responds favorably to oils and ointments. Lamellar ichthyosis (recessive) seems to improve with the oral administration of synthetic retinoids, which may prove quite useful in management (Marks and DyFes, 1978). Caution needs to be exercised with the use of these potent new agents, however, as there are reports of significant hypertriglyceridemia with treatment (Katz et al., 1980). In addition, retinoids may well be potent human teratogens (Rosa, 1983). Patients with X-linked ichthyosis do not respond to vitamin A derivatives and in fact their condition may deteriorate somewhat during therapeutic trials. However, recent clinical experiments with new buffered lactic acid preparations or with topical cholesterol therapy may offer some hope for improved management in the near future (Lykkesfeldt and Hoyer, 1983).

Due to the frequency of X-linked ichthyosis, the clearly established pattern of inheritance, and the existence of numerous pedigrees with multiple affected individuals in several generations, a number of workers have undertaken linkage studies of X-linked ichthyosis and other X-chromosome markers. Evaluation of these pedigrees demonstrates no obvious reduction in genetic fitness for either hemizygous affected males or heterozygous females. Linkage with the G6PD and color blindness loci was readily excluded, but strong evidence for linkage with the Xg locus has been established in a number of laboratories (Adam et al., 1966, 1969; Filippi and Khan, 1968; Kerr and Wells, 1964; Shapiro et al., 1978b; Wells et al., 1966; Went et al., 1969). The aggregate lod score with $\theta \simeq 0.10$ is greater than 17.

Although ichthyosis was not originally appreciated as a clinical feature of steroid sulfatase deficiency, two groups subsequently noted the presence of ichthyosis in several family members under study (Koppe et al., 1978; Shapiro et al., 1978b). Subsequent investigation of a large number of families with classical X-linked ichthyosis has shown that all are associated with steroid sulfatase deficiency (Shapiro et al., 1978a). This observation, plus the abnormalities in stratum corneum lipids to be described below, makes it seem virtually certain that steroid sulfatase deficiency is the primary biochemical etiology of X-linked ichthyosis.

Further credence is added to support this notion from consideration of patients with multiple sulfatase deficiency. As previously described, such patients have steroid sulfatase deficiency due to a poorly understood autosomal recessive mutation affecting expression of a number of sulfatases (Murphy *et al.,* 1971). These individuals have ichthyosis and have increased levels of cholesterol sulfate in their stratum corneum (E. Bergner and L. J. Shapiro, unpublished results). This finding excludes the formal possibility that steroid sulfatase deficiency and X-linked ichthyosis are closely linked genetic disorders in linkage disequilibrium, or are the result of a deletion of linked loci. The recognition of the pathogenetic role of steroid sulfatase deficiency in X-linked ichthyosis has done much to improve the diagnosis, treatment, and basic understanding of this condition.

Testicular Abnormalities

Patients with steroid sulfatase deficiency seem to enjoy relatively good health with few coincident abnormalities postnatally other than their skin disease. Many patients in their 70s have been observed. Recently, however, two groups have raised the possibility of additional causally related abnormalities of testicular dysfunction and neoplasia in some patients with this condition. In general, testicular function has been thought to be normal in this syndrome due to the presence of normal pubertal development, virilization, and fertility. In addition, measurements of testosterone, androstenedione, LH, and FSH have been normal in several adult subjects studied (Shapiro, 1982). However, Traupe and Happle (1983) found cryptorchidism in seven of 25 subjects with steroid sulfatase deficiency in their clinic. The reason for this surprisingly high incidence of cryptorchidism in X-linked ichthyosis is unknown. Previous summaries have not mentioned similar findings. These workers may have in some way identified a unique subset of patients with steroid sulfatase deficiency. Lykkesfeldt *et al.* (1983) reported two STS-deficient subjects with testicular tumors. One of these had a seminoma and another had an embryonal carcinoma and a seminoma discovered 5 years apart. A third patient with testicular cancer and steroid sulfatase deficiency is known to me. At present, it is difficult to say whether these observations represent true associations between such testicular abnormalities and steroid sulfatase deficiency, or chance events. A theoretical basis for such abnormalities will, however, be considered below.

Steroid Metabolism in STS Deficiency

As might be anticipated, the levels of a number of sulfated metabolites are increased in maternal urine (Taylor, 1982; Taylor and Shackleton, 1979) and amniotic fluid of affected pregnancies (Braumstein et al., 1976; Oakey et al., 1974; Osathanondh et al., 1976). In contrast, with the exception of cholesterol sulfate (CS) (Bergner and Shapiro, 1981; Epstein et al., 1981a), levels of sulfated steroids in neonatal urine (Taylor and Shackleton, 1979), cord blood (France et al., 1973, Tabei and Heinrichs, 1976; Taylor and Shackleton, 1979), and postnatal plasma from affected infants and adults are generally normal (Ruokonen et al., 1980). One group observed striking elevation of cord blood DHEAS in a single child, which returned to normal by 6 months of age (Osathanondh et al., 1976). In at least 11 other infants, cord DHEAS levels were near normal. Furthermore, the levels of DHEA in both cord blood and in postnatal plasma are generally normal. Perfusion studies have indicated that the human fetus as a whole has a very active sulfokinase activity toward a variety of free steroids, but relatively little steroid sulfatase function (Dicfalusy, 1969). In contrast, the perfused placenta rapidly hydrolyzes steroid sulfates, but has relatively little sulfokinase activity.

The finding of normal DHEAS and DHEA levels in patients with steroid sulfatase deficiency suggests that desulfation may not be terribly important quantitatively for the homeostasis of either compound. Alternatively there may be other mechanisms to achieve desulfation of DHEAS. Some DHEA is of course the result of direct adrenal secretion. It has been proposed that DHEA is an important hormone and has its peripheral circulating concentration regulated by a pituitary peptide hormone dubbed CASH (corticotropin-androgen stimulating hormone) (Parker and Odell, 1979). It is tempting to speculate that in situations where DHEAS → DHEA conversion is impaired, this system comes into play to increase the direct adrenal secretion of DHEA. Alternative explanations for these results must be considered. First, since no autopsy study of STS-deficient patients has ever been done, it is possible that the mutation in STS deficiency affects enzyme activity in some but not all tissues and that discrete STS isozymes exist in some organs. This possiblility cannot be assessed directly, for obvious reasons. A second theory is that some anatomic site might contain a "transconjugase" activity capable of direct conversion of steroid sulfates to glucuronides without the need of a free steroid intermediate. There is no precedent for such an enzymatic mechanism. A third theoretical possibility is that there is a physiological enterohepatic circulation of DHEAS with desulfation by intestinal bacteria and either further metabolism or reabsorption of free steroid. Such a role for intestinal flora now has very ample precedent. Recent studies indicate that deoxycorticosterone sulfate in humans (Casey and MacDonald, 1982) and estrogen sulfates in humans and rats may well be metabolized by such a pathway (Adlercreutz *et al.*, 1976; Back *et al.*, 1981). Preliminary data suggest that such a route of intestinal bacterial desulfation exists in at least one patient with STS deficiency given a tracer dose of ^{3}H-DHEAS (E. Bergner and L. J. Shapiro, unpublished results). This subject was able to desulfate appreciable amounts of DHEAS prior to but not following oral ampicillin administration. Furthermore, steady state plasma levels of free DHEA fell from normal to a subnormal range following antibiotic administration. Another subject apparently failed to desulfate the tracer even under basal conditions, however. In any event, circulating DHEA and DHEAS levels do not seem to be very much disrupted by this disease.

The most consistent substrate abnormality in STS-deficient subjects is a striking elevation in cholesterol sulfate in plasma and red blood cell membranes. This results in CS levels of 15- to 30-fold greater than normal and is already present in cord blood (Bergner and Shapiro, 1981). Fifty percent of daily CS disposal is thought to occur via the biliary route, although enterohepatic recirculation of CS was not considered in these calculations. If reabsorption of intact CS takes place to any significant extent, this may be a gross overestimate. The majority of CS appears to be bound to plasma LDL. The relatively large amount of CS associated with LDL in STS deficiency confers increased electronegativity and altered electrophoretic mobility on this lipoprotein (Epstein *et al.*, 1981*a*). Whether a significant fraction of cholesterol sulfate might normally be metabolized via the LDL receptor pathway and what the impact of the increased negative charge of LDL is on its interaction with receptor in STS deficiency have not been determined. As mentioned previously, it has been speculated that the alterations in lipid composition of the stratum corneum in STS-deficient subjects are responsible for their ichthyosis (Williams and Elias, 1981). Whether such changes reflect increased cholesterol sulfate directly or some secondary abnormalities remains to be determined. Interestingly, mitochondria from the fetal adrenal cortex appear to preferentially utilize cholesterol sulfate as a substrate for the desmolase enzyme while the adult adrenal uses cholesterol almost exclusively (Korte *et al.,* 1982). Thus, in fetal life, CS may be a principal precursor for adrenal steroidogenesis.

In summary, it is not clear why plasma CS is elevated in STS-deficient subjects while other sulfated steroids are present in normal levels, and the physiological impact of this alteration is not known. CS has a slightly more favorable K_m for rat liver and human placental STS than does DHEAS, but it seems unlikely that this accounts for the differences observed. Rather, the association of CS with LDL and of DHEAS with other serum proteins probably determines their differential tissue partitioning and extraction. Further work should clarify such issues. It seems safe to conclude that normal CS disposal is more dependent on the activity of the steroid sulfatase system than is DHEAS.

Testicular Metabolism in STS Deficiency

As noted previously, the recently recognized incidence of cryptorchidism and testicular tumors dictates a reexamination of the impact of STS deficiency on testicular function. If in fact these associations are ultimately found to have statistical validity, at least two potential kinds of mechanisms might be suggested to account physiologically for these findings. Since many patients with steroid sulfatase deficiency are fertile, normally virilized, and have normal testosterone production as adults, either the patients described above have very subtle alterations in testicular physiology, or they could have some sequelae of disordered metabolism *in utero.* Alternatively, they could be a unique subset of STS-deficient subjects. One hypothesis that can be considered in more detail is that *some* STS⁻ patients have small Xp deletions, which result in the loss of some X-chromosome genes in addition to STS. These genes might represent necessary functions for testicular descent or may mitigate the development of tumors. Alternatively, since the distal X is thought to pair with the Y during meiosis, discernible deletions of Xp might result in disordered germ cell development. Another possible mechanistic relationship between STS mutations and testicular abnormalities is that steroid sulfatase deficiency *per se* might negatively impact on testicular steroidogenesis and lead to cryptorchidism or tumors by this route. The relative importance of the Δ^4 and the Δ^5 pathways in testicular testosterone production is still subject to some debate, and little information is available regarding the specific utilization of these pathways prenatally. Furthermore, whatever the extent to which the Δ^5 pathway is employed, the role of sulfate 3-β-hydroxy-Δ^5-steroids is unknown. As described above, the fetal adrenal gland may preferentially utilize cholesterol sulfate as a substrate for steroidogenesis, particularly as compared to the adult adrenal. Similar developmentally regulated alterations in testosterone biosynthetic pathways may be operative as well. In addition, it is possible that genetically determined polymorphism exists regarding the flux among these various alternative pathways. Thus, although no gross disruption of androgen production is attendant to steroid sulfatase deficiency, perhaps more subtle abnormalities, including the intratesticular accumulation of sulfated intermediates, play some role in these recently appreciated clinical features of steroid sulfatase deficiency.

GENETICS OF STEROID SULFATASE

With the development of methods to accurately assay STS activity in cultured fibroblasts, leukocytes, and other tissues, it became possible to quickly identify STS-deficient individuals in pedigrees. The recognition of X-linked ichthyosis as a clinical concomitant of STS deficiency has made it obvious that a gene related to STS expression is located on the human X chromosome. However, it should be pointed out that other autosomal genes may be involved in STS expression. Since STS is a glycoprotein (Noel *et al.*, 1983; L. J. Shapiro, unpublished results) and since it must presumably be situated in an appropriate intracellular compartment in order to function, it is quite conceivable that alterations in posttranslational processing or in other functions could affect ultimate STS expression. Evidence in support of this view derives from observations of patients with the autosomally inherited multiple sulfatase deficiency disorder (MSDD) (Murphy *et al.*, 1971). They have a profound reduction of STS activity as well as the activity of other sulfatases (Basner, 1979). These individuals often have clinically apparent ichthyosis, elevation of cholesterol sulfate levels, and impaired placental estrogen biosynthesis. This defect in a single gene results in the concomitant reduction of activities of at least nine distinct sulfatases known to be encoded on different chromosomes. Most of these (except STS) are lysosomal in location. Cell culture conditions can modulate the levels of enzyme expressed (Fluharty *et al.*, 1978, 1979), and the amount of immunoreactive enzyme varies with the amount of enzyme activity present (Fiddler *et al.*, 1979). The biochemical basis of this condition is not known, but it clearly illustrates the ability of nonstructural genes to influence the apparent level of STS. It will be important to recall this point when discussing some of the data regarding the genetics of STS expression in the mouse (see below).

Somatic Cell Studies

Confirmation that the STS structural gene(s) resides on the X chromosome derives from somatic cell genetic studies. It has been fortunate for purposes of these analyses that mouse A9 cells lack detectable STS activity when assayed with a variety of substrates. Many permanent rodent cell lines have somewhat reduced STS specific activity as compared to human fibroblasts, and several mouse L-cell derivatives seem to be totally devoid of enzyme expression. Whether this is a result of an alteration acquired in culture or the fact that the C3H/An mouse substrain from which L cells are allegedly derived are STS deficient in many of their organs and tissues remains to be seen (Balazs *et al.*, 1979). In addition to this system, human STS activity can be investigated in interspecific hybrids by electrophoretic analysis and visualization of activity in gels stained with the fluorogenic substrate 4-methylumbelliferyl sulfate or by use of species-specific anti-STS antibodies. Analysis of mouse–human and hamster–human hybrids carrying normal human X chromosomes and human X chromosomes derived from patients with X/autosome translocations have verified that the human STS gene is on the short arm distal to Xp22 (Mohandas *et al.*, 1979; Muller *et al.*, 1980c). With regard to the previously raised questions about the number of steroid sulfatase enzyme molecular types that might exist, it is of note that all of the enzyme activities map to the same region, so that if multiple steroid sulfatase structural genes exist, they would appear to be located in a single portion of the genome.

Deletion Mapping

Further evidence for the distal Xp location of the STS gene has come from the study of patients with a variety of Xp translocations or deletions. Tiepolo *et al.* (1980) described a moderately retarded patient with an unbalanced X/Y translocation and a variety of physical abnormalities, including ichthyosis. Further study has documented that this patient was nullisomic for Xp22.3 → Xpter and was steroid sulfatase deficient. Subsequently, a number of other males with X/Y translocations and deletions of approximately the same extent have been reported with similar findings (Akesson *et al.,* 1980; Allderdice *et al.,* 1983; Bernstein *et al.,* 1978; Borgaonkar *et al.,* 1974; Boyd *et al.,* 1981; Ferguson-Smith *et al.,* 1983; Heath *et al.,* 1980; Khudr *et al.,* 1973; Magenis *et al.,* 1982; Metaxotou *et al.,* 1983; Tiepolo *et al.,* 1977; van den Berge *et al.,* 1977; Zuffardi *et al.,* 1982). Some of these X/Y translocations are sporadic and some are familial. In most, the translocation chromosomes do not appear to be functional in male sex determination, in that 46Xt(X:Y) individuals are female and 46Yt(X:Y) subjects are male. However, two cases, apparently with very distal breakpoints, have resulted in translocation chromosomes that seem to carry this male sex determination information (Bernstein *et al.,* 1978, 1980). Clearly, the resolution of cytogenetic techniques is not adequate to map these various breakpoints, and molecular methods and markers will be required to more precisely characterize the nature and genesis of these chromosomal aberrations. Significantly, most subjects studied to date with X/Y translocations in which the translocation chromosome was the sole X material present in the males [with the exception of the patients described by Bernstein *et al.* (1978, 1980)] have been STS deficient. While inactivation of the STS gene by a position effect is a formal possibility since the reciprocal translocation product cannot be studied, actual deletion of the STS gene seems more likely, coinciding with the cytogenetic observations. From these findings and those described below, it would seem that distal Xp nullisomy is reasonably well tolerated.

Two additional families that provide information on the location of the STS gene have recently been encountered. Curry *et al.* (1984) have described an X-linked form of chondrodysplasia punctata characterized by mild mental retardation, short stature, stippled epiphyses early in life, and ichthyosis. Four males in two unrelated kindreds were identified with

this constellation of abnormalities, and all had STS deficiency and elevated levels of plasma cholesterol sulfate. On careful study, each had a
very small deletion of distal Xp involving the Xp22.3 subband. Heterozygous carrier females could also be recognized both cytologically and
biochemically and were significantly shorter than their noncarrier female
sibs. One additional piece of evidence supporting the assignment of STS
to the distal human short arm derives from studies of so-called XX
males. This condition will be discussed below (p. 369) in more detail.
Recent evidence suggests that such individuals may have cytologically
undetectable X/Y translocations, probably involving the distal X short
arm (de la Chapelle *et al.,* 1984; Guellaen *et al.,* 1984). While some XX
males appear to have normal steroid sulfatase activity (Ropers *et al.,*
1981*b*), two have been observed in dosage studies to have reduced STS
levels compatible with a deletion of the STS locus from one of the two
chromosomes (Pierella *et al.,* 1981; Wieacker *et al.,* 1983). In one of these
patients, this finding was confirmed by segregating the two X chromosomes in somatic cell hybrids and showing that one of them was found
in hybrids devoid of human STS activity. Thus, the collective data
involving X/autosome translocations in hybrids and deletion mapping
using X/Y translocations, Xp- pedigrees, and XX males leave little doubt
regarding the assignment of the human STS gene to Xp22.3 → Xpter.

STS in Other Species

The location of the STS gene in other species is less clear than in
humans, although some data regarding this point have appeared in the
literature. Ropers and Wiberg (1982) reported a gene dosage effect with
X-chromosome number in wood lemmings. Gartler and Rivest (1983)
found a dosage effect in ooctyes in X0 and XX mice, suggesting that STS
was X-linked in the mouse. Interestingly, however, this differential
expression is not reflected in somatic tissues from X0 and XX mice.
Their hypothesis is that the steroid sulfatase gene may be X-linked in the
mouse and *is* subject to X inactivation in somatic tissues (Crocker and
Craig, 1983; Gartler and Rivest, 1983), but in the oocyte, a gene dosage
effect is observed because of the known activity of both X chromosomes
in this cell type. Several other workers have suggested that one or more
autosomal loci are important in the control of steroid sulfatase expression
in the mouse. They have studied quantitative variation in STS activity

in various strains of inbred mice (Erickson *et al.*, 1983; Keinanen *et al.*, 1983; Nelson and Daniel, 1979; Nelson *et al.*, 1983). Genetic analysis was consistent with autosomal inheritance of a single Mendelian factor accounting for these strain-specific differences. However, the variability studied related to absolute levels of STS activity and was not associated with either altered kinetic or electrophoretic properties of the enzyme. Thus, the genes in question do not necessarily reflect the structural locus for the STS enzyme. Other investigators have studied a near complete deficiency of STS activity in a substrain of C3H/An mice (Balazs *et al.*, 1979). However, this genetic variant may not be reflected in all tissues (L. J. Shapiro *et al.*, unpublished results). This trait behaves like a single-gene autosomal marker in genetic studies, although location within a defined mouse linkage group has not yet been possible (M. Siniscalco, personal communication).

Cooper *et al.* (1984) have recently argued that STS is not X-linked in marsupials. This is based on studies of rodent–marsupial somatic cell hybrids that contain a complete marsupial X chromosome. None of these hybrids expressed the electrophoretically separable form of marsupial steroid sulfatase. Unfortunately, it is not clear that any positive hybrids expressing marsupial steroid sulfatase were identified to prove that in fact marsupial steroid sulfatase could be identified in such experiments. Nonetheless, Cooper and colleagues feel that their results are consistent with the fact that the "basic" marsupial X chromosome is smaller than the basic eutherian X and that the X and Y seem to lack a pairing segment in marsupials. Clearly, further research with molecular probes will be required to establish the actual location of steroid sulfatase genes in other mammalian species. If in fact the STS locus in humans is a relatively recent arrival to the X chromosome in an evolutionary sense, it will be of interest to see whether this reflects some unique functional requirements for STS expression or is just a chance event.

SOME GENES ON THE HUMAN X-CHROMOSOME SHORT ARM ARE NOT INACTIVATED

Mann *et al.* (1962) described the red cell Xg antigen system using serum from a multiply transfused male to detect its presence. This antigen has turned out to be a relatively weak immunogen, giving rise to low-titer antibodies in a relatively small number of exposed individuals. Furthermore, consistent expression has been observed only in red blood cells. Nonetheless, work carried out with such serologic reagents, primarily in the laboratory of Race and Sanger (1975), has added enormously to the understanding of the regulation of the X chromosome. This chromosomal locus has been referred to as Xg with alternative alleles Xg^a and Xg. The corresponding phenotypes are Xg(a+) and Xg(a−). Although Xg antigent (Xg^a) positivity is clearly inherited as an X-linked trait, expression of Xg^a is somewhat anomalous. Since the early to mid-1960s, strong evidence has been accumulated to support the concept that the Xg locus escapes X inactivation. Anti-Xg^a antibody is not able to recognize two populations of red cells in obligate Xg^a/Xg heterozygotes (Gorman *et al.*, 1963). Data derived from several studies established the autonomous production of Xg^a at the individual red cell level. A twin pair was studied in which both individuals were blood chimeras and had both type O and type AB cells in their peripheral circulation. These cells were separated by immunological means and the type O cells were found to be Xg(a+) and the type AB cells Xg(a−) in these individuals (Ducos *et al.*, 1971). This demonstrates that it is physically possible for both Xg(a+) and Xg(a−) cells to survive in the circulation of an individual and excludes the formal possibility of an extraerythrocytic origin for Xg^a, which could explain the apparent presence of Xg^a on all red cells in female heterozygotes.

Several additional kinds of evidence support the notion that Xg escapes inactivation. In addition to the lack of mosaicism mentioned above, the frequencies of Xg(a+) and Xg(a−) phenotypes differ significantly between males and females. Furthermore, studies of patients with chronic myelocytic leukemia (CML) have provided important information (Fialkow *et al.*, 1970; Lawler and Sanger, 1970). Cytogenetic investigation using the characteristic Philadelphia chromosome marker and isozyme studies in female patients who were G6PD heterozygotes have established a clonal origin of erythroid precursors as well as myeloid precursors in CML patients. Studies of the frequency of Xg(a+) and Xg(a−) phenotypes in a large number of women with CML showed a frequency of Xg^a positivity in this population, which was characteristic of normal females and distinct from that of normal males. If X inactivation is operative at the Xg locus, one might have expected each clonally derived cell line to be equivalent to males with a single X chromosome and Xg gene and thus reflect the male or chromosome specific gene frequency.

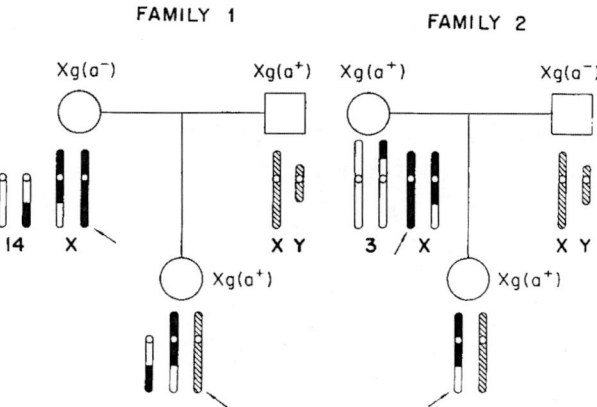

Fig. 4. Evidence for noninactivation of *Xg* from two X-autosome translocations. In family 1, an Xg(a−) balanced female carrier of an X/14 translocation chromosome had a daughter who was a balanced carrier as well. The girl's father was Xg(a+). As is often the case, the structurally normal chromosome (carrying the *Xg^a* allele) was prefentially inactivated, but the daughter was still Xg(a+). In family 2, an unbalanced translocation carrier with preferential inactivation of the abnormal X appeared to express Xg^a antigen from the inactive X.

    Three additional lines of evidence support the escape of inactivation of the *Xg* locus. Females doubly heterozygous for *Xg^a/Xg* and for hereditary X-linked sideroblastic anemia have also been informative (Weatherall *et al.,* 1970). Such women have two red cell populations, which are physically separable by their size into cells that have either the paternally derived X active, or the maternally derived X as the active X chromosome. Both populations expressed Xg^a equally. Studies of women doubly heterozygous for the Lesch–Nyhan syndrome *(HPRT$^+$/HPRT$^-$)* and *Xg^a/Xg* have also been informative (Fialkow, 1970). Due to strong selective pressure in circulating erythroid cells, only the paternally derived *(HPRT$^+$)* X chromosome is found to be active in red blood cell progenitors and normal levels of erythrocyte HPRT activity are seen. In three informative women in whom the phase relationship could be determined, it was possible to conclude that Xg^a was being expressed in their erythrocytes from an inactive X chromosome. Finally, two pedigrees in which X/autosome translocations were identified also gave information (Pearson, 1978). In one balanced female translocation carrier and in one unbalanced individual the preferential pattern of inactivation typically observed made it possible to conclude that the *Xg* gene was being transcribed from an otherwise inactive X (Fig. 4).

STS Is Not Inactivated

As mentioned previously, several linkage studies have convincingly demonstrated the genetic proximity of the X-linked ichthyosis *STS* locus to *Xg*. For these reasons, it became of interest to assess the function of the human STS gene with regard to X-chromosome inactivation. Initial studies focused on the expression of STS in fibroblast clones derived from obligate heterozygotes for STS deficiency. No STS-deficient clones were identified in preliminary experiments, but the possibility that selection exists against STS cells either *in vivo* or *in vitro* was an alternative interpretation of the data. Subsequently, fibroblasts were cloned from skin biopsies taken from women doubly heterozygous for G6PD variants and STS deficiency (Migeon *et al.,* 1982; Shapiro *et al.,* 1979). Two of these women carried the Mediterranean G6PD trait and two were heterozygous for A/B electrophoretic variants. Clones with either the maternally or paternally derived X chromosome active could thus be identified with certainty, and still STS activity was always present. Thus it appears that, like *Xg,* the *STS* locus escapes inactivation.

Further credence for this model has been obtained from somatic cell hydrid studies. Using as parental cell lines in a fusion experiment human fibroblasts from female patients with balanced X/autosome translocations, it has been possible to construct a number of human–rodent hybrid lines that retain a structurally normal, but inactive human X chromosome as their only human X material. Such cell lines maintain the X chromosome in an inactive state, as can be concluded from the lack of expression in human HPRT, G6DP, PGK, and α-galactosidase A, and from the late replication pattern of the chromosome visualized with a BrdU/acridine orange staining protocol. However, human steroid sulfatase continues to be produced by these hybrid cells (Mohandas *et al.,* 1980).

A final line of evidence supporting the lack of inactivation of the human STS locus comes from gene dosage studies. Although data from X-aneuploid individuals have been inconsistent, it seems clear that there is an STS dosage difference between males and females in a number of tissues, including fibroblasts, leukocytes, and placenta (Bedin *et al.,* 1981; Chance and Gartler, 1983; Dancis *et al.,* 1983; Epstein and Leventhal, 1981; Lykkesfeldt *et al.,* 1981; Muller *et al.,* 1980*a* and 1980*b*). However, it is equally clear that the ratio of female to male specific activities is less than two and on the average approximates 1.6. These results, along with more careful fibroblast cloning studies, makes it seem likely that some partial dosage compensation occurs at the STS locus and that this is achieved by down regulating one of the two STS loci in females.

The MIC2X and MIC2Y Loci

One additional gene has been mapped to the same region on the X chromosome in which *STS* and *Xg* are located. This is a gene called *MIC2X* (Goodfellow *et al.*, 1980). It specifies a ubiquitously distributed human specific cell surface antigen of unknown function recognized by a monoclonal antibody termed 12E7 (Levy *et al.*, 1979). Goodfellow and co-workers have used somatic cell hybrids to map this gene to the X chromosome and studies of hybrids containing the Xp- (delXp22.3 → Xpter) chromosome previously described indicate that *MIC2X* is located in this terminal region of Xp. By studying 12E7 expression in mouse–human hybrids retaining only the inactive human X, it has been shown that, like *STS* and *Xg*, the *MIC2X* locus excapes X-chromosome inactivation (Goodfellow *et al.*, 1984). Thus, these three genes, which map to the same portion of distal Xp, are all regulated in a similar fashion. There is some circumstantial data to suggest that *MIC2X* and *Xg* might be distal to *STS*, but the gene order is clearly uncertain at this point (Wieacker *et al.*, 1984). The *MIC2X* gene differs from *Xg* and *STS* in one important regard, however. That is that there appears to be a functional homologue of the *MIC2X* gene, dubbed *MIC2Y*, which is situated on the Y chromosome (Goodfellow *et al.*, 1983). This has been established by study of 12E7 expression in human–rodent hybrids having a Y chromosome, but lacking a human X. Furthermore, intact fibroblasts from the 46XY(Xp-) patient expressed 12E7, while, as just described, the Xp- chromosome isolated in hybrids does not direct the production of 12E7 (Curry *et al.*, 1984). The demonstration of *MIC2X* and *MIC2Y* represents an important theoretical contribution in considering the evolution and the function of the X and Y.

Inactivation and Structurally Abnormal X Chromosomes

The status of X inactivation for distal Xp on structurally abnormal X chromosomes is somewhat less certain. Polani *et al.* (1970) studied Xg blood groups in patients with deletions of the X-chromosome long arm.

They found three females who were $Xg(a-)$ daughters of $Xg(a^+)$ fathers. Each should have inherited an Xg^a allele from their fathers and thus been phenotypically $Xg(a^+)$. It was therefore argued that the aberrant X must have been paternally derived, and, as it was the preferentially inactive X in these individuals, that the inactivation must have included the Xg locus. However, nonpaternity and mosaicsim could not be excluded in all of the cases. Both Polani *et al.* (1970) and Sanger *et al.* (1977) observed that the distribution of $Xg(a+)$ and $Xg(a-)$ phenotypes in patients with structural abnormalities of the X chromosome was comparable to that seen in a normal male population and differed significantly from the frequency in the female population, again suggesting that the Xg locus had been inactivated on these abnormal X chromosomes. Ropers *et al.* (1981*a*) followed up these studies with a quantitative assessment of STS levels in two female subjects with structural aberrations of the X chromosome. These two individuals were found to have STS activities in the range observed in male controls. Chance and Gartler (1983) made a similar observation in a single patient. In evaluating these results, however, it should be pointed out that there is a fairly broad normal range for STS enzyme activity both in leukocytes and cultured fibroblasts with considerable overlap between normal males and females.

While the data described above would support the notion that *STS* and *Xg* might in fact be inactivated when situated on the structurally *abnormal* X chromosomes, other information refutes these findings. Pearson *et al.* (1978) showed that a girl who inherited a preferentially inactivated X/3 translocation chromosome (Xpter–Xq26::3q21–3qter) expressed Xg^a from this otherwise inactivated chromosome. This could be shown since the X/3 chromosome was late replicating in all cells, as would be expected in females with an unbalanced X/autosome translocation, and because this girl was $Xg(a+)$ while her father, who donated a structurally normal X, was $Xg(a-)$. Recently, Imken *et al.* (in press) have used somatic cell hybrid studies of STS expression to show that *STS* (and *MIC2X*) escape inactivation on at least two different abnormal inactive X chromosomes. They isolated somatic cell hybrids that retained these structurally aberrant inactive chromosomes as their only human X-derived material. These hybrid lines expressed both STS and 12E7. It is not yet possible to reconcile all of these observations, but it is clearly *possible* for *STS, MIC2X,* and *Xg* to escape inactivation both on structurally normal and abnormal X chromosomes. Whether these genes invariably behave in this fashion is uncertain.

STS and Studies of X Inactivation

Further studies of the STS gene and correlation of expression with gene and chromatin structure and methylation patterns should aid substantially in understanding the process of X-chromosome inactivation. The biology of this developmentally regulated pattern of gene expression has been recently reviewed (Gartler and Riggs, 1983). In particular, the role of DNA methylation in the control of gene expression on the X chromosome has been intensively investigated (Jones *et al.*, 1982; Lester *et al.*, 1982; Liskay and Evans, 1980; Mohandas *et al.*, 1981; Razin and Riggs, 1980; Shapiro and Mohandas, 1983; Wolf and Migeon, 1982; Yen *et al.*, 1984). Several points merit reemphasis, however. First, the process of initiation of inactivation is likely to be mechanistically different from the process of maintenance of the inactivated state. Furthermore, there may be more than one type of X inactivation. The initiation of X inactivation must almost surely have a chromosomal basis to explain the *cis* regulation of such a large number of genes. However, inactivation of somatic tissues and cells is clearly maintained at a much more localized level. This conclusion is supported by DNA-mediated gene transfer studies, which indicate that the information necessary to control expression is located with a finite (approximately 100 kb) region containing a given structural gene (Chapman *et al.*, 1982; Kratzer *et al.*, 1983; Liskay and Evans, 1980; Taylor, 1982). In addition, experiments implicating DNA methylation in the maintenance of X inactivation support a more localized control. For example, in experiments in which genes on an inactive X chromosome are reactivated by 5-azacytidine, individual genes are observed to be reexpressed, rather than the chromosome as a whole (Jones *et al.*, 1982; Mohandas *et al.*, 1981, 1982). Finally, the inactivation that takes place in extraembryonic membranes and in the yolk sac endoderm appears to take place somewhat earlier in embryogenesis, to involve preferential inactivation of the paternal X chromosome, and not to be associated with the same kind of DNA modification observed in X inactivation in somatic cells (Kratzer *et al.*, 1983; Takagi and Sasaki, 1975; West *et al.*, 1977). This latter feature is manifested by the ability of the *inactive* X-derived *HPRT* gene to function in a gene transfer assay when the DNA is taken from mouse embryo yolk sac endoderm as opposed to somatic tissues. Thus there appear to be at least two types of X inactivation and perhaps two phases of inactivation (with chromosomal and DNA sequence modification components) in somatic tissues. Further studies of STS expression and methylation in various embryonic tissues and at various times in development should help clarify some of these issues.

A second point is that there does not seem to be any fundamental difference in underlying structure between genes that are inactivated and those that are not. Since one and only one X is maintained in an active configuration and this is true regardless of how similar in DNA sequence the two X chromosomes might be [as, for example, in inbred mice or in parthenogenetically derived mouse embryos (Rastan *et al.*, 1980)] only one X is inactivated and the other is expressed. In addition, in X/autosome translocation chromosomes that are inactivated, inactivation can spread for variable lengths into the adjacent autosomal segment (Eicher, 1970; Mohandas *et al.*, 1982). Thus, there appears to be nothing unique about X-chromosome DNA sequences that renders them susceptible to X inactivation. Exactly how and why the *STS, Xg,* and *MIC2X* genes escape from this inactivation needs to be clarified. It is possible that this unique pattern of regulation is related to the role of this region (distal Xp) in X/Y pairing and recombination.

PAIRING AND RECOMBINATION OF X AND Y CHROMOSOMES

It has been proposed both from evolutionary considerations and cytological observations that a region of the human X chromosome is homologous to a portion of the Y chromosome (Burgoyne, 1982; Lyon, 1974; Ohno, 1967; Polani, 1982; Solari, 1974). Presumably, the early sex chromosomes were quite homologous to one another, but the genes required to specify the heterogametic sex became concentrated on one of the two chromosomes. Since strong selective pressure would obviously exist to favor the concomitant inheritance of all of the sex-determining factors, mechanisms probably evolved to suppress recombination between the ancestral X and Y, at least in the region of these important genes. It has been suggested that X inactivation may take place and have its earliest evolutionary antecedent in male spermatogenesis. Arguments have been set forth to indicate that the single X chromosome in males must undergo inactivation in order to achieve functional spermatogenesis (Lifschytz and Lindsley, 1972). Evidence to support this contention has been garnered in *Drosophila,* mouse, and man. Supernumerary X chromosomes disrupt spermatogenesis in all of these species. Furthermore, balanced X/autosome translocations result in male sterility in these animals as well (Lucchesi, 1973). Teleologically this is either because the autosomal gene sequences in some way interfere with the requisite X inactivation necessary for functional spermatogenesis, or because X inactivation spreads into the adjacent autosomal genes, rendering the germ cell functionally monosomic for some critical functions. Further support for the existence of X inactivation in male germ cells comes from the study of mice carrying a mutation called sex reversal *(Sxr).* XX Sxr individuals are phenotypically male, but are sterile, while X0 Sxr animals have spermatogenesis (Cattanach *et al.,* 1982).

If indeed the male X undergoes inactivation during spermatogenesis and X/Y recomination needs to be suppressed, it is interesting to speculate on the mechanistic connection between these two events. Furthermore, the relationship between paternal X inactivation during spermatogenesis and the preferential inactivation of the paternal X in extraembryonic tissues of eutherian mammalian embryos and of marsupials as a whole remains to be elucidated. In any case, it appears that with evolutionary time, X/Y recombination has largely been surpressed, leading to the genetic isolation of most of these two chromosomes. Most of the genes related to functions other than sex determination appear to have been lost from the Y. The resulting "inequity" in gene dosage between males and females and the need for balance between X-encoded and autosomally encoded gene products requires rectification and probably provided the selective pressure to permit the emergence of X inactivation in mammals. *Drosophila* have developed a different solution to this evolutionary problem and achieve dosage compensation by coordinately regulating the transcription of both female X chromosomes to be equal to the transcription of the genes on the single X of *Drosophila* males (Lucchesi, 1973, 1983). This latter process may involve the action of diffusible *trans*-acting positive regulators present in limiting amounts to enhance transcription of the single active X in males.

In some way opposing this need to genetically isolate the X and Y through suppression of recombination is the potential requirement for X/Y pairing during male meiotic division in order to ensure appropriate chromosome segregation. This theory was originally espoused by Koller and Darlington nearly 50 years ago (Koller and Darlington, 1934). Cytological data clearly support the notion of X/Y pairing, and electron microscopic observations in many mammalian species provide physical evidence of synaptonemal complexes in such situations. The physical portions of the human chromosomes that appear to engage in this pairing are, of course, the distal part of Xp and most of Yp. As noted above, the recent work of Goodfellow and colleagues has provided direct evidence for the homology of these portions of the genome (Goodfellow *et al.,* 1983). They have shown that functional loci (*MIC2X* and *MIC2Y*) exist in these two areas and that each can specify production of the cell surface antigen 12E7 as determined by an indirect radioimmunoassay. Since the antigenic specificity recognized by the 12E7 monoclonal antibody is unique to humans and is not even shared with most other primates, Goodfellow has argued that the 12E7 antigen must have arisen relatively recently in an evolutionary sense, and that at least one X/Y exchange must have taken place subsequent to the divergence of *Homo sapiens.* As will be discussed, such recombinational events may be very common.

Genetic evidence to support recombination between X and Y chromosomes in mammals has comes from studies of the Sxr mouse previously described. Jones and Singh (1981) and Sing *et al.,* (1980) have identified a moderately repetitive sequence, which they have termed Bkm because it represents a minor sex-specific satellite DNA component of the Banded Krait. This sequence has been highly conserved in evolution and is predominantly associated with the heterogametic sex in all species studied (Singh *et al.,* 1981). Y-Chromosome-specific Bkm sequences have been found in humans and in mice. While these genes are apparently transcribed, their function and role in sex determination is unknown. Due to their abundance, Bkm sequences can be readily localized by *in situ* hybridization methods. Singh and Jones (1982), Cattanach *et al.* (1982), Evans *et al.* (1982), and McLaren and Monk (1982) have shown that Bkm sequences are normally localized to the pericentromeric region of the mouse Y chromosome. In XY males who carry the Sxr trait, however, an additional area of hybridization is seen on the distal part of the Y. By studying meiotic preparations, actual transfer of the Bkm sequences from the abnormal Y to an X could be visualized. Following this exchange some of the X chromosomes now carried Bkm material. Presumably these X chromosomes were incorporated into gametes that gave rise to the XX progeny with a male phenotype, and, indeed, the Bkm hybridizing material is seen on one of the X chromosomes in such XX individuals. Since X/Y recombinational events were observed in most of the meioses that could be examined, it is suggested by extrapolation that such X/Y interchange occurs as an obligatory event during meiotic division in normal males as well. If such exchanges also take place in humans, the pairing region that cytologically encompasses the *STS, Xg,* and *MIC2X* loci may be involved. Further work should clarify the converging observations regarding X/Y homology, X/Y recombination, and escape of inactivation of these three genes.

If recombination between the X and Y chromosomes of man does occur at some appreciable frequency, the site of this recombination is also of great interest (Fig. 5). Is recombination obligatory and does it occur at

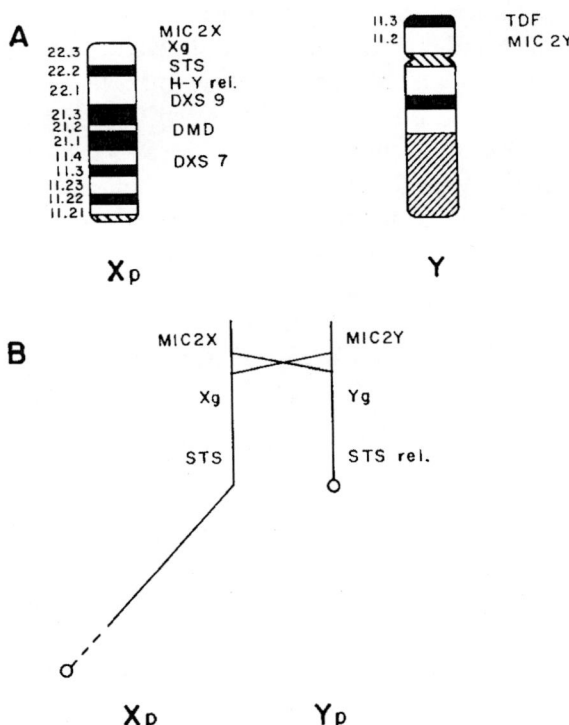

Fig. 5. The short arm of the human X chromosome and the human Y chromosome. (A) Known genes and cloned DNA segments. (B) The presumed pairing segments of X and Y. The presence of a nonfunctional *STS* gene on the Y chromosome is speculative (see text). The site of obligatory or frequent crossing over is shown. Since *Xg* and *STS* functional gene copies are not found on the Y, this site must be distal to these two genes. While there is some evidence that *STS* is proximal to *Xg*, this is not established. The situation of *MIC2X* and *MIC2Y* distal to the site of recombination is similarly arbitrary, but is supported by presumptive exchange of these two loci.

a reasonably constant and defined site on the X? If X/Y exchange took place at a reasonably precise location, genes located distally to this area should have homologues on the Y and should show "pseudoautosomal" or "partial sex-linked" inheritance (Burgoyne, 1982; Polani, 1982). That is, it might be possible to demonstrate linkage of such genes with other X-linked markers when only female meiotic events are scored, but that an absence of sex linkage would be found in the offspring of studied males, with male-to-male transmission of specific markers observed in addition to father-to-daughter transmission. If the site of X/Y recombination were not rigidly fixed, however, one might see exchange of loci between X and Y for some genes at a somewhat lower frequency. There is no evidence of a functional locus on the human Y chromosome corresponding to *STS* either from somatic cell genetic studies or pedigree analysis in families with STS deficiency. It is important to recognize that this conclusion is based on sampling of a relatively small number of Y chromosomes. When molecular probes for the STS gene become available, it will be of considerable interest to see whether a nonfunctioning homologue of *STS* can be found on the Y and to assess how far it has diverged from the X-linked *STS* gene and thus derive some assessment of the extent and duration of the genetic isolation of these two loci. As noted previously, the presence of functional genes on both X and Y that lead to the production of 12E7 argues that at least once (and probably much more commonly) in evolutionary history X/Y interchange proximal to these loci has occurred.

These considerations discussed above lead to a reevaluation of the genetic basis of STS deficiency in man. As previously indicated, the incidence of this disorder is about one in 5000–6000 males. This disease frequency has been found in numerous and diverse ethnic groups and geographic locations. No obvious selective advantage has been identified for individuals either heterozygous or hemizygous for an *STS⁻* allele. One possible explanation for this seemingly high prevalence of STS deficiency is that the disorder may be appearing at a rate considerably greater than could be accounted for by classical mutational mechanisms. It seems plausible that the *STS⁻* state may occasionally arise from either an unequal X/Y recombinational event or one that occurs proximal to the *STS* gene and results in loss of the X-linked *STS* locus (and generation of a deletion) or exchange of the X-linked *STS* copy for a nonfunctional Y homologue. Such a model would predict the generation of another product of meiosis, which would be a Y chromosome bearing the X-linked *STS* locus as well as other X material. While *STS*-bearing Y chromosomes have not been observed, they might be difficult to detect (Fig. 5).

Support for this type of occasional aberrant X/Y recombination has recently been derived from several clinical observations. More than a dozen sporadic cases of cytologically apparent X/Y translocations have been reported in the medical literature. Furthermore, a number of publications dealing with familial cases of X/Y translocations have appeared (Akesson *et al.*, 1980; Allderdice *et al.*, 1983; Bernstein *et al.*, 1978, 1980; Borgaonkar *et al.*, 1974; Boyd *et al.*, 1981; Ferguson-Smith *et al.*, 1983; Hecht *et al.*, 1980; Khudr *et al.*, 1973; Magenis *et al.*, 1982; Metaxotou *et al.*, 1983; Tiepolo *et al.*, 1977, 1980; van den Berge *et al.*, 1977; Yamada *et al.*, 1982; Zuffardi *et al.*, 1982). In all cases, the X-chromosome breakpoint has been in the distal Xp22 region. In most instances, the male sex determining genes were not transferred to the X chromosome, but virtually all of the identified males were nullisomic for *STS*, and had ichthyosis and short stature. Females heterozygous for such translocations may be shorter than expected. These observations have been verified through the study of patients with apparent deletions of Xp22.3–Xpter (without the detectable Y translocations) (Curry *et al.*, 1982). Studies of spontaneous pregnancy loss in such pedigrees suggest that, as is the case with Turner syndrome, nullisomy for distal Xp may be poorly tolerated in fetal life but may not have dire consequences postnatally (Curry *et al.*, 1984). One additional interesting observation is that nullisomy for Xp may predispose to X-chromosome aneuploidy (Curry *et al.*, 1984).

About one in 20,000 phenotypic males is born with an XX karyotype. The etiology of this form of sex reversal has been elusive for some time. Recently, two groups have presented molecular and functional evidence for submicroscopic transfer of a piece of Y material to one of the X chromosomes in XX males (Burgoyne, 1984; de la Chapell *et al.*, 1984; Guellaen *et al.*, 1984). In some instances, anomalous inheritance of Xg blood groups suggests that actual X/Y interchange may have occurred with consequent loss of Xp material (de la Chapelle *et al.*, 1971). Other investigators have shown that in some, but not all, XX males the loss of X material includes the STS locus, even though cytologically no X material seems to be missing (Pierella *et al.*, 1981; Wieacker *et al.*, 1983). XX males are well known in cattle and goats (Burgoyne, 1984), and in at least one pedigree of cocker spaniels in which both XX males and XX true hermaphrodites occur (Selden *et al.*, 1978). Most true hermaphrodites in humans have XX karyotypes. One of several potential explanations for all of these observations is that these events are caused by translocation of Y sequences to one of the X chromosomes. The variability in phenotype from one individual to the next and between ovarian and testicular tissue could indicate either differences in which X is inactivated, or the extent to which inactivation has spread into the putative adjacent Y sequences. A corollary is that the high frequency of STS deficiency in human populations is due to the measurable frequency with which meiotic errors occur in this region, resulting in loss of the functional STS gene from the X. With application of molecular methods, this is a testable hypothesis.

CONCLUSION

The study of steroid sulfatase deficiency, a relatively uncommon inborn error of metabolism, has led to a marked increase in our understanding of sulfated steroid and hormone metabolism. The pathways of estriol biosynthesis and the interconversion of DHEAS and DHEA are being clarified by investigations of this disorder, as are the contributions of sulfated intermediates to intratesticular testosterone production. Study of patients with steroid sulfatase deficiency has permitted identification of the critical role of cholesterol sulfate in epidermal metabolism and should lead in the future to a more detailed understanding of keratinization. Studies of the STS gene have enabled delineation of a region of the human X chromosome that escapes X inactivation and seems to participate in X/Y pairing and recombination. The relationship between pairing and escape of inactivation is unclear. Finally, studies of steroid sulfatase expression have allowed the recognition and more precise definition of normal and abnormal recombinational events on the X and Y chromosomes. These are considerable dividends for a modest investment in research.

ACKNOWLEDGMENTS.   In the preface to this series, the editors have indicated that these reviews are to reflect the individuality of the author. This chapter certainly conforms to that design, and I apologize for the necessary selectivity that was required with regard to both discussion and citation. I would like to thank all of my colleagues and collaborators in this area over the past several years, and in particular T. Mohandas, for many helpful suggestions and thoughts. In addition, I am most grateful to N. Hitt for assistance in preparation of this manuscript. My own research work cited here has been supported by grants from the National Institutes of Health and the March of Dimes Birth Defects Foundation.

REFERENCES

Adam, A., Ziprkowski, L., Feinstein, A., Sanger, R., and Race, R. R., 1966, Ichthyosis, Xg blood groups, and protan, *Lancet* i:877.

Adam, A., Ziprkowski, L., Feinstein, A., Sanger, R., Tippett, P., Gavin, J., and Race, R. R., 1969, Linkage relations of X-borne ichthyosis to the Xg blood groups and to other markers of the X in Israelis, *Ann. Hum. Genet. (Lond.)* 32:323–332.

Adlercreutz, H., Martin F., Pulkkinen, M., Dencker, H., Rimer, U., Sjoberg, N. O., and Tikkanen, M. J., 1976, Intestinal metabolism of estrogens, *J. Clin. Endocrinol. Metab.* 43:497–505.

Akesson, H. O., Hagberg, B., and Wahlstrom, J., 1980, Y-to-X chromosome translocation observed in two generations, *Hum. Genet.* 55:39–42.

Allderdice, P. W., Aveling, J. V., Eales, B. A., Lewis, M. J., McAlpine, P. J., Ross, J. B., and Simms, R. J., 1983, Familial t(X:y)(p223qll) associated with short stature in 4 male and 5 female carriers, and with X-linked ichthyosis and anhydrosis in 4 male carriers, *Am. J. Hum. Genet.* 34:124A.

Anderson, P. C., and Martt, J. M., 1965, Myotonia and keratoderma induced by 20,25 diazacholesterol, *Arch. Dermatol.* 92:181–183.

Back, D. J., Chapman, C. R., May, S. A., and Rowe, P. H., 1981, Absorption of oestrone sulphate from the gastrointestinal tract of the rat, *J. Stern. Biochem.* 14:347–356.

Baden, H. D., Hooker, P. H., Kubilus, J., and Tarascio, A., 1980, Sulfatase activity of keratinizing tissues in X-linked ichthyosis, *Pediatr. Res.* 14:1347–1348.

Balazs, I., Fillippi, G., Rinaldi, A., Grzeschik, K. H., and Siniscalco, M., 1979, Studies on human X-linked ichthyosis and steroid sulfatase in man, mice, and their hybrids, *Cytogenet. Cell Genet.* 25:133.

Basner, R., von Figura, K., Glossl, J., Klein, U., and Kresse, H., 1979, Multiple deficiency of mucopolysaccharide sulfatases in mucosulfatidosis, *Pediatr. Res.* 13:1316–1318.

Beastall, G. H., Kelly, A. M., England, P., Rao, L. G. S., MacGregor, M. W., and Paterson, M. L., 1976, Urinary estrogen and plasma human placental lactogen as initial screening tests for a placental sulfatase deficiency, *Scott. Med. J.* 21:106–108.

Bedin, M., Weil, D., Fournier, T., Cedar, L., and Frezal, J., 1981, Biochemical evidence for the non-inactivation of the steroid sulfatase locus in human placenta and fibroblasts, *Hum. Genet.* 59:256–258.

Bergner, E., and Shapiro, L. J., 1981, Increased cholesterol sulfate in plasma and red blood cell membranes of steroid sulfatase deficient patients, *J. Clin. Endocrinol. Metab.* **53:**221–223.

Bernstein, R., Wagner, J., Isdale, J., Norse, G. T., Lane, A. B., and Jenkins, T., 1978, X–Y translocation in a retarded phenotypic male, *J. Med. Genet.* **15:**466–474.

Bernstein, R., Pinto, M. R., Almeida, M., Solarsh, S. M., Meck, J., and Jenkins, T., 1980, X–Y translocation in an adolescent mentally normal phenotypic male with features of hypogonadism, *J. Med. Genet.* **17:**437–443.

Bleau, G., and Van den Heuvel, W. J. A., 1974, Desmosteryl sulfate and desmosterol in hamster epididymal spermatozoa, *Steroids* **24:**549–55.

Bleau, G., Chapdelaine, A., and Roberts, K. D., 1971, Studies on mammalian and molluscasn steroid sulfatase. Solubilization and properties, *Can J. Biochem.* **49:**234.

Bleau, G., Bodley, F. H., Longpre, J., Chapdelaine, A., and Roberts, K. D., 1974, Cholesterol sulfate 1. Occurrence and possible biological function as an amphipathic lipid in the membrane of the human erythrocyte. *Biochim. Biophys. Acta* **352:**1–9.

Bleau, G., Lalumiere, G., Chapdelaine, A., and Roberts, K. D., 1975, Red cell surface structure, stabilization by cholesterol sulfate as evidenced by scanning electron miscroscopy, *Biochim. Biophys. Acta* **375:**220–223.

Borgaonkar, D. S., Sroka, B. M., and Flores, M., 1974, Y-to-X translocation in a girl. *Lancet* i:68–69.

Boyd, E., Ferguson-Smith, M. A., Ferguson-Smith, M. E., Jamieson, M. E., Russell, J. E., and Aiktken, D. A., *et al.,* 1981, A case of X:Y translocation which maps the *Xg* locus to Xp24 → pter, *J. Med. Genet.* **18:**224.

Braunstein, G. D., Ziel, F. H., Allen, A., van de Velde, R., and Wade, M. E., 1976, Prenatal diagnosis of a placental steroid sulfatase deficiency, *Am. J. Obstet. Gynecol.* **126:**716–719.

Burgoyne, P. S., 1982, Genetic homology and crossing over in the X and Y chromosomes of mammals, *Hum. Genet.* **61:**85–90.

Burgoyne, P., 1984, The origins of men with two X chromosomes, *Nature* **307:**109.

Calvin, H. I., van de Wiele, R. L., and Lieberman, S., 1963, Evidence that steroid sulfates serve as biosynthetic intermediates: *In vivo* conversion of pregnenolone-sulfate-S^{35} to dehydroiso-androsterone-S^{35}, *Biochemistry* **2:**648.

Casey, M. L., and MacDonald, P. C., 1982, Metabolism of deoxycorticosterone and deoxycorticosterone sulfate in men and women, *J. Clin. Invest.* **70:**312–319.

Cattanach, B. M., Evans, E. D., Burtenshaw, M. D., and Barlow, J., 1982, Male, female and intersex development in mice of identical chromosome constitution, *Nature* **300:**445–446.

Chance, P. F., and Gartler, S. M., 1983, Evidence for a dosage effect at the X-linked steroid sulfatase locus in human tissues, *Am. J. Hum. Genet.* **35:**234–240.

Chapdelaine, A., MacDonald, P. C., Gonzales, O., Gurpide, E., van de Wiele, R. L., and Lieberman, S., 1965, Studies on the secretion and interconversion of the androgens. IV. Quantitative results in a normal man whose gonadal and adrenal function were altered experimentally, *J. Clin. Endocrinol. Metab.* **25:**1569.

Chapman, V. M., Kratzer, P. G., Siracusa, L. D., Quarantillo, B. A., Evans, R., and Liskay, R. M., 1982, Evidence for DNA modification in the maintenance of X chromosome inactivation in adult mouse tissue, *Proc. Natl. Acad. Sci. USA* **79:**5357–5361.

Cockayne, E. A., 1933, *Inherited Abnormalities of the Skin and Its Appendages,* Oxford Press, London.

Cooper, D. W., McAllan, B. M., Donald, J. A., Dawson, G., Dobrovic, A., and Graves, J. A. M., 1984, Steroid sulphatase is not detected on the X chromosome of Australian marsupials, *Cytogenet. Cell Genet.* **37**:439.

Crawfurd, M. A., 1982, Review: Genetics of steroid sulfatase deficiency and X-linked ichthyosis, *J. Inherited Metab. Dis.* **5**:153–163.

Crocker, M., and Craig, I., 1983, Variation in regulation of steroid sulphatase locus in mammals, *Nature* **303**:721–722.

Curry, C. J. R., Lanman, J. T., Magenis, R. E., Brown, M. G., Bergner, E. A., and Shapiro, L. J., 1982, X-linked chondrodysplasia punctata with ichthyosis: Chromosomal localization to Xp, *Am. J. Hum. Genet.* **34**:122A.

Curry, C. J. R., Lanman, J. T., Tasai, J., O'Lague, P., Magenis, R. E., Brown, M., Goodfellow, P., Mohandas, T., Bergner, E. A., and Shapiro, L. J., 1984, Chondrodysplasia punctata due to a deletion of the short arm of the X chromosome, *N. Engl. J. Med.* **311**:1010–1014.

Dancis, J., Jansen, V., and Hutzler, J., 1983, Hair root analysis in X-linked ichthyosis, *J. Inherited Metab. Dis.* **6**:173–177.

DeGroot, W. P., Jobsis, A. C., Marinkovic-Ilsen, A., Koppe, J. G., and De Bruijn, H. W. A., 1980, Sex-linked ichthyosis and placental sulphatase C deficiency, *Br. J. Dermatol.* **103**:73–79.

De la Chapelle, A., Simila, S., Lanning, M., Kontturi, M., and Johansson, C. J., 1971, Two further males with female karyotypes, *Hum. Genet.* **11**:286–294.

De la Chapelle, A., Tippett, P. A., Wetterstrand, G., and Page, D., 1984, Genetic evidence of X–Y interchange in a human XX male, *Nature* **307**:170–171.

De Luca, C., Brown, J. H., and Shows, T. B., 1979, Lysosomal arylsulfatase deficiences in humans: Chromosome assignment of arylsulfatase A and B, *Proc. Natl. Acad. Sci. USA* **76**:1957–1961.

De Peretti, E., and Forest, M. G., 1978, Patterns of plasma dehydroepiandrosterone sulfate levels in humans from birth to adulthood and evidence for testicular production, *J. Clin. Endocrinol. Metab.* **47**:572.

Dicfalusy, E., 1969, Steroid metabolism in the human foetoplacental unit, *Acta Endocrinol.* **61**:649–664.

Dominguez, O. V., Valencia, S. A., and Loza, A. C., 1975, On the role of steroid sulfates in hormone biosynthesis, *J. Ster. Biochem.* **6**:301–309.

Drayer, N. M., and Lieberman, S., 1965, Isolation of cholesterol sulfate from human blood and gallstones, *Biochem. Biophys. Res. Commun.* **18**:126.

Drayer, N. M., and Lieberman, S., 1967, Isolation of cholesterol sulfate from human aortas and adrenal tumors, *J. Clin. Endocrinol. Metab.* **27**:136.

Ducos, J., Marty, Y., Sanger, R., and Race, R. R., 1971, Xg and X chromosome inactivation, *Lancet* **ii**:219–220.

Eicher, E. M., 1970, X-Autosome translocations in the mouse: Total inactivation versus partial inactivation of the X chromosome, *Adv. Genet.* **15**:175–259.

Elias, P. M., 1981, Epidermal lipids, membranes, and keratinization, *J. Dermatol.* **20**:1–19.

Epstein, E. H., and Bonifus, J. M., 1984, Purification of steroid sulfatase from normal human placenta, *Clin. Res.* **32**:138A.

Epstein, E. H., and Leventhal, M. E., 1981, Steroid sulfatase of human leukocytes and epidermis and the diagnosis of recessive X-linked ichthyosis, *J. Clin. Invest.* **67**:1257–1262.

Epstein, E. H., Krauss, R. M., and Shackleton, C. H. L., 1981*a*, X-linked ichthyosis: Increased blood cholesterol sulfate and electrophoretic mobility of low-density lipoprotein, *Science* **214**:659–660.

Epstein, E. H., Williams, M. L., and Elias, P. M., 1981*b*, Steroid sulfatase, X-linked ichthyosis, and stratus corneum cell cohesion, *Arch. Dermatol.* **117**:761–763.

Erickson, R. P., Harper, K., and Kramer, J. M., 1983, Identification of an autosomal locus affecting steroid sulfatase activity among inbred strains of mice, *Genetics* **105**:181–189.

Evans, E. P., Burtenshaw, M. D., and Catanach, B. M., 1982, Meiotic crossing-over between the X and Y chromosomes of male mice carrying the sex-reversing (Sxr) factor, *Nature* **300**:443–445.

Ferguson-Smith, M. A., Sanger, R., Tippett, P., Aitken, D. A., and Boyd, E., 1983, A familial t(X:Y) translocation which assigns the Xg blood group locus to the region Xp22.3 → pter, *Cytogenet. Cell Genet.* **32**:273–274.

Fialkow, P. J., 1970, X-Chromosome inactivation and the *Xg* locus, *Am. J. Hum. Genet.* **22**:460–463.

Fialkow, P. J., Lisker, R., Giblett, E. R., and Zavala, C., 1970, *Xg* locus: Failure to detect inactivation in females with chronic myelocytic leukaemia, *Nature* **226**:367–368.

Fiddler, M. B., Vine, D., Shapira, E., and Nadler, H. L., 1979, Is multiple sulfatase deficiency due to defective regulation of sulphohydrolase expression? *Nature* **282**:98–100.

Filippi, G., and Khan, P. M., 1968, Linkage studies on X-linked ichthyosis in Sardinia, *Am. J. Hum. Genet.* **20**:564–569.

Fluharty, A. L., Stevens, R. L., Davis, L. L., Shapiro, L. J., and Kihara, H., 1978, Presence of arylsulfatase A in multiple sulfatase deficiency disorder fibroblasts, *Am. J. Hum. Genet.* **30**:249–255.

Fluharty, A. L., Stevens, R. L., de la Flor, S. D., Shapiro, L. J., and Kihara, H., 1979, Arylsulfatase A modulation with pH in multiple sulfatase deficiency disorder fibroblasts, *Am. J. Hum. Genet.* **31**:574–580.

France, J. T., 1979, Steroid sulphatase deficiency, *J. Ster. Biochem.* **11**:647–651.

France, J. T., and Liggins, G. C., 1969, Placental sulfatase deficiency, *J. Clin. Endocrinol Metab.* **29**:138–141.

France, J. T., Seddon, R. J., and Liggins, G. C., 1963, A study of a pregnancy with low estrogen production due to placental sulfatase deficiency, *J. Clin. Endocrinol. Metab.* **36**:1–9.

France, J. T., Downey, J. A., McNaught, R. W., Seddon, R. J., and Liggins, G. C., 1976, Placental sulfatase deficiency, in: *Proc. V. International Congress of Endocrinology*, Vol. 2 (V. H. T. James, ed.), Excerpta Medica, Amsterdam.

French, A. P., and Warren, J. C., 1967, Properties of steroid sulphatases and arylsuphatase activities of human placenta, *Biochem. J.* **105**:233–241.

Gartler, S. M., and Riggs, A. D., 1983, Mammalian X-chromosome inactivation, *Annu. Rev. Genet.* **17**:155–190.

Gartler, S. M., and Rivest, M., 1983, Evidence for X-linkage of steroid sulfatase in the mouse: Steroid sulfatase levels in oocytes of XX and XO mice, *Genet.* **103**:137–141.

Gauthier, R., Vigneault, N., Bleau, G., Chapdelaine, A., and Roberts, K. D., 1978, Solubilization and partial purification of steroid sulfatase of human placenta, *Steroids* **31**:783–798.

Goodfellow, P., Banting, G., Levy, R., Povey, S., and McMichael, A., 1980, A human X-linked anigen defined by a monoclonal antibody, *Somat. Cell Genet.* **6**:777–787.

Goodfellow, P., Banting, G., Sheer, D., Ropers, H. H., Caine, A., Ferguson-Smith, M. A., Povey, S., and Voss, R., 1983, Genetic evidence that a Y-linked gene in man is homologous to a gene on the X chromosome. *Nature* **302**:346–349.

Goodfellow, P., Pym, B., Mohandas, T., and Shapiro, L. J., 1984, The *MIC2X* locus escapes X inactivation, *Am. J. Hum. Genet.***36**:777–782.

Gorman, J. G., Kire, J., Treacy, A. M., and Cahan, A., 1963, The application of -Xg^a antiserum to the question of red cell mosaicism in female heterozygotes, *J. Lab. Clin. Med.* **61**:642–649.

Guellaen, G., Casanova, M., Bishop, C., Geldwerth, D., Andre, G., Fellous, M., and Weissenbach, J., 1984, Human XX males with Y single-copy DNA fragments, *Nature* **307**:172–173.

Hameister, H., Wolff, G., Lauritzen, C. H., Lehmann, W. O., Hauser, A., and Ropers, H. H., 1979, Clinical and biochemical investigations on patients with partial deficiency of placental steroid sulfatase. *Hum. Genet.* **46**:199–207.

Hecht, T., Cooke, H. J., Cerrillo, M., Meer, B., Reck, G., and Hameister, H., 1980, A new case of Y to X translocation in a female, *Hum. Genet.* **54**:303–307.

Horton, R., and Tait, J. F., 1967, *In vivo* conversion of dehydroisoandrosterone and testosterone in man, *J. Clin. Endocrinol. Metab.* **27**:79.

Huhtaniemi, I., 1977, Studies on steroidogenesis and its regulation in human fetal adrenal and testis, *J. Ster. Biochem.* **8**:491–497.

Imken, L., Mohandas, T., Sparkes, R. S., and Shapiro, L. J., in press, The steroid sulfatase locus on structurally abnormal X chromosomes is expressed, *Am. J. Hum. Genet.*

Iwamori, M., Moser, H. W., and Kishimoto, Y., 1976, Solubilization and partial purification of steroid sulfatase from rat liver: Characterization of estrone sulfatase, *Arch. Biochem. Biophys.* **174**:199–208.

Jobsis, A. C., DeGroot, W. P., Tigges, A. J., 1980, DeBruijn, H. W. A., Rijken, Y., Meijer, A. E. F. H., and Marinkovic-Ilsen, A., X-linked ichthyosis and X-linked placental sulfatase deficiency: A disease entity, *Am. J. Pathol.* **99**:279–290.

Jones, K. W., and Singh, L., 1981, Conserved DNA sequences in vertebrate sex chromosomes, *Hum. Genet.* **58**:46–53.

Jones, P.A., Taylor, S. M., Mohandas, T., and Shapiro, L. J., 1982, Cell cycle specific reactivation of an inactive X chromosome locus by 5-azadeoxycytidine, *Proc. Natl. Acad. Sci. USA* **79**:1215–1219.

Katz, R. A., Jorgensen, H., and Nigra, T. D., 1980, Elevation of serum triglyceride levels from oral isotretinoin in disorders of keratinization, *Arch. Dermatol.* **116**:1369–1372.

Keinanan, B. M., Nelson, K., Daniel, W. L., and Roque, J. M., 1983, Genetic analysis of murine arylsulfatase C and steroid sulfatase, *Genetics* **105**:191–206.

Kerr, C. B., and Wells, R. S., 1964, X-Linked ichthyosis and the Xg groups, *Lancet* i:1369–1370.

Kerr, C. B., and Wells, R. S., 1965, Sex-linked ichthyosis, *Ann. Hum. Genet. Lon.* **29**:33–50.

Khudr, G., Benirschke, K., Judd, H. L., and Strauss, J., 1973, Y to X translocation in a woman with reproductive failure: A new arrangement, *J. Am. Med. Assoc.* **226**:544–549.

Koller, P. D., and Darlington, C. D., 1934, The genetical and mechanical properties of the sex chromosomes of *Rattus norvegicus, J. Genet.* **29**:159–173.

Kolodny, E. H., and Moser, H. W., 1983, Sulfatide lipidosis: Metachromatic leukodystrophy, in: *The Metabolic Basis of Inherited Disease* (J. Stanbury, J. B. Wyngaarden, D. S. Frederickson, J. L. Goldstin, and M. S. Brown, eds.), 5th ed., pp. 881–905, McGraw-Hill, New York.

Koppe, J. G., Marinkovic-Ilsen, A., Rijken, Y., DeGRoot, W. P., and Jobsis, A. C., 1978, X-linked ichthyosis, a sulphatase deficiency, *Arch. Dis. Child.* **53**:803–806.

Korte, K., Hemsell, P. G., and Mason, J. I., 1982, Sterol sulfate metabolism in the adrenals of the human fetus, anencephalic newborn and adult, *J. Clin. Endocrinol. Metab.* **55:**671–675.

Korth-Schutz, S., Levine, L. S., and New, M. I., 1976, Dehydroepiandrosterone sulfate levels, a rapid test for abnormal androgen secretion, *J. Clin. Endocrinol. Metab.* **42:**1005.

Kratzer, P. G., Chapman, V. M., Lambert, H., Evans, R. E., and Liskay, R. M., 1983, Differences in the DNA of the inactive X chromosome of fetal and extraembryonic tissues of mice, *Cell* **33:**37–42.

Kubilus, J., Tanascio, A. J., and Baden, H. P., 1979, Steroid sulfatase deficiency in sex-linked ichthyosis, *Am. J. Hum. Genet.* **31:**50–53.

Lakshima, S., and Balasubramanian, A. S., 1981, The distribution of estrone sulfatase, dehydroepiandrosterone sulfatse, and arylsulphatase C in the primate *(Macaca radiata)* brain and pituitary, *J. Neurochem.* **37:**358–362.

Lalumiere, G., Bleau, G., Chapdelaine, A., and Roberts, K. D., 1976, Cholesteryl sulfate and sterol sulfatase in the human reproductive tract, *Steroids* **27:**247–260.

Lalumiere, G., Longpre, J., Trudel, J., Chapdelaine, A., and Roberts, K. D., 1975, Cholesterol sulfate II. Studies on its metabolism and possible function in canine blood, *Biochimica Biophys. Acta* **394:**120–128.

Langlais, J., Zollinger, M., Plante, L., Chapdelaine, A., Bleau, G., and Roberts, K. D., 1981, Localization of cholesteryl sulfate in human spermatozoa in support of a hypothesis for the mechanism of capactitation, *Proc. Natl. Acam. Sci. USA* **78:**7266–7270.

Lawler, S. D., and Sanger, R., 1970, Xg blood groups and clonal-origin theory of chronic myeloid leukaemia, *Lancet* **1970:**584–585.

Legault, Y., Bleau, G., Chapdelaine, A., and Roberts, K. D., 1979, The binding of sterol sulfates to hamster spermatozoa, *Steroids* **34:**89.

Lester, S. C., Korn, N. J., and DeMars, R., 1982, Derepression of genes on the human inactive X chromosome: Evidence for differences in locus-specific rates of derepression and rates of transfer of active and inactive genes after DNA-mediated transformation, *Somat. Cell Genet.* **8:**265–284.

Levy, R., Dilley, J., Fox, R. I., and Warnke, R., 1979, A human thymus-leukemia antigen defined by hybridoma monoclonal antibodies, *Proc. Natl. Acad. Sci. USA* **76:**6552–6556.

Lifschytz, E., and Lindsley, D. C., 1972, The role of X-chromosome inactivation during spermatogenesis, *Proc. Natl. Acad. Sci. USA.* **69:**182–186.

Liscum, L., Cummings, R. D., Anderson, R. G. W., DeMartino, G. N., Goldstein, J. L., and Brown, M. S., 1983, 3-Hydroxy-3-methylglutaryl-CoA reductase: A transmembrane glycoprotein of the endoplasmic reticulum with 14-linked "high mannose" oligosaccharides, *Proc. Natl. Acad. Sci. USA* **80:**7165–7169.

Liskay, R. M., and Evans, R. J., 1980, Inactive X chromosome DNA-mediated cell transformation for the hypoxanthine phosphoribosyl transferase gene, *Proc. Natl. Acad. Sci. USA* **77:**4895–4898.

Lucchesi, J. C., 1973, Dosage compensation in *Drosophila, Annu. Rev. Genet.* **7:**225–237.

Lucchesi, J. C., 1983, Dosage compensation in *Drosophila,* in: *Isozymes: Current Topics in Biological and Medical Research. Vol. 9: Gene Expression and Development* (M. Ratazzi, ed.), pp. 179–183, Alan R. Liss, New York.

Lykkesfeldt, G., and Hoyer, H., 1983, Topical cholesterol treatment of recessive X-linked ichthyosis, *Lancet* **II:**1337–1338.

Lykkesfeldt, J., Bock, E., and Lykkesfeldt, A. E., 1981, Sex specific difference in placental steroid sulphatase activity (Letter to the Editor) *Lancet* **1981:**

Lykkesfeldt, G., Hoyer, H., Lykkesfeldt, A. E., and Skakkebaer, N. E., 1983, Steroid sulphatase deficiency associated with testis cancer, *Lancet* **ii:**1456.

Lyon, M. F., 1974, Evolution of X chromosome inactivation in mammals, *Nature* 250:651–653.

MacDonald, P. C., Chapdelaine, A., Gonzales, O., Gurpide, E., van de Wiele, R. C., and Lieberman, S., 1965, Studies on the secretion and interconversion of the androgens. III Results obtained after the injection of several radioactive C_{19} steroids, singly or as mixtures, *J. Clin. Endocrinol. Metab.* 25:1557.

Magenis, R. E., Webb, M. J., McKean, R. S., et al., 1982, Translocation (X:y) (p22.33; pp11.2) in XX males: Etiology of male phenotype, *Hum. Genet.* 62:271–276.

Mann, J. D., Cahan, A., Gelb, H. G., Fisher, N., Hamper, J., Tippett, P., Sanger, R., and Race, R. R., 1962, A sex-linked blood group, *Lancet* I:8.

Marks, R., and DyFes, P. J., 1978, *The Ichthyoses,* S.P. Medical Books, New York.

Mathew, J., and Balasubramanian, A. S., 1982, Arylsulphatase C and estrone sulphatase of sheep hypothalamus, preoptic area, and midbrain: Separation by hydrophobic interaction chromatography and evidence for differences in their lipid environment, *J. Neurochem.* 39:1205–1209.

McKusick, V. A., and Neufeld, E. F., 1983, The mucopolysaccharide storage diseases, in: *The Metabolic Basis of Inherited Disease,* (J. Stanbury, J. B. Wyngaarden, D. S. Frederickson, J. L. Goldstin, and M. S. Brown, eds.), 5th ed., pp.751–777, McGraw-Hill, New York.

McLaren, A., and Monk, M., 1982, Fertile females produced by inactivation of an X chromosome of 'sex-reversed' mice, *Nature* 300:446–448.

McNaught, R. W., and France, J. T., 1980, Studies of the biochemical basis of steroid sulphatase deficiency: Preliminary evidence suggesting a defect in membrane–enzyme structure, *J. Ster. Biochem.* 13:363–373.

Metaxotou, C., Ikkos, D., Panagiotopoulou, P., Alevizaki, A., Mavrou, A., Tsenghi, C., and Matsaniotis, N., 1983, A familial X/Y translocation in a boy with ichthyosis, hypogonadism and mental retardation. *Clin. Genet.* 24:380–383.

Meyer, J. C. Grundmann, H. P., and Schnyder, U. W., 1979, Determination of arylsulfatase C in hair follicles, *Arch. Dermatol. Res.* 266:95–97.

Migeon, B. R., Shapiro, L. J., Norum, R. A., Mohandas, T., Axelman, J., and Dabora, R. C., 1982, Differential expression of the steroid sulfatase locus on the active and inactive human X chromosome, *Nature* 299:838–840.

Mohandas, T., Shapiro, L. J., Sparkes, R. S., and Sparkes, M. C., 1979, Regional assignment of the steroid sulfatase-X-linked ichthyosis locus: Implications for a non-inactivated region on the short arm of the human X-chromosome. *Proc. Natl. Acad. Sci. USA* 76:5779–5783.

Mohandas, T., Sparkes, R. S., Hellkuhl, B., Grzeschik, K. H., and Shaprio, L. I., 1980, Expression of an X-linked gene from an inactive human X-chromosome in mouse–human hybrid cells: Further evidence for the non-inactivation of the steroid sulfatase locus in man, *Proc. Natl. Acad. Sci. USA* 77:6759–6763.

Mohandas, T., Sparkes, R. S., and Shapiro, L. J., 1981, Reactivation of an inactive human X chromosome: Evidence for X-inactivation by DNA methylation, *Science* 211:393–396.

Mohandas, T., Sparkes, R. S., and Shapiro, L. J., 1982, Genetic evidence for the inactivation of a human autosomal locus attached to an inactive X chromosome, *Am. J. Hum. Genet.* 34:811–817.

Moser, H. W., Moser, A. B., and Orr, J. C., 1966, Preliminary observations on the occurrence of cholesterol sulfate in man, *Arch. Biochem. Biophys.* 116:146.

Muller, C. R., Migl, B., Ropers, H. H., and Happle, R., 1980, Heterozygote detection in steroid sulfatase deficiency, *Lancet* ii:546–547.

Muller, C. R., Migl, B., Traupe, H., and Ropers, H. H., 1980b, X-linked steroid sulfatase: Evidence for different gene-dosage in males and females, *Hum. Genet.* **54**:197–199.

Muller, C. R., Westerveld, A., Migl, B. S., Franke, W., and Ropers, H. H., 1980c, Regional assignment of the gene locus for steroid sulfatase, *Hum. Genet.* **54**:201–204.

Munson, P. L., Gallagher, T. F., and Kock, F. C., 1944, Isolation of dehydroisoandrosterone sulfate from normal male urine, *J. Biol. Chem.* **152**:67.

Murphy, J. V., Wolfe, H. J., Balazs, I., and Moser, H. W., 1971, A patient with deficiency of arylsulfatases A,B,C, and steroid sulfatase associated with storage of sulfatide, cholesterol sulfate, and glycosaminoglycans, in: *Lipid Storage Diseases: Enzymatic Defects and Clinical Implications* (J. Bernsohn and H. J. Grossman, eds.), p. 67, Academic Press, New York.

Nelson, K., and Daniel, W. L., 1979, Interstrain variation of murine arylsulfatase C, *Experientia* **35**:309–310.

Nelson, K., Keinanen, B. M., and Daniel, W. L., 1983, Murine arylsulfatase C: Evidence for two isozymes. *Experientia* **39**:740–742.

Noel, H., Beauregard, G., Potier, M., Bleau, G., Chapdelaine, A., and Roberts, K. D., 1982a, The target sizes of the *in situ* and solubilized forms of human placental steroid sulfatase as measured by radiation inactivation, *Biochim. Biophys. Acta* **758**:88–90.

Noel, H., Plante, L., Bleau, G., Chapdelaine, A., and Roberts, K. D., in preparation, Human placental steroid sulfatase: Purification and properties.

Notation, A. D., 1975, Regulatory interactions for the control of steroid sulfate metabolism, *J. Ster. Biochm.* **6**:311–316.

Oakey, R. E., Cawood, M. L., and MacDonald, P. R., 1974, Biochemical and clinical observations in a pregnancy with placental sulphatase and other enzyme deficiencies, *Clin. Endocrinology* **3**:131–148.

Ohno, S., 1967, *Sex Chromosomes and Sex-linked Genes,* Springer-Verlag, Berlin.

Osanthanondh, R., Canick, J., Ryan, K. J., and Tulchinsky, D., 1976, Placental sulfatase deficiency: A case study, *J. Clin. Endocrinol. Metab.* **43**:208–214.

Parker, L. N., and Odell, W. D., 1979, Evidence for the existence of cortical androgen stimulating hormone, *Am. J. Physicol.* **236**:616–620.

Payne, A. H., 1980, Testicular steroid sulfotransferases: Comparison to liver and adrenal steroid sulfotransferases of the mature rat, *Endocrinol.* **106**:1365–1370.

Pearson, P. L., Witterland, W. F., Meera-Khan, P., Dewitt, J., and Babrow, M., 1978, Reinvestigation of two X/autosome translocations: Segregation in hybrids, *Cytogenet. Cell Cenet.* **22**:534–537.

Pierella, P., Craig, I., Barbrow, M., and de la Chappelle, A., 1981, Steroid sulphatase levels in XX males, including observations on two affected cousins, *Hum. Genet.* **59**:87–88.

Polani, P. E., 1982, Pairing of X and Y chromosomes, non-inactivation of X-linked genes, and the maleness factor, *Hum Genet.* **60**:207–211.

Polani, P. E., Angell, R., Giannelli, F., de la Chapelle, A., Race, R. R., and Sanger, R., 1970, Evidence that the *Xg* locus is inactivated in structurally abnormal X chromosomes, *Nature* **227**:613–616.

Race, R. R., and Sanger, R., 1965, *Blood Groups in Man,* 6th ed., pp. 578–635, Blackwell Scientific, Oxford.

Rastan, S., Kaufman, M. H., Handyside, A. H., and Lyon, M. F., 1980, X-Chromosome inactivation in extraembryonic membranes of diploid parthenogenetic mouse embryos demonstrated by differential straining, *Nature* **288**:172–173.

Razin, A., And Riggs, A. D., 1980, DNA methylation and gene function, *Science* **210**:604–610.

Reiter, E. O., Fouldauer, V. G., and Root, A. W., 1977, Secretion of the adrenal androgen, dehydroepiandrosterone sulfate during normal infancy, childhood, and adolescence, in sick infants, and in children with endocrinologic abnormalities, *J. Pediatr.* **90**:766.

Roberts, K. D., and Lieberman, S., 1970, The biochemistry of the 3β-hydroxyl-Δ^5 steroid sulfates, in: Chemical and Biological Aspects of Steroid Conjugation (S. Bernstein and S. Soloman, Eds.), p. 219, Springer-Verlag, New York.

Roberts, K. D., Bandi, L, Calvin, H. J., Drucker, W. D., and Lieberman, S., 1964, Evidence that steroid sulfates serve as biosynthetic intermediates. IV. Conversion of cholesterol sulfate *in vivo* to urinary C_{19} and C_{21} steroidal sulfates, *Biochemistry* **3**:1983–1988.

Ropers, H. H., and Wiberg, V., 1982, Evidence for X-linkage and non-inactivation of steroid sulphatase locus in wood lemmings, *Nature* **296**:766–767.

Ropers, H. H., Migl, B., Zimmer, J., Fraccaro, M., Maraschio, P. P., and Westerveld, A., 1981a, Activity of steroid sulfatase in fibroblasts with numerical and structural X chromosome aberrations, *Hum. Genet.* **57**:354–356.

Ropers, H. H., Migl, B., Zimmer, J., and Muller, C. R., 1981b, Steroid sulfatase activity in cultured fibroblasts of XX males, *Cytogenet. Cell Genet.* **30**:168–173.

Rosa, F. W., Teratogenicity of isotretinoin, 1983, *Lancet* **ii**:513.

Rose, F. A., 1982, The mammalian sulphatases and placental sulfatase deficiency in man, *J. Inherited Metab. Dis.* **5**:145–152.

Rosenfeld, R. S., Hellman, L., and Gallagher, T. F., 1982, Metabolism and interconversion of dehydroisoandrosterone and dehydroisoandrosterone sulfate, *J. Clin. Endocrinol. Metab.* **35**:187.

Roy, A. B., 1970, Enzymological aspects of steroid conjugation, in: *Chemical and Biological Aspects of Steroid Conjugation,* (S. Bernstein and S. Solomon, eds.), p. 74, Springer-Verlag, New York.

Ruiter, M., and Meyler, L, 1960, Skin changes after therapeutic administration of nicotinic acid in large does, *Dermatol.* **120**:139–144.

Ruokonen, A., and Oikarinen, A., 1981, Steroid sulphatase activity in the skin biopsies of various types of ichythyosis, *Br. J. Dermatol.* **105**:291–295.

Ruokonen, A., Oikarinen, A., Palatsi, R., and Huhtaniemi, I., 1980, Serum steroid sulphates in ichthyosis, *Br. J. Dermatol.* **102**:245–248.

Sanger, R., Tippett, P., Gavin, J., Teesdale, P., and Daniels, G. L., 1977, Xg blood groups and sex chromosome abnormalities in people of northern European ancestry. An Addendum, *J. Med. Genet.* **14**:210–213.

Schachter, B., and Marrian, G. F., 1938, The isolation of estrone sulfate from the urine of pregnant mares, *J. Biol. Chem.* **126**:663.

Sedgwick, W., 1863, On the influence of sex in hereditary disease, *Br. Foreign Med-Chiurg. Rev.* **31**:445.

Selden, J. R., Wachtel, S. S., Koo, G. C., Haskins, M. E., and Patterson, D. F., 1978, Genetic basis of XX male syndrome and XX true hermaphroditism: Evidence in the dog, *Science* **201**:644–646.

Sever, R. J., Frost, P., and Weinstein, G., 1968, Eye changes in ichthyosis. *J. Am. Med. Assoc.* **206**:2283–2286.

Shapiro, L. J., 1982, Steroid sulfatase deficiency and X-linked ichthyosis, In: *The Metabolic Basis of Inherited Disease* (J. B. Stanbury, J. B. Syngaarden, D. S. Fredrickson, J. L. Goldstein, and M. S. Brown, eds.), 5th ed., pp. 1027–1037, McGraw-Hill, New York.

Shapiro, L. J., and Mohandas, T., 1980, Molecular genetics of X-linked ichthyosis, *Pediatr. Res.* **14**:527.

Shapiro, L. J., and Mohandas, T., 1983, DNA methylation and the control of gene expression on the human X chromosome, *Cold Spring Harbor Symp. Quant. Biol.* **XLVII**:631–638.

Shapiro, L. J., Cousins, L., Fluharty, A. L., Stevens, R. L., and Kihara, H., 1977, Steroid sulfatase deficiency, *Pediatr. Res.* **11**:894–897.

Shapiro, L. J. Mohandas, T., Weiss, R., and Romeo, G., 1979, Non-inactivation of an X chromosome locus in man, *Science* **204**:1224–1226.

Shapiro, L. J., Weiss, R., Buxman, M. M., Vidgoff, J., Dimond, R. L., Roller, J.A., and Wells, R. S., 1978*a*, Enzymatic basis of typical X-linked ichthyosis, *Lancet* **ii**:756–757.

Shapiro, L. J., Weiss, R., Webster, D., and France, J. T., 1978*b*, X-Linked ichthyosis due to steroid sulfatase deficiency, *Lancet* **i**:70–72.

Siiteri, P. K., and Macdonald, P. C., 1963, The utilization of circulating dehydroisoandrosterone sulfate for estrogen synthesis during human pregnancy, *J. Clin. Endocrinol. Metab.* **26**:751.

Siiteri, P. K., and Wilson, J. D., 1974, Testosterone formation and metabolism during male sexual differentiation in the human embryo, *J. Clin. Endocrinol. Metab.* **38**:113–125.

Siiteri, P. K., and MacDonald, P. C., 1966, Placental estrogen biosynthesis during human pregnancy, *J. Clin. Endocrinol. Metab.* **26**:751.

Simpson, G. H., Blair, J. H., and Cranswick, E. H., 1964, Cutaneous effects of a new butyrophenone drug, *Clin. Pharm. Ther.* **5**:310–321.

Singh, L., and Jones, K. W., 1982, Sex reversal in the mouse is caused by a recurrent nonreciprocal crossover involving the X and an aberrant Y chromosome, *Cell* **28**:205–216.

Singh, L., Purdom, I. F., and Jones, K. W., 1980, Sex chromosome associated satellite DNA: Evolution and conservation, *Chromosoma* **79**:137–157.

Singh, L., Purdom, I. F., and Jones, K. W., 1981, Conserved sex chromosome-associated nucleotide sequences in eukaryotes, *Cold Spring Harbor Symp. Quant. Biol.* **45**:805–813.

Smith, W. P., Christensen, M. S., Nacht, S., and Gans, E. H., 1980, Effects of polar lipids on the barrier function of the stratum corneum, *Fed. Proc.* **39**:286.

Solari, A. J., The behavior of the XY pair in mammals, 1974, *Int. Rev. Cytol.* **38**:273–317.

Steinmann, B., Mieth, D., and Gitzelmann, R., 1981, A newly recognized cause of low urinary estriol in pregnancy: multiple sulfatese deficiency of the fetus, *Gynecol. Obstet. Invest.* **12**:107–109.

Stern, C., 1973, *Human Genetics,* 3rd ed., pp. 484–485, W. H. Freeman, San Francisco.

Tabei, T., and Heinrichs, L., 1976, Diagnosis of placental sulfatase deficiency, *Am. J. Obstet. Gynecol.* **124**:409–414.

Takagi, N., and Sasaki, M., 1975, Preferential inactivation of the paternally derived X chromosome in the extraembryonic membranes of the mouse, *Nature* **256**:640–642.

Taylor, N. F., 1982, Review: Placental sulphatase deficiency, *J. Inher. Metab. Dis.* **5**:164–176.

Taylor, N. F., and Shackleton, C. H. L., 1979, Gas chromotographic steroid analysis for diagnosis of placental sulfatase deficiency: A study of nine patients, *J. Clin. Endocrinol. Metab.* **49**:78–86.

Tiepolo, L., Zuffardi, O., and Rodewald, A., 1977, Nullisomy for the distal portion of Xp in a male child with a X/Y translocation, *Hum. Genet.* **39**:277–281.

Tiepolo, L., Zuffardi, O., Fraccaro, M., di Natale, D., Gargantini, L., Muller, C. R., and Ropers, H. H., 1980, Assignment by deletion mapping of the steroid sulfatase X-linked ichthyosis locus to Xp223, *Hum. Genet.* **54**:205–206.

Traupe, H., and Happle, R., 1983, Clinical spectrum of steroid sulfatase deficiency: X-linked recessive ichthyosis, birth complications and cryptorchidism, *Eur. J. Pediatr.* **140**:19–21.

Van den Berge, H., Petit, P., and Fryns, J. P., 1977, Y to X translocation in man, *Hum. Genet.* **36**:129–141.

Vihko, R., and Ruokonen, A., 1974, Regulation of steroidogenesis in testis, *J. Ster. Biochm.* **5**:843–848.

Vihko, R., and Ruokonen, A., 1975, Steroid sulphates in human adult testicular steroid synthesis, *J. Ster. Biochem.* **6**:353–356.

Warren, J. C., and Timberlake, C. E., 1964, Biosynthesis of estrogens in pregnancy: Precursor role of plasma dehydroisoandrosterone, *Obstet. Gynecol.* **23**:689.

Weatherall, M. E., Pembrey, M. E., Hall, E. G., Sanger, R., Tippett, P., and Gavin, J., 1970, Familial sideroblastic anemia: Problem of Xg and X chromsome inactivation, *Lancet* **1970**:744–748.

Wells, R. S., and Jennings, M. C., 1967, X-linked ichthyosis and ichthyosis vulgaris, *J. Am. Med. Assoc.* **202**:485–488.

Wells, R. S., and Kerr, C. B., 1965, Genetic classification of ichthyosis, *Arch. Dermatol.* **92**:1–6.

Wells, R. S., and Kerr, C. B., 1966a, Clinical features of autosomal dominant and sex-linked ichthyosis in an English population, *Br. Med. J.* **L**:947–950.

Wells, R. S., and Kerr, C. B., 1966b, The histology of ichthyosis, *J. Invest. Dermatol.* **46**:530–535.

Wells, R. S., Jennings, M. C., Sanger, R., and Race, R. R., 1966, Xg blood groups and ichthyosis, *Lancet* **i**:493–494.

Went, L. N., DeGroot, W. P., Sanger, R., Tippett, P., and Gavin, J., 1969, X-Linked ichthyosis: Linkage relationship with the Xg blood groups and other studies in a large Dutch kindred, *Ann. Hum. Genet. (Lond.)* **32**:333–345.

West, J. D., Freis, W. I., Chapman, V. M., and Papaioannou, V. E., 1977, Preferential expression of the materially derived X chromosome in the mouse yolk sac, *Cell* **12**:873–882.

Wieacker, P., Voiculescu, J., Muller, C. R., and Ropers, H. H., 1983, An XX male with a single STS gene dose, *Cytogenet. Cell Genet.* **35**:72–74.

Wieacker, P., Wienker, T. F., Merorah, B., Dallapiccola, B., Vavies, K. E., and Ropers, H. H., 1984, Linkage relationship between Xg, steroid sulfatase (STS) and retinoschisis (RS), respectively, and a cloned DNA sequence from the distal short arm of the X chromosome, *Cytogenet. Cell Genet.* **37**:608.

Williams, M. C., and Elias, P. M., 1981, Stratum corneum lipids in disorders of cornification. I. Increased cholesterol sulfate content of stratum corneum in recessive X-linked ichthyosis, *J. Clin. Invest.* **68**:1404–1410.

Winkelmann, R. J., Perry, H. O., Achor, R. W. P., and Kirby, T. J., 1963, Cutaneous syndromes produced as side effects of triparanol therapy, *Arch. Dermatol.* **190**:372–377.

Wolf, S. F., and Migeon, B. R., 1982, Studies of X chromosome DNA methylation in normal human cells, *Nature* **295**:667–671.

Yamada, K., Nanko, S., Hattori, S., and Isurugi, K., 1982, Cytogenetic studies in a Y to X translocation observed in three members of one family, with evidence of infertility in male carriers, *Hum. Genet.* **60**:85–90.

Yen, P. Y., Patel, p., Chinault, C., and Shapiro, L J., 1984, Methylation of HPRT genes on active and inactive human X chromosomes, *Proc. Natl. Acad. Sci. USA.* **1759**–1763.

Zuckerman, N. G., and Hagerman, D. D., 1966, The hydrolysis of estrone sulfate by rat kidney microsomal sulfatase, *Arch. Biochem. Biophys.* **135**:410–415.

Zuffardi, O., Maraschio, P., LoCurto, F., Muller, V., Giarola, A., and Perotti, L., 1982, The role of Yp in sex determination: New evidence from X/Y translocations, *Am. J. Med. Genet.* **12**:175–184.

Addenda

CHAPTER 3: GENETIC MUTATIONS AFFECTING HUMAN LIPOPROTEIN METABOLISM

Vassilis I. Zannis and Jan L. Breslow

1. Synthesis, intra and extracellular modifications, and genetic mutations of apolipoproteins.

The DNA sequence of full length apolipoprotein cDNA clones has shown that the signal peptide sequence of human apo A-II,[509-511] apo C-II[512,513] and apo C-I[514] consists of 18, 22, and 26 amino acids, respectively. Both human apo C-II and apo C-I have been mapped on chromosome 19.[512 and Breslow *et al.*, unpublished data] It has been shown that the liver contains high levels of apo C-I mRNA and apparently represents the major site of apo C-I synthesis.[514]

Pulse chase experiments of hepatoma cell cultures (HepG2) have shown that the cleavage of the apo A-II prosegment AlaLeuValArgArg occurs mostly extracellularly. The processing enzyme is a thiol protease which is secreted by the HepG2 cells.[515] Recent studies have demonstrated the existence of a metalloprotease activity in normal as well as in Tangier plasma, which slowly converts the proapo A-I to mature apo A-I.[516,517] Contrary to previous expectations, these observations suggest a normal proapo A-I to apo A-I conversion in Tangier disease.[517] We must bear in mind, however, that the conversion experiments were performed with crude plasma fractions. Therefore, they must be interpreted with caution until the results are duplicated with purified enzyme preparations. The other leading hypothesis of a possible structural apo A-I gene mutation in Tangier patients has not been substantiated. DNA sequence of the apo A-I gene of a patient with Tangier disease has shown that the corresponding Tangier apo A-I protein sequence is normal.[518] Thus, the molecular defect underlying Tangier disease remains elusive. Since this condition is characterized by low levels of plasma apo A-I and HDL, future research should be directed toward protein factors which may be involved in the formation, as well as in the catabolism, of the HDL particle.

Using gel isoelectric focusing techniques, additional electrophoretic apo E variants have been observed that focus in the E5 and E7 region of the gel.[519] These variants were found with higher frequency in patients with arteriosclerosis and suggest that aberrant apo E phenotypes may contribute to the development of arteriosclerosis disease.

Two dimensional gel electrophoresis and immunoblot analysis of apo C-II obtained from three different kindred with apo C-II deficiency revealed trace concentrations of electrophoretic variants of apo C-II, either with more basic[520,521] or more acidic[521] isoelectric points as compared to normal apo C-II. These observations suggest that some of the apo C-II deficiencies may result from structural apo C-II gene mutations that result either in decreased apo C-II synthesis or in the synthesis of unstable forms of apo C-II that are hypercatabolized in plasma.

The rat apo A-IV sequence has been deduced from the DNA sequence of full length apo A-IV cDNA clone.[522] The protein has 391 amino acids including a 20 amino acid long signal peptide. Similar to human apo A-I and apo E, the rat apo A-IV DNA sequence contains 13 tandemly repeated 66 nucleotide regions that may have originated from internal gene duplications. In addition, high sequence homology has been observed among the repeated sequences of rat apo A-I, apo A-IV, and apo E.[523] These findings suggest that apo A-I, apo E, and apo A-IV may have evolved from a common ancestral precursor.

2. Progress in our understanding of the lipoprotein receptors.

The amino acid sequence of the human LDL receptor has been deduced from the nucleotide sequence of a full length LDL cDNA clone.[524] The primary translation product of LDL receptor mRNA consists of 860 amino acids and contains a 21 amino acid long signal peptide. Computer analysis of the 839 amino acid long mature receptor protein indicates that the receptor can be divided into five domains. Starting at the amino terminus, the first domain consists of approximately 322 amino acids. Fifteen percent of the amino acids of this domain are cysteins that are linked in disulfide bridges. This domain contains eight highly homologous repeated sequences. Four of the eight residues of the carboxy terminal of these repeated regions are acidic amino acids and there is evidence suggesting that they may correspond to the ligand binding site of the receptor. The second domain consists of approximately 350 residues and contains five repeated sequences, 25 amino acids in length. This domain may contain the two N linked glycosylation sites of the LDL receptor.[525]

The third domain consists of 48 amino acids, 18 of which are either serines or threonines. Existing evidence suggests that these residues are the sites of O-linked glycosylation of the LDL receptor. The fourth domain consists of 22 hydrophobic amino acids that are believed to form the membrane spanning region of the receptor. Finally, the fifth domain consists of 50 amino acids of the carboxyterminal region that are located in the cytoplasmic side of the plasma membrane.

The apo E receptor has been recently purified from canine liver membranes by using an HDLc-sepharose affinity column as the final purification step.[526] The purified apo E receptor is a protein of 66,000 MW which cross reacts with anti-LDL antibodies. The purified receptor displays the ligand specificity and affinity that has been assigned to unfractionated membrane preparations.[237 and Table III]

REFERENCES

509. Sharpe, C. R., Sidoli, A., Shelley, C. S., Lucero, M. A., Shoulders, C. C., and Baralle, F. E. Human apolipoproteins AI, AII, CII. cDNA sequences and mRNA abundance, *Nucleic Acid Res.* **12**:3917 (1984).

510. Knott, R. J., Priestley, L. M., Urdea, M., and Scott, J., Isolation and characterization of a cDNA encoding the precursor for human apolipoprotein AII. *Biochem. Biophys. Res. Commun.* **120**:734 (1984).

511. Lackner, K. J., Simon, W. L., and Brewer, H. B., Jr., Human apolipoprotein A-II: Complete nucleic acid sequence of preproapo A-II, *FEBS Lett.* **175**:159 (1984).

512. Jackson, C. L., Bruns, G. A. P., and Breslow, J. L., Isolation and sequence of a human apolipoprotein CII cDNA clone and its use to isolate and map to human chromosome 19 the gene for apolipoprotein CII, *Proc. Natl. Acad. Sci. USA.* **81**:2945 (1984).

513. Fojo, S. S., Law, S. W., and Brewer, H. B., Jr., Human apolipoprotein C-II: Complete nucleic acid sequence of preapolipoprotein C-II, *Proc. Natl. Acad. Sci. USA.* **81**:6354 (1984).

514. Knott, T. J., Robertson, M. E., Priestley, L. M., Urdea, M., Wallis, S., and Scott, J., Characterisation of mRNAs encoding the precursor for human apolipoprotein CI, *Nucleic Acids Res.* **12**:3909 (1984).

515. Gordon, J. I., Sims, H. F., Edelstein, C., Scanu, A. M., and Strauss, A. W., Human proapolipoprotein AII is cleaved following secretion from HEP G2 cells by a thiol protease, *Circulation* **70II**:142 (1984).

516. Edelstein, C., Gordon, J. I., Toscas, K., Sims, H. F., Strauss, A. W., and Scanu, A. M., In vitro conversion of proapoprotein A-I to apoprotein A-I, *J. Biol. Chem.,* **258**:11430 (1984).

517. Bojanovski, D., Gregg, R. E., and Brewer, H. B., Jr., In vitro conversion of pro apo A-I_Tangier to mature apo A-I_Tangier, *J. Biol. Chem.* **259**:6049 (1984).

518. Zannis, V. I., Breslow, J. L., Ordovas, J., and Karathanasis, S. K., Isolation and sequence of Tangier apo A-I gene, *Circulation* **70II**:8 (1984).

519. Yamamura, T., Yamamoto, A., Sumiyoshi, T., Hiramori, K., Nishioeda, Y., and Nambu, S., New mutants of apolipoprotein E associated with atherosclerotic diseases but not to type III hyperlipoproteinemia, *J. Clin. Invest.* **74**:1229 (1984).

520. Fojo, S. F., Law, S., Baggio, G., Gregg, R. E., and Brewer, H. B., Jr., Complete nucleic acid sequence of preapolipoprotein C-II and an analysis of the apolipoprotein (apo) C-II gene in apo C-II deficient patients, *Circulation* **70II**:8 (1984).

521. Little, J. A., Maguire, G. F., Kakis, G., and Breckenridge, C. W., Apolipoprotein (apo) CII deficiency associated with nonfunctional mutant forms of apo C-II, *Circulation* **70II**:119 (1984).

522. Boguski, M. S., Elshourbagy, N., Taylor, J. M., and Gordon, J. I., Rat apolipoprotein A-IV contains 13 tandem repetitions of a 22-amino acid segment with amphipathic helical potential, *Proc. Antl. Acad. Sci. USA.* **81**:5021 (1984).

523. Boguski, M. S., Elshourbagy, N., Taylor, J. M., Birkenmeier, E., and Gordon, J. I., Comparative analysis of repeated sequences in rat HDL-associated apolipoproteins A-I, A-IV and E, *Circulation* **70II**:7 (1984).

524. Yamamoto, T., David, C. G., Brown, M. S., Schneider, W. J., Casey, M. L., Goldstein, J. L., and Russell, D. W., The human LDL receptor: A cysteine-rich protein with multiple alu sequences in its mRNA, *Cell.* **39**:27 (1984).

525. Cummings, R. D., Kornfeld, S., Schneider, W. J., Hobgood, K. K., Tolleshaug, H., Brown, M. S., and Goldstein, J. L., Biosynthesis of the N- and O-linked oligosaccharides of the low density lipoprotein receptor, *J. Biol. Chem.* **258**:15273 (1983).

526. Hui, D. Y., Brecht, W., Lorenz, T., Friedman, G., Innerarity, R. L., and Mahley, R. W., Purification of the hepatic apo-E receptor, *Circulation* **70II**:311 (1984).

CHAPTER 4: GLUCOSE-6-PHOSPHATE DEHYDROGENASE

L. Luzzatto and G. Battistuzzi

The methylation of the *Gd* gene has been extensively investigated, but only with respect to the 3′ end of the gene. In the active X-chromosome of both males and females, certain specific sites are reproducibly methylated and others are reproducibly unmethylated, while in the inactive X-chromosome of females, at least two additional sites are methylated

(Toniolo *et al.*, 1984b). In different male tissues the methylation of certain other sites correlates positively with the level of G6PD activity, which suggests transcriptional regulation (Battistuzzi *et al.*, 1985). Thus, the methylation pattern is specific and distinctively different when it relates to all or none regulation (X-inactivation) or to tissue-specific expression. It remains to be seen whether this is generally true for housekeeping genes. The timing of replication of *Gd* is early during the S-phase in HeLa cells, similar to what is found for a variety of other housekeeping genes (Goldman *et al.*, 1984).

With respect to the mechanism of malaria resistance, it has been shown recently that *P. falciparum* does produce its own G6PD when grown *in vitro* in G6PD-deficient RBC, but not in normal RBC. This would explain effective adaptation of the parasite to the former cell type, and therefore lack of protection of G6PD(−) hemizygotes. At the same time, it shows that the enzyme is essential for the parasite and would therefore explain the mechanism of protection in heterozygous mosaics, in whom adaptation cannot take place effectively (E. A. Usanga and L. Luzzatto, unpublished).

ADDITIONAL REFERENCES

Battistuzzi, G., D'Urso, M., Toniolo, D., and Luzzatto, L., 1985, Tissue-specific levels of human glucose 6-phosphate dehydrogenase correlate with methylation of specific sites at the 3′ end of the gene, *Proc. Natl. Acad. Sci. USA.* (in press).

Beutler, E., 1978, *Hemolytic Anemia in Disorders of Red Cell Metabolism*, Plenum Medical Book Company, New York and London.

De Leon, P. A. M., Wolf, S. F., Persico, M. G., Toniolo, D., and Migeon, B. R. Localization of the G6PD locus in mouse and man by *in situ* hybridization: Further evidence for an inverted order of homologous X-linked genes, *Somatic Cell Genetics.* (in press).

Fincham, J. R. S., Day, P. R., and Radford, A., 1979, *Fungal Genetics*, 3rd ed., Blackwell Scientific Publications, Oxford.

Galiano, S., Ferraris, A. M., Giuntini, P., and Gaetani, G. F., 1982, Regulation of glucose-6-phosphate dehydrogenase, in: *Advances in Red Cell Biology* (D. J. Weatherall, G. Fiorelli, and S. Gorino, eds.) pp. 357–363, Raven Press, New York.

Goldman, M. A., Holmquist, G. P., Gray, M. C., Caston, L. A., and Nag, A., 1984, Replication timing of genes and middle repetitive sequences, *Science*, 224:686–692.

Kirkman, H. N., and Gaetani, G. F., 1984, Catalase: A tetrameric enzyme with four tightly bound molecules of NADPH, *Proc. Natl. Acad. Sci. USA.* (in press).

Littlefield, J. W., 1964, The selection of hybrid mouse fibroblasts, *Cold Spring Harbor Symp. Quant. Biol.*, 29:161–166.

Schröter, W., and Tillman, W., 1977, The relationship between metabolic defects and the red cell membrane. *IV Meeting of the International Society for Haematology, Istanbul, Turkey,* Abstracts, p. 564.

Seeler, R. A., 1978, Extreme hyperbilirubinemia in patients with sickle cell disease, *J. Pediatr.,* **92:**171.

Szabo, P., Purrello, M., Rocchi, M., Archidiacono, N., Alhadeff, B., Filippi, G., Toniolo, D., Martini, G., Luzzatto, L., and Siniscalco, M., (1984), Cytological mapping of the human G6PD gene distally to the fragile-X site suggests a high rate of meiotic recombination across this site, *Proc. Natl. Acad. Sci. USA.* (in press).

CHAPTER 5: STEROID SULFATASE DEFICIENCY AND THE GENETICS OF THE SHORT ARM OF THE HUMAN X CHROMOSOME

Larry J. Shapiro

Several recent studies have focused attention on cloned DNA probes which identify sequences with striking homology on the human X and Y chromosomes. While studies of these sequences on the Y have revealed either a Y short arm or a Y long arm localization, mapping of the X sequences has shown that many are situated on the long arm of the X well outside of the pairing region. Sequencing studies of one of these X/Y pairs indicate identity over more than 1000 base pairs of DNA (Cooke et al., 1984). Detailed restriction mapping of another set shows greater than 99% homology over 36 kb (Page et al., 1984). This degree of homology would predict either strong selection for the specific nucleotide sequences in question, or an evolutionarily recent exchange between the human X and Y. This latter interpretation is supported by the finding of an X-linked copy of one of these genes in chimpanzees, orangutans, and gorillas, without a Y-linked copy. Thus, the Y-linked versions must have arrived in this location subsequent to the divergence of these species. These results suggest that X/Y pairing and recombination may be even more complex than originally contemplated (Erickson and Goodfellow, 1984).

REFERENCES

Cooke, H. J., Brown, W. A. R., and Rappold, G. A., 1984. Closely related sequences on human X and Y chromosomes outside the pairing region. *Nature,* **311**:259–261.

Erickson, R. P. and Goodfellow, P. N., 1984. Sex chromosome evolution: Sharing outside of pairing. *Nature,* **311**:106–107.

Page, D. C., Harper, M. E., Love, J. and Botstein, D., 1984. Occurrence of a transposition from the X-chromosome long arm to the Y-chromosome short arm during human evolution. *Nature,* **311**:119–123.

Index